HYPERCHOLESTEROLEMIA

Edited by **Sekar Ashok Kumar**

Hypercholesterolemia
http://dx.doi.org/10.5772/58487
Edited by Sekar Ashok Kumar

Contributors

Sigrid Mennickent, Jeannie Chan, John L. VandeBerg, Laura A. Cox, Genesio M. Karere, Yew Keong Choong, Takao Kato, Lorenzo Iughetti, Patrizia Bruzzi, Barbara Predieri, Safila Naveed, Lucía Cid Conde, José López-Castro, Elba Leiva, Olivier Descamps, Lale Tokgozoglu, Eric Bruckert, Avia Rosenhouse-Dantsker, Anna Bukiya, Ludmila Vladimirova-Kitova

Published by InTech
Janeza Trdine 9, 51000 Rijeka, Croatia

Publishing Process Manager Iva Simcic
Technical Editor InTech DTP team
Cover InTech Design team

First published September, 2015
Printed in Croatia

Additional hard copies can be obtained from orders@intechopen.com

Hypercholesterolemia, Edited by Sekar Ashok Kumar
p. cm.
ISBN 978-953-51-2169-5

For EU product safety concerns:
IN TECH d.o.o., Prolaz Marije Krucifikse Kozulić 3, 51000 Rijeka, Croatia,
info@intechopen.com or visit our website at intechopen.com.

Meet the editor

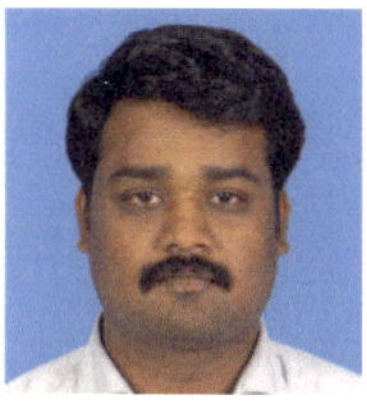

Dr. S. Ashok Kumar is an Assistant Professor at the Centre for Biotechnology, Anna University, Chennai, Tamil Nadu, India. He has done doctoral research on hypercholesterolemia and obtained his PhD from the University of Madras. Later, he joined as a postdoctoral fellow at CancerCare Manitoba, University of Manitoba. At present, as an Assistant Professor at Anna University, he is actively involved in the research field of hypercholesterolemia and targeting signaling pathways in metabolic disorder. Dr. Kumar's research work has been supported by grants from national funding agencies such as UGC and DST-SERB. His research findings were published in nine international journals and a book chapter. Dr. Kumar is an active Member of the Board of Studies in Biotechnology and Member of the Editorial Board of Scientific Publication.

Contents

Preface

Increased dietary intake of fat has received considerable attention in the past few decades because of its link with an increased risk of atherosclerosis and subsequent cardiovascular disease. Apart from dietary origin, there are several other factors such as genetic factors and hormonal changes that play a vital role in hypercholesterolemia-induced cardiovascular disease. A number of risk factors have been identified for the development of atherosclerosis, among which, hypercholesterolemia is a well-recognized primary risk factor for cardiovascular disease. A strong relationship between hypercholesterolemia and cardiovascular disease has been established through epidemiological, experimental, and clinical trial data. Understanding and targeting hypercholesterolemia becomes important since it is an earlier stage in the pathogenesis of atherosclerosis and can also be managed with appropriate treatment.

This book describes the basic information on the causes, diagnosis, consequences, and treatment strategies for hypercholesterolemia. InTech has invited experts in the related field from different countries to take part in this book. The chapters contain more updated and wide information, and indeed, some chapters take a practical approach towards the management of hypercholesterolemia. This book is a collection of information on hypercholesterolemia from different authors in order to present a vast and clear knowledge about hypercholesterolemia to readers.

Dr. Sekar Ashok Kumar
Assistant Professor
Centre for Biotechnology
Anna University Chennai
Chennai, Tamil Nadu, India

Section 1

Hypercholesterolemia- Basic Information, Animal Models, Consequences and Approaches to Treatment

Chapter 1

Animal Models of Diet-induced Hypercholesterolemia

Jeannie Chan, Genesio M. Karere, Laura A. Cox and
John L. VandeBerg

Additional information is available at the end of the chapter

http://dx.doi.org/10.5772/59610

1. Introduction

Cholesterol is a component of the cell membrane and metabolites of cholesterol, such as bile acids, steroid hormones and vitamin D, serve important biologic functions in vertebrates. Cholesterol is synthesized primarily in the liver and transported to cells throughout the body by lipoproteins via the blood, even though all nucleated cells in the body are capable of synthesizing cholesterol. Whole-body cholesterol homeostasis is determined by cholesterol absorption, cholesterol synthesis and cholesterol excretion, and losing control of any of these processes leads to an increase in plasma cholesterol. Liver and intestine are the major sites that control cholesterol homeostasis. The liver synthesizes cholesterol for secretion in nascent lipoproteins when blood levels of cholesterol are low, and removes excess cholesterol from the blood by taking up chylomicron remnants, high density lipoprotein (HDL), very low density lipoprotein (VLDL) and low density lipoprotein (LDL) particles. It converts cholesterol into bile acids, and secretes cholesterol and bile acids into bile for elimination from the body. The intestine regulates influx of cholesterol from the lumen and efflux of cholesterol back into the lumen to control the amount of cholesterol that enters the body [1].

Hypercholesterolemia is characterized by LDL cholesterol exceeding 159 mg/dl [2]. Many developed countries have a high prevalence of hypercholesterolemia. According to an estimate based on data from the 2005-2008 National Health and Nutrition Examination Survey, the Centers for Disease Control and Prevention reported that 33.5% of US adults aged 20 or older had high levels of LDL cholesterol [3]. Diets containing high levels of cholesterol and high levels of fat (HCHF) are frequently the culprit in causing hypercholesterolemia. In addition, genetic factors influence susceptibility to diet-induced hypercholesterolemia.

Hypercholesterolemia is a complex disorder often due to multiple genetic defects and rarely due to a single genetic defect as in the case of familial hypercholesterolemia [4]. Because hypercholesterolemia is associated with risk of developing atherosclerosis, much research has been devoted to understanding the genetic variants and environmental factors that contribute to elevated blood LDL cholesterol. There are several challenges to investigating gene-diet interactions in humans. It is difficult to control the diet and environment of human subjects for long periods of time, and ethical constraints limit access to tissue samples. These problems can be circumvented by using animals to study the effects of diets on cholesterol homeostasis and atherosclerosis because animals can be fed the same diet and kept under the same laboratory conditions for long periods of time, and because access to tissue samples from animals is less restricted. Numerous animal species have been used as animal models for investigating hypercholesterolemia, including rabbits [5,6], mice [7], guinea pigs [8], minipigs [9], laboratory opossums [10] and nonhuman primates [11-15]. Nonhuman primates are more similar to humans than other animals, but ethical issues, facilities and high cost limit studies with nonhuman primates. Non-primate animal models have other limitations. However, extensive use of the collage of primate and non-primate models has provided considerable insights into the genes and molecular mechanisms that control plasma cholesterol in response to diets.

In this chapter, we discuss mouse, laboratory opossum and nonhuman primate models of hypercholesterolemia. Mice lipoprotein profiles differ from humans and they are resistant to developing hypercholesterolemia and atherosclerosis, but genetic engineering tools have been used effectively to alter their lipoprotein profiles. A commonly used mouse model in which the apolipoprotein E gene *(apoE)* is disrupted exhibits a lipoprotein profile similar to that of humans. In addition, *apoE* knockout mice become hypercholesterolemic and have a propensity to develop atherosclerosis [16,17]. Mice have also been used extensively to elucidate mechanisms that regulate cholesterol homeostasis. Cholesterol excretion is one of the major processes that can be targeted to reduce hypercholesterolemia. A nonbiliary pathway for disposal of cholesterol termed transintestinal cholesterol excretion (TICE) was first described in mice almost a decade ago [18]. A growing body of evidence for TICE has since been gathered using genetically modified and normal mice [19,20]. The discovery of TICE has opened a new avenue of research into the role of the intestine in cholesterol excretion [21].

The laboratory opossum is a model of diet-induced hypercholesterolemia developed at Texas Biomedical Research Institute that does not require genetic manipulation to knock out or overexpress specific genes to elevate LDL cholesterol [22,23]. Through many generations of inbreeding and selection for plasma cholesterol response to an HCHF diet, high and low responding strains of opossums were produced. All strains have normal levels of plasma cholesterol on a basal diet. However, high responding opossums exhibit an extremely high LDL cholesterol response when fed an HCHF diet compared to low responding opossums. Hypercholesterolemia in high responding opossums is caused by mutations in at least two genes. One of the causative genes has been identified as *ABCB4;* mutations in the *ABCB4* gene impair biliary cholesterol secretion [24]. The *ABCB4* gene has not been shown previously to be associated with hypercholesterolemia. The opossum model provides an opportunity to investigate genes that interact with *ABCB4* to regulate cholesterol homeostasis.

Nonhuman primates are utilized as models of hypercholesterolemia because of their physiologic and genetic similarities with humans [25]. In addition, nonhuman primates naturally develop hypercholesterolemia and atherosclerosis, both of which can be exacerbated by HCHF diets to mimic diet-induced hypercholesterolemia and atherosclerosis in humans [11,15,26]. Because of these characteristics, nonhuman primates including baboon (*Papio hymadryas*), rhesus macaque (*Macaca mulatta*), green monkey (*Chlorocebus aethiops*) and cynomolgus monkey (*Macaca fascicularis*) have been used as animal models for biomedical research aimed at understanding diet-induced hypercholesterolemia in humans. Nonhuman primates exhibit species and individual variations in plasma cholesterol in response to HCHF diets. Studies using pedigreed baboons and high-throughput sequencing technology have identified genetic factors that influence plasma cholesterol response to HCHF diets [13,27].

2. Mouse models

2.1. Mouse models of cholesterol metabolism

Mouse models are the most widely used animal models because of several advantages such as ease of breeding, large litter size, a short generation time of 9 months and economies of colony maintenance. An additional advantage of mice is the availability of tools to add exogenous genes to the germ line to create transgenic mice, or to disrupt endogenous genes by homologous recombination in murine embryonic stem cells to create knockout mice. Although there are important differences between mice and humans in lipoprotein and cholesterol metabolism, genetic manipulation has provided mouse models that resemble some aspects of hypercholesterolemia in humans.

Non-genetically modified mice have high levels of HDL cholesterol and low levels of LDL cholesterol, whereas humans have high levels of LDL cholesterol and low levels of HDL cholesterol. The difference in lipid profiles between mice and humans is due to absence of the cholesteryl ester transfer protein (CETP) in mice [28,29]. CETP is an enzyme that transfers cholesterol ester from HDL to VLDL and LDL in exchange for triglycerides [30]. In normal mice lacking CETP, more than 80% of plasma cholesterol is carried on HDL, so mice with high levels of HDL cholesterol are resistant to hypercholesterolemia and atherosclerosis. To overcome this problem to using mice as models for research aimed at understanding cholesterol metabolism in humans, several genetically engineered strains of mice were generated to alter the distribution of plasma cholesterol from HDL to VLDL and LDL. The genetically modified mice include CETP transgenic, apoE knockout and LDL receptor knockout mice.

CETP transgenic mice. Transgenic mice carrying human and cynomolgus monkey versions of the *CETP* gene were studied to investigate the effects of CETP on distribution of plasma lipoprotein cholesterol. Transgenic mice expressing high levels of human CETP showed a small decrease in HDL cholesterol and a small increase in VLDL and LDL cholesterol on the basal (chow) diet [29]. Transgenic mice expressing high levels of cynomolgus monkey CETP showed greater responsiveness than nontransgenic mice when challenged with an HCHF diet. Total plasma cholesterol of *CETP* transgenic mice averaged 250 mg/dl whereas those of nontransgenic mice averaged 163 mg/dl. Furthermore, *CETP* transgenic mice showed that CETP activity was inversely associated with apoA-I, but positively associated with apoB [28]. These observations demonstrated that human and monkey CETP can interact with mouse lipoproteins to mediate its effects in lipoprotein metabolism.

ApoE deficient mice. ApoE is a 34 kD glycoprotein produced primarily in the liver and to a lesser extent in other tissues. With the exception of LDL particles, apoE is a structural component of all lipoprotein particles and chylomicrons. It binds to the LDL receptor and to the LDL receptor-related protein to remove VLDL and chylomicron remnants from the plasma [31]. Using gene targeting to disrupt the *apoE* gene, mutant mice developed severe hypercholesterolemia as expected from a defect in lipoprotein clearance from plasma. Total plasma cholesterol levels were highly elevated in homozygous apoE deficient (*apoE-/-*) mice (400-500 mg/dl) compared with normal mice (80 mg/dl) on a chow diet with 0.01% cholesterol and 4.5% fat. A more dramatic increase in plasma cholesterol was observed in *apoE-/-* mice (1800 mg/dl) fed an HCHF diet with 0.15% cholesterol and 20% fat. Plasma cholesterol concentrations in the VLDL and intermediate density lipoprotein (IDL) fractions were increased on both diets. The *apoE-/-* mice were highly susceptible to atherosclerosis, even on chow diet, as a result of the increase in plasma cholesterol concentrations [16,17].

LDL receptor deficient mice. The LDL receptor is a cell surface receptor expressed in many cell types. In the liver, the LDL receptor regulates plasma cholesterol by binding to apoB and apoE on the surface of lipoprotein particles and removes these particles from the plasma [32]. Patients with familial hypercholesterolemia [33] and Watanabe-heritable hyperlipidemic rabbits [34] develop elevated levels of LDL cholesterol due to mutations in the LDL receptor. Based on this knowledge, LDL receptor knock out (*LDLR-/-*) mice were generated to increase plasma LDL cholesterol concentrations. The loss of functional LDL receptors elevated total plasma cholesterol in *LDLR-/-* mice, but the effect was more moderate compared to *apoE-/-* mice. The mean total plasma cholesterol on a chow diet was 293 mg/dl and on a diet enriched with cholesterol (0.2%) and fat (19%) was 425 mg/dl. The increase in plasma cholesterol in *LDLR-/-* mice was attributed to increases in IDL and LDL cholesterol [35]. Compared with familial hypercholesterolemia patients (receptor-negative homozygotes) who have plasma cholesterol levels over 700 mg/dl, the effect of LDL receptor deficiency is less severe in mice. This is due to the fact that mice produce VLDL particles containing both apoB-48 and apoB-100, whereas humans only produce VLDL particles containing apoB-100 [36]. In mice, VLDL particles containing apoB-48 can be cleared from the plasma by the chylomicron remnant receptor in addition to the LDL receptor, so fewer VLDL particles are converted to LDL particles. Therefore, LDL receptor deficiency in mice does not increase plasma cholesterol to the same extent as in humans.

2.2. Mouse models of atherosclerosis

Disruption of the *apoE* gene causes hypercholesterolemic *apoE* knockout mice to develop atherosclerotic lesions spontaneously [16,17]. Foam cell lesions were observed in chow-fed *apoE-/-* mice 10 weeks after birth and the lesions progress to fibrous plaques by 20 weeks of age. An HCHF diet accelerates all stages of lesion formation and increases the size of lesions;

thus, formation of atherosclerotic lesions in *apoE-/-* mice is responsive to diet as in humans. Because of the short period of time for lesion formation in apoE-/- mice, they have been used extensively to study dietary and genetic factors affecting atherosclerosis and mechanisms of atherogenesis, as well as to assess efficacy of pharmacologic agents on lesion size. Progression of early lesions to advanced lesions in *apoE-/-* mice is similar to that in humans; lesions often develop at vascular branch points and progress rapidly to foam cells with fibrous plaques and necrotic lipid cores [37]. The major difference from humans is a low incidence of ruptured plaques that leads to thrombosis and arterial occlusion. Plaque rupture is the event that causes a heart attack in humans. A higher incidence of ruptured plaques was obtained by feeding a diet enriched with 0.15% cholesterol and 21% fat to *apoE-/-* mice. After 8 weeks of feeding the HCHF diet to *apoE-/-* mice, acute plaque ruptures were observed in the brachiocephalic arteries of more than half of the animals [38].

2.3. Mouse models of cholesterol excretion

Hepatobiliary cholesterol excretion. The human body cannot degrade cholesterol, but it can convert cholesterol to bile acids in the liver. Fecal excretion is the major route for the body to remove cholesterol as bile acids or neutral sterols (cholesterol and its metabolites formed by bacteria in the intestine). Diet-induced hypercholesterolemia can be mitigated by increasing the loss of cholesterol in feces. Fecal excretion of cholesterol and bile acids depends on transporting these molecules from the liver into bile. The ABCG5/G8 [39] and ABCB11 [40] proteins transport cholesterol and bile acids, respectively. The ABCB4 protein transports phospholipids (mainly phosphatidylcholine), which is essential for secretion of cholesterol into bile [41,42]. ABCB11 plays a central role in hepatobiliary secretion as bile flow is the driving force for biliary secretion of cholesterol and phospholipids [43].

Many studies have been carried out using transgenic and knockout mouse models to further our knowledge of the physiologic pathways and molecular mechanisms that control cholesterol excretion. Transgenic mice expressing the human *ABCG5* and *ABCG8* genes directed by their own regulatory DNA sequences (*hG5G8Tg* mice) had higher levels (5-fold) of biliary cholesterol and higher levels (3- to 6-fold) of fecal neutral sterol compared with nontransgenic mice, providing evidence that ABCG5 and ABCG8 function as cholesterol transporters [44]. Moreover, cholesterol absorption in these transgenic mice was reduced by 50% because the proteins encoded by *ABCG5* and *ABCG8* genes are also expressed in the small intestine and they transport cholesterol from the intestine into the lumen [44]. In another study, *Abcg5* and *Abcg8* double knockout (*G5G8-/-*) mice were created to investigate the effects of disrupting these genes on biliary cholesterol secretion. *G5G8-/-* mice were more diet-responsive than normal mice on a 2% cholesterol diet. Plasma cholesterol increased 2-fold in *G5G8-/-* mice, but not in normal mice. Hepatic cholesterol was markedly increased in *G5G8-/-* mice (18-fold) compared with normal mice (3-fold). Accordingly, expression of the cholesterol synthesis genes HMG-CoA synthase and HMG-CoA reductase was lower in *G5G8-/-* mice than normal mice. Fecal neutral sterol was reduced by 36% in *G5G8-/-* mice relative to that in normal mice. The findings using double knockout mice also supported ABCG5 and ABCG8 function in cholesterol transport [45].

Another series of experiments was conducted to investigate the role of phospholipids in secretion of biliary cholesterol. Disruption of the *Abcb4* (also known as *Mdr2*) gene in mice led to a severe liver disease. Phospholipids were undetectable in the bile of homozygous *Abcb4* knockout (*Abcb4-/-*) mice, while the levels in heterozygous *Abcb4* knockout (*Abcb4+/-*) mice were half of those in nontransgenic mice. Interestingly, *Abcb4-/-* mice secreted extremely low levels of cholesterol into bile, but cholesterol levels in flowing bile from *Abcb4+/-* mice were similar to those in nontransgenic mice [41]. Langheim et al. [46] investigated whether overexpression of ABCG5 and ABCG8 could restore biliary cholesterol secretion in *Abcb4-/-* mice by breeding *Abcb4-/-* mice with *hG5G8Tg* mice to generate *Abcb4-/-;hG5G8Tg* mice. The *Abcb4-/-;hG5G8Tg* mice also secreted very low levels of biliary cholesterol, which were similar to the levels in *Abcb4-/-* mice. Taken together, these results indicate that biliary cholesterol secretion requires a minimal concentration of phospholipids in the bile. Biliary phospholipid secretion in the liver serves two purposes. One is to protect the canalicular membrane of hepatocytes exposed to high concentrations of bile acids from damage by the detergent action of bile acids. Secretion of phospholipids by the liver into the bile reduces bile salt micelles to extract phospholipids from the membranes of hepatocytes. The other is to make phospholipids available for incorporation into pure bile salt micelles to form bile salt mixed micelles. Solubility of cholesterol in bile salt mixed micelles is greater than that in pure bile salt micelles, thus phospholipid secretion prevents formation of gallstones [47].

Nonbiliary cholesterol excretion. Hepatobiliary secretion is known to be the main pathway for eliminating cholesterol from the body, but an increasing body of evidence suggests that plasma cholesterol is also eliminated by a nonbiliary pathway in mice. As mentioned above, *G5G8-/-* mice did not show a dramatic reduction in fecal neutral sterol excretion despite they had extremely low levels of biliary cholesterol. Normal or even increased fecal neutral sterol excretion was observed in other mouse models (*Abcb4-/-*, *Npc1l1*$^{\text{-LiverTg}}$) that are severely impaired in hepatobiliary cholesterol secretion [20]. This observation suggests the existence of an alternate route, known as TICE, which does not involve biliary cholesterol secretion. Plasma cholesterol is transported via blood to intestinal cells and eventually secreted into the intestinal lumen for disposal in feces [20]. It should be mentioned that a nonbiliary cholesterol excretion pathway has also been postulated to explain fecal neutral sterol loss in bile-diverted dogs [48, 49] and bile-diverted rats [50].

Intestinal perfusion studies [19] and *in vivo* stable isotope studies [51] in mice that have an intact hepatobiliary secretion and enterohepatic cycling system revealed that TICE accounted for ~30% of fecal cholesterol excretion. The site of action of TICE is the proximal small intestine [19,52]. It is thought that TICE involves plasma lipoproteins to deliver cholesterol to the intestine, then cholesterol is taken up by receptors at the basolateral membrane of enterocytes and traverses the enterocytes to the apical membrane where it is excreted into the intestinal lumen. There are still many gaps in our understanding of the molecular mechanism of TICE. HDL is ruled out as the lipoprotein that delivers cholesterol to the intestine because TICE was not diminished in *Abca*1 knockout mice having extremely low concentrations of plasma HDL [53,54]. Evidence to support VLDL remnants or LDL as the plasma cholesterol carrier came from studies using antisense oligonucleotides (ASO) to knockdown expression of proteins critical for production of VLDL and alter plasma VLDL cholesterol concentrations. ASO-mediated knockdown of acyl-CoA:cholesterol acyltransferase activity 2 (ACAT2) in mice fed a high cholesterol diet resulted in an increase in both VLDL cholesterol and fecal neutral sterol excretion [55]. Conversely, ASO-mediated knockdown of microsomal triglyceride transfer protein resulted in a decrease in both VLDL cholesterol and fecal neutral sterol excretion [56]. As for the receptor that takes up cholesterol at the basolateral membrane, it is not likely to be the LDL receptor nor scavenger receptor BI (SR-BI) because neutral sterol excretion was not affected in *LDLR-/-* mice [57] and SR-BI-/- mice [58,59]. It may involve other members of the LDL receptor or a novel receptor. Lastly, Abcg5/Abcg8 and Abcb1 participate in the secretion of cholesterol from enterocytes into the intestinal lumen [57].

A study in patients with complete biliary obstruction revealed they still excreted substantial amounts of neutral sterol into feces [60]. Data from these patients showed that ~20% to 30% of neutral sterols were excreted by TICE, which is similar to that excreted by TICE in normal mice. However, the relevance of TICE for disposal of cholesterol in humans without biliary obstruction has yet to be established. A recent *ex vivo* study showed that human and mouse intestinal (duodenual) explants mounted on Ussing chambers were capable of effluxing cholesterol, providing evidence for the activity of TICE in humans [57].

3. Laboratory opossum model

3.1. Characteristics of laboratory opossums

The gray short-tailed opossum (*Monodelphis domestica*) is a docile, nocturnal marsupial native to Brazil and adjacent countries. It is the only marsupial species that has adapted to breeding in captivity to produce large numbers of animals [61]. In addition to being able to breed in captivity throughout the year, *Monodelphis* have a short generation time of 6 months and produce large litters (typically 6-13). Breeding colonies have been established in the United States, Brazil, Germany, United Kingdom, Japan, and Australia. Opossums in captive colonies are quite different genetically from their wild counterparts due to selection that has undoubtedly taken place while the animals were bred in isolated colonies for many generations; therefore laboratory stocks of this species are referred to as laboratory opossums. Adult laboratory opossums weigh 70-150 g, which is intermediate between mice (20-30 g) and rats (250-300 g). They are maintained in polycarbonate rodent cages, and the standard laboratory diet is commercial pelleted fox food provided *ad libitium*. Owing to its physical characteristics as a laboratory animal and economic production in captivity, *Monodelphis domestica* has become the most widely used marsupial in biomedical research. Furthermore, it was the first marsupial species to have its genome sequenced and analyzed [62]. The availability of genome sequence data has accelerated progress on genetic aspects of research involving *Monodelphis*.

The opossum model has advantageous characteristics for understanding cholesterol homeostasis. *Monodelphis* is omnivorous like humans, and its natural diet includes cholesterol derived from the consumption of insects and small vertebrates. Therefore, laboratory opossums and humans are likely to have many similarities in lipoprotein and cholesterol metabolism. Unlike genetically modified (transgenic and knockout) mouse models, the opossum model provides an opportunity to identify naturally occurring variants of genes and to study how interactions among gene variants lead to development of hypercholesterolemia. Some partially inbred strains of opossums have inbreeding coefficients in excess of 0.95, and strains with high or low responses to an HCHF diet have inbreeding coefficients in excess of 0.8. Since more than 80% of the genes in each partially inbred strain have alleles that are identical by descent, the work required to identify genes that cause diet-induced hypercholesterolemia in the opossum model is substantially reduced.

3.2. Development of partially inbred strains

Nine wild-caught animals were imported from Brazil into the United States in 1978 by the National Zoo in Washington, D.C. The founders of the breeding colony of laboratory opossums at Texas Biomedical Research Institute were comprised of 20 first and second generation descendants of those nine founders, together with 17 additional wild-caught opossums from Brazil and two from Bolivia. After several generations of inbreeding, some individuals were fed a high cholesterol (0.6% by weight) and high fat (17% by weight) diet for 6 months, and total blood cholesterol was measured after an overnight fast. Low and high responses were observed among opossums, with few animals exhibiting an intermediate response, i.e. the phenotypes are clustered at the high and low ends of the range. Low responding opossums had blood cholesterol levels ranging from 62-171 mg/dl whereas high responding opossums had levels of 215-932 mg/dl [22]. Furthermore, analysis of lipoprotein particles by gradient gel electrophoresis showed elevated levels of LDL particles in high responding opossums [22]. Subsequently, inbreeding and selection for either low responsiveness or high responsiveness to the HCHF diet led to development of two related low responding partially inbred strains (designated ATHE and ATHL) and a high responding partially inbred strain (designated ATHH) that show extreme difference (>5-fold) in plasma cholesterol concentrations in response to the HCHF diet. These strains are being used to identify genetic variants and molecular mechanisms that cause diet-induced hypercholesterolemia.

3.3. Hypercholesterolemia in high responders

Dietary challenge and plasma cholesterol response. Studies were conducted to compare lipoprotein characteristics of low responders from the ATHE strain and high responders from the ATHH strain. The standard laboratory diet is the basal diet, which contains 0.04% cholesterol and 8.1% fat, by weight. Plasma cholesterol concentrations of low and high responders do not differ on this diet. Most of the plasma cholesterol is carried by HDL, and ~30% of total plasma cholesterol is carried by LDL [10]. After consuming the HCHF diet for at least 4 weeks, total plasma cholesterol increases slightly (< 2-fold) in low responders, but dramatically in high responders (>5-fold). HDL cholesterol levels of low and high responders show small (< 2-fold) but significant increases. The increase in plasma cholesterol in high responders is mainly due to an increase in VLDL and LDL (V+LDL) cholesterol such that the percentage of total plasma cholesterol carried by V+LDL is increased to ~85% in response to diet. The increase in V+LDL cholesterol on the HCHF diet alters the plasma lipid profile of high responding opossums to resemble more closely that of humans. Plasma triglyceride concentrations are relatively low in low and high responders on the basal diet, and they are not responsive to dietary challenge. The major lipoprotein is apoA-I and the minor lipoprotein is apoE in HDL particles from low and high responders on both diets. ApoB is the major lipoprotein in V+LDL particles from low and high responders on the basal diet and low responders on the HCHF diet. The V+LDL particles from high responders on the HCHF diet are more heterogeneous, and they carry apoE in addition to apoB [10].

Cholesterol absorption. Additional studies were conducted to determine whether low and high responders differ in cholesterol absorption, which is one of the physiologic processes that govern cholesterol homeostasis. Cholesterol absorption was measured by the fecal isotope ratio method. On the basal diet, the percentage of cholesterol absorbed through the intestine was ~60% in low and high responding opossums. On the HCHF diet, low responders reduced the percentage of absorbed cholesterol by 50%, whereas high responders did not [63]. Several genes that play a role in cholesterol absorption were analyzed to determine whether their expression differed between low and high responders on the HCHF diet. Dietary cholesterol increased expression of *ABCG5* and *ABCG8* in the small intestine of low and high responders to limit absorption of cholesterol by transporting cholesterol from enterocytes to the intestinal lumen; the extent of increase was similar in both strains of opossums. The *NPC1L1* gene transports cholesterol from the lumen into enterocytes, and the *ACAT2* and *MTP* genes facilitate chylomicron formation and secretion in the small intestine. These genes were expressed at similar levels in low and high responders. Therefore, the difference in cholesterol absorption between low and high responders is not due to differences in expression of genes that regulate influx and efflux of cholesterol in the small intestine [64].

Bile acid synthesis. Liver is the other major site that controls cholesterol homeostasis. In the liver, cholesterol is converted to bile acids, and bile acids and free cholesterol are secreted into bile for disposal via fecal excretion. Bile acids are synthesized by two pathways, the classic pathway and the alternate pathway. The rate-limiting enzyme in the classic pathway is 7α-hydroxylase. The enzyme sterol 27-hydroxylase initiates bile acid synthesis in the alternate pathway and catalyzes several oxidation reactions in the classic and alternate bile acid synthesis pathways [65]. Low and high responders on the HCHF diet had similar 7α-hydroxylase activities but differed in sterol 27-hydroxylase activities. Low responders had higher activity of hepatic sterol 27-hydroxylase (14.1 ± 0.8 pmol/mg protein/min) compared with high responders (10.1 ± 0.8 pmol/mg protein/min; $P<0.01$) [66]. Sterol 27-hydroxylase is encoded by the *CYP27A1* gene. Expression of the *CYP27A1* gene was also higher (2-fold) in low responders fed a high cholesterol diet [64]. Given that sterol 27-hydroxylase catalyzes several reactions in the classic and alternate pathways of bile acid synthesis, a reduction in enzyme activity was consistent with lower concentrations of total bile acids in gall bladder bile of high responders (194 ± 19 mol/ml for high responders versus 244 ± 15 mol/ml for low responders; $P=0.05$) [66].

Biliary cholesterol and biliary phospholipids. Bile samples collected from gall bladders were analyzed to determine whether there are any differences in the secretion of cholesterol into bile by low and high responders fed the HCHF diet. The results revealed differences in biliary cholesterol concentration and biliary phospholipid concentration in gall bladder bile. Cholesterol concentration in the bile of low responders (5.7 ± 1.3 mg/ml) was higher than that of high responders (1.3 ± 0.7 mg/ml; $P<0.05$). Similarly, phospholipid concentration in the bile of low responders (29.7 ± 3.7 mg/ml) was also higher than that of high responders (6.9 ± 5.5 mg/ml for high responders; $P<0.05$) [24]. Biliary cholesterol secretion is mediated by ABCG5, ABCG8 and NPC1L1. ABCG5 and ABCG8 transport cholesterol from the liver into bile [45] whereas NPC1L1 transports cholesterol from the bile back into the liver [67]. Biliary phospholipid secretion is mediated by ABCB4 [41,42]. The difference in biliary cholesterol and biliary phospholipid secretion prompted an investigation of the expression of these genes in response to dietary challenge in low and high responders. *ABCG5* and *ABCG8* mRNA levels did not differ between low and high responding opossums, whereas *NPC1L1* mRNA levels were down-regulated in high responders [68]. There was no significant difference in *ABCB4* mRNA levels between low and high responders on the two diets [69]. Therefore, expression of cholesterol and phospholipid transporter genes cannot explain differences in biliary lipid concentrations.

Association of ABCB4 with hypercholesterolemia. Development of a genetic linkage map of *Monodelphis* [70], coupled with the *Monodelphis* genome sequence [62], facilitated the identification of genes that predispose high responders to develop hypercholesterolemia on the HCHF diet. Genome-wide linkage analyses on data from pedigreed opossums located two quantitative trait loci (QTL) influencing V+LDL cholesterol levels. The QTL on chromosome 1 influences V+LDL cholesterol on the basal diet, and the QTL on chromosome 8 influences V+LDL cholesterol on the HCHF diet [69]. One gene in the chromosome 8 QTL is *ABCB4*. Since ABCB4 plays a role in biliary secretion of phospholipids and cholesterol, lower levels of biliary lipids in high responding opossums could be due to an impairment of ABCB4 function. We tested this hypothesis by sequencing the *ABCB4* gene to identify mutations and found two single nucleotide polymorphisms (SNPs) that cause missense mutations in exons 2 and 7 of the *ABCB4* gene from high responders. In exon 2, Gly at amino acid 29 in allele 1 is substituted by Arg in allele 2. In exon 7, Leu at amino acid 235 in allele 1 is substituted by Ile in allele 2. Allele 1 is predominant in the high responding strain, whereas allele 2 is predominant in the two low responding strains [24,69].

Using a pedigree-based genetic association approach, matings of high responders with low responders were carried out to produce F2 progeny in two different crosses (designated JCX and KUSH6) to determine whether ABCB4 has an effect on response to dietary cholesterol. Animals from both crosses were genotyped for the ABCB4 Ile235Leu polymorphism and subjected to measured genotype analysis using plasma cholesterol data from a basal diet and from a 4-week HCHF diet. The average concentration of plasma total cholesterol and V+LDL cholesterol on the HCHF diet was highest in JCX animals homozygous for the *ABCB4* '1' allele, intermediate in animals with the *ABCB4* '1/2' genotype, and lowest in animals homozygous for the *ABCB4* '2' allele. A similar pattern was observed in animals from the KUSH6 cross. The results showed that genetic variation in *ABCB4* had a significant effect on variation in V+LDL cholesterol levels in response to the HCHF diet, and implicated defects in biliary phospholipid and biliary cholesterol secretion in causing diet-induced hypercholesterolemia in the opossum model. However, it was apparent from the analysis that there is at least one additional gene that influences diet-induced hypercholesterolemia because some opossums that are homozygous for the missense mutations are not high responders [24,69].

Variations in the *ABCB4* gene have not been shown previously to be associated with variations in plasma LDL cholesterol in response to diet in other experimental animals or humans. ABCB4 mutations affect secretion of phospholipids, and clinical symptoms are due to production of bile with a low phospholipid content which cannot prevent bile salts from damaging the membranes of cells lining the bile ducts. Moreover, the phospholipid deficient bile has a high cholesterol saturation index. In humans, *ABCB4* variants that have a severe effect are associated with progressive familial intrahepatic cholestasis type 3, a liver disease that often develops in the first year of life. *ABCB4* variants that have a moderate effect are associated with a gallstone disease in adults known as low-phospholipid associated cholelithiasis, and a reversible form of cholestasis known as intrahepatic cholestasis of pregnancy that develops in women during the third trimester of pregnancy and resolves after delivery of their babies [71]. *ABCB4* knockout mice lacking phospholipid transport function develop sclerosing cholangitis, which progresses to metastatic liver cancer [72,73]. Mutations in the opossum A*BCB4* gene do not have a severe effect as high responders exhibit no adverse symptoms when the animals are fed the basal diet. The reduction in biliary cholesterol and biliary phospholipids associated with *ABCB4* mutations leads to an increase in plasma V+LDL cholesterol when high responders are challenged with the HCHF diet. However, a gene whose identity is still unknown seems to be able to compensate for the reduction in biliary cholesterol secretion and rescues high responders that are homozygous for the *ABCB4* mutations from developing diet-induced hypercholesterolemia. Identification of this gene will lead to a better understanding of the process involving *ABCB*4 in controlling plasma LDL cholesterol concentration in response to dietary cholesterol.

3.4. Pathologic features of high responders

Fatty livers. Dysregulated cholesterol homeostasis causes high responders to develop fatty livers and atherosclerotic lesions. Cholesterol accumulates in the livers of high responders as a result of impaired biliary cholesterol secretion. After 4 weeks of HCHF diet, serum levels of liver enzymes (alanine aminotransferase, aspartate aminotransferase, and γ–glutamyltransferase) and bilirubin were significantly elevated, indicating high responders had liver injury. Histology revealed steatosis, inflammation and ballooned hepatocytes in their livers after 8 weeks of HCHF diet. The pathologic condition in the liver worsened as high responders continued to consume the HCHF diet. In one study in which high and low responders were fed the HCHF diet for 24 weeks, livers of high responders were markedly enlarged compared to those of low responders. The enlarged livers had an increase in free cholesterol (2-fold), esterified cholesterol (11-fold) and triglycerides (2-fold), but no significant increase in free fatty acids. Low responders did not display any significant morphological changes in the liver after 24 weeks on the HCHF diet. Prolonged HCHF dietary challenge caused high responders to develop fibrosis in addition to steatosis, inflammation and ballooned cells. Liver fibrosis is a characteristic feature of the severe form of nonalcoholic fatty liver disease known as nonalcoholic steatohepatitis.

Expression of a set of hepatic genes associated with inflammation, oxidative stress and fibrogenesis was up-regulated in high responders, and the gene expression pattern was consistent with the histopathological features in the livers of high responders [74].

Atherosclerotic lesions. Similar to humans, hypercholesterolemia leads to development of atherosclerotic lesions in the arteries of high responding opossums. Low responding opossums whose V+LDL cholesterol was below 75 mg/dl did not develop gross or histologically detectable lesions after consuming the HCHF diet for one year. In contrast, high responding opossums whose V+LDL cholesterol was over 500 mg/dl developed gross and histologically detectable lesions after 40 weeks of HCHF diet. The opossum lesions were similar in histologic characteristics to those observed in cholesterol-fed mouse models of atherosclerosis [23].

4. Non-human primate models

Non-human primate models stand out as the most biologically similar to humans in physiologic and genetic characteristics of hypercholesterolemia [25]. This is because nonhuman primates and humans share similar biochemical, anatomical and physiological characteristics, including lipid synthesis and metabolism. Both humans and primates exhibit spontaneous and diet-induced hypercholesterolemia [15] and develop atherosclerosis [11,75]. Commonly used nonhuman primates include African green monkey (green monkey), rhesus monkey, cynomolgus monkey and baboon. These species not only have a high degree of physiological similarity with humans, but also have many of the same genes underlying relevant phenotypes. The size of nonhuman primates by comparison to mice enables the collection of tissue and organ samples of equivalent sizes to humans, including arteries and hearts. It is important to mention that great apes share greater similarities to humans than other nonhuman primates. However, cost and ethical considerations prohibit use of great apes for most human disease studies.

4.1. Nonhuman primate responses to HCHF diet

Nonhuman primates respond to HCHF diet as do humans. Most nonhuman primates respond to HCHF diet by an increase in average total plasma cholesterol concentration ranging from 200-800 mg/dl with no change in weight [11,15]. Total plasma cholesterol levels positively correlate with LDL cholesterol, VLDL cholesterol and triglyceride levels with no change in HDL cholesterol levels. In addition, triglyceride concentration is positively correlated with VLDL cholesterol and LDL cholesterol concentrations [15,25]. However, there are differences among species and among individuals in response to HCHF diet in nonhuman primates.

Variation among species. Nonhuman primate species differ in their response to HCHF diet challenges by exhibiting variation in plasma cholesterol [11,76]. Baboons and green monkeys display moderate response with an average plasma cholesterol concentration of 204 and 275 mg/dl, respectively, while cynomolgus monkeys and rhesus macaque have the highest response, 307 and 467 mg/dl, respectively [11,15,76]. The response of baboons is similar to that of humans [11].

In addition, green monkeys and baboons show unusual increases in HDL cholesterol levels in response to HCHF diet compared to most nonhuman primate species [11,76]. The mechanisms underlying the marked difference in response to HCHF diet for green monkeys and baboons are not well understood. Sorci-Thomas et al. [76] compared the responses of green and cynomolgus monkeys to HCHF diet. Because green monkeys develop modest hypercholesterolemia compared to cynomolgus monkeys when challenged with HCHF diet, green monkeys were fed diet with more cholesterol than cynomolgus monkeys to induce equivalent extent of hypercholesterolemia in both species. Surprisingly green monkeys still had 2-3-fold higher plasma HDL cholesterol and apoA-I concentrations than cynomolgus monkeys, indicating that higher plasma HDL cholesterol in green monkeys was due to factors independent of level of dietary cholesterol. Further investigation indicated that green monkey hepatic apoA-I and mRNA expression levels were respectively 2-fold and 3.7-fold higher, and intestinal *apoA-I* mRNA level was 3.7-folder higher than in cynomolgus monkeys. These observations indicate that factors that regulate mRNA transcription and post-transcription, including microRNA (miRNA) gene regulation, may be determinants of resistance to HCHF diet.

Variation among individuals. Similar to humans, nonhuman primates display variation among individual animals of the same species in response to HCHF diet [77-80]. This variation is one of the important features of nonhuman primate models that enables us to identify genetic variants that predispose individuals to develop hypercholesterolemia.

a. *Plasma lipoprotein cholesterol levels.* The response of plasma cholesterol level to HCHF diet differs among individuals. Baboons challenged with HCHF diet for 2 years exhibited an increase in plasma cholesterol levels from 5 to 197 mg/dl [81]. Based on these observations, McGill et al. selectively bred two lines of baboons with extreme plasma cholesterol levels; low responders and high responders to HCHF diet. Subsequent studies have shown that low and high responders differed in LDL cholesterol levels when challenged with HCHF diet. High responders had approximately 2-fold higher plasma cholesterol than low responders [11,80]. In addition, LDL *apoB* concentrations were 2-3-fold higher in high responders compared with low responders [11]. This difference was due to higher production of apoB in high responders. However, apoB mRNA levels did not differ between low and high responders on HCHF diet, suggesting that apoB production is regulated at the post-transcriptional level and is influenced by plasma cholesterol levels, which differ between low and high responders.

McGill et al. [82] examined the effect of cholesterol or saturated fat on plasma cholesterol response in low and high responders. The study revealed that high responders challenged with diet containing high cholesterol (1.7 mg/kcal) displayed a higher percent increase of LDL and VLDL cholesterol levels than low responders, and that there was no difference in HDL cholesterol levels between high and low responders. The type of saturated fat, corn or coconut oil in the diet did not influence plasma cholesterol variation between the two lines of baboons. Genetic analysis revealed that genetic factors explained 57% of the response to dietary cholesterol. These findings indicated that dietary cholesterol, and not saturated fat, drives variation in plasma cholesterol in baboons.

b. *Expression of 27-hydroxylase.* Nonhuman primates exhibit individual variation in the synthesis of bile acids from cholesterol. Sterol 27-hydroxylase is an important enzyme for bile acid synthesis in both the classic and alternate pathways. Kushwaha et al. [83] measured plasma and hepatic 27-hydroxycholesterol levels, hepatic 27-hydroxylase activity and mRNA levels in 12 low and 12 high responding baboons. Low responders displayed higher 27-hydroxycholesterol levels, 27-hydroxylase activities and mRNA levels than high responders when fed the HCHF diet but not when fed the chow diet. These parameters were negatively correlated with LDL and VLDL cholesterol concentrations in low responders. These findings indicate that sterol 27-hydroxylase is induced by HCHF diet and that the induction is higher in low responding baboons, resulting in higher bile acid synthesis. Thus, the ability to induce sterol 27-hydroxylase influences LDL cholesterol variation in baboons.

c. *ApoE levels and LDL receptor expression.* The liver clears excess plasma lipoprotein cholesterol through the LDL receptor and the LDL receptor-related protein. ApoE is a component of chylomicrons and most of the lipoproteins, and aids in receptor mediated-clearance of plasma lipoprotein cholesterol [31]. A study in cynomolgus and green monkeys fed an HCHF diet demonstrated that apoE concentrations were positively correlated with total plasma cholesterol concentrations, plasma LDL cholesterol concentrations and LDL particle size [12]. Since apoE is a high-affinity ligand for the LDL receptor and the LDL receptor-related protein, plasma cholesterol clearance by the liver is expected to increase when apoE levels are elevated, but this is not the case. A possible explanation is that LDL receptors are down-regulated in hypercholesterolemic monkeys, and clearance of VLDL and LDL particles is impeded. ApoE-enriched LDL particles accumulate in the plasma of hypercholesterolemic animals because VLDL particles are metabolized to LDL particles rather than being removed from the circulation by the LDL receptor as in monkeys with normal plasma cholesterol concentrations [12].

Together, these findings suggest that plasma cholesterol variation in nonhuman primates may be influenced by the level of sterol 27-hydroxylase activity in the liver. A decrease in conversion of cholesterol to bile acids may lead to an increase in plasma cholesterol, which in turn decreases LDL receptor expression. As a consequence, the rate of clearance of plasma VLDL and LDL cholesterol is reduced and circulating levels of LDL cholesterol are elevated.

4.2. Genetic mechanisms that influence individual variation in plasma cholesterol levels

Baboon genetic resources to study lipid metabolism. The baboon is the most commonly used primate model for genetic studies of complex traits and susceptibility to complex diseases [14]. The Southwest National Primate Research Center (SNPRC) at Texas Biomedical Research Institute maintains approximately 1,500 living baboons for biological research. These baboons have been used to develop nonhuman primate genomic resources to study responses to environmental factors, such as diet, and how these factors interact with genomic factors in causing complex diseases or disorders. In addition, SNPRC maintains an extensive pedigree database consisting of 16,000 baboons across seven generations. This is the largest nonhuman primate pedigree in the world. The pedigreed population includes approximately 384 founders of olive

(*P. h. anubis*) and yellow (*P. h. cynocephalus*) baboons, and their hybrid descendants. These resources provided a unique opportunity to map baboon genes, resulting in the first ever nonhuman primate linkage map [84,85]. In addition, tissues and blood samples have been collected from 8,000 baboons, and DNA, serum and buffy coats from 4,000 animals [14].

Genetic factors for hypercholesterolemia in baboons. Baboon response to HCHF diet is modest, similar to the response of humans. Because of this similarity as well as other baboon characteristics that mimic human characteristics, numerous studies have utilized baboon resources available at SNPRC to understand how genetic variation influences lipoprotein cholesterol in response to diet. This initiative started more than three decades ago when scientists at the Texas Biomedical Research Institute observed differential response of baboons to HCHF diet [81]. These observations led to selective breeding and characterization of distinct phenotypes of baboons and revealed that differential response to HCHF diet is heritable [86,87].

Attempts to find the major genes influencing plasma cholesterol in response to dietary challenge revealed that polymorphisms in the LDL receptor gene contributed only 6% of the variation [88], suggesting that lipid response to HCHF diet is multigenic. Hypercholesterolemia is a complex disorder plausibly influenced by complex genetic networks. Therefore, to elucidate the mechanisms that underlie cholesterol variation, a system biological approach is most appropriate. Using available pedigree and genotypic information for more than 2,400 baboons, important lipid/lipoprotein-related QTL have been identified [27,89,90]. In addition, improved Next Gen Sequencing techniques for RNA and DNA sequencing and genetic network analyses have enabled understanding of genes encoding these QTL.

Studies were undertaken to interrogate the QTL to discover gene, genetic variants and functional mechanisms that influence variation in response to diet in baboons. In one study, four novel candidate genes (*TENC1, ACVR1B, ERBB3, DGKA*) were identified that encode a QTL for LDL cholesterol concentration variation. This QTL overlaps multiple other QTL for LDL related traits, including particle size, suggesting that these genes have pleiotropic effects [13]. *TENC1* was downregulated while *ACVR1B, ERBB3* and *DGKA* were upregulated in response to HCHF diet. The protein products of all four genes are central molecules for a single pathway, affirming that multiple genes influence LDL cholesterol variation. Interestingly these genes are associated with cancer in the *AKT/GSK3B* signaling pathway [91]. Several studies have alluded a link between cancer, hypercholesterolemia and atherosclerosis [92-95], but the link is not well understood. One aspect that is clear is that cholesterol is intertwined in the etiology of cancer and atherosclerosis. In addition, tumorigenesis thrives by the ability to alter important biological processes, including regulation of cholesterol levels. For cancer cells to proliferate uncontrollably, essential cell components, such as cholesterol must be available for plasma membrane synthesis. In order to meet the demand for cholesterol, pathways regulating cellular cholesterol homeostasis are altered in cancer cells.

Other studies have investigated the role of miRNA in LDL cholesterol variation in baboons [13,80]. miRNAs were hypothesized to regulate genes encoding variation in LDL cholesterol in response to HCHF diet. Hepatic miRNA expression profiling in low and high LDL cholesterol half–sibling baboons by RNA sequencing revealed 226 miRNAs were differentially expressed (160 downregulated and 66 upregulated) between low and high responders in response to HCHF diet. In order to identify molecular mechanisms that may regulate LDL cholesterol variation, these miRNAs were overlaid onto gene networks that differ between low and high baboon responders. Seven miRNAs were inversely expressed with respect to the four candidate genes. Together, these findings demonstrate that hepatic miRNAs are responsive to diet, and that response differs among baboons with different plasma LDL cholesterol levels.

4.3. Nonhuman primates and atherosclerosis, the clinical endpoint of hypercholesterolemia

Atherosclerosis, a complex progressive disease, is the leading cause of mortality and morbidity in developed countries [96,97]. The clinical end-point of atherosclerosis is cardiovascular disease primarily caused by thickening and/or occlusion of coronary arteries. Atherosclerotic heart disease is the leading cause of death in the world and is projected to remain the single leading cause of death by 2030 [98].

Atherogenesis is similar in nonhuman primates and humans. Atherogenesis is a multifactorial process. Initial events during atherogenesis include deposition of modified or oxidized cholesterol (ox-cholesterol) in the artery wall, resulting in endothelial dysfunction; adhesion of circulating monocytes onto the endothelium; entry of ox-cholesterol and monocytes into the intima layer of the artery; engulfment of ox-cholesterol by monocytes and transformation into macrophages and foam cells; production of pro-inflammatory cytokines and connective matrix; conversion and proliferation of smooth muscle cells; cell apoptosis; and intima thickening. During these processes, atherosclerotic lesions, which are grossly and microscopically heterogeneous, develop on the intimal arterial surface. In nonhuman primates, as in humans, the initial lesions are flat fatty streaks, which are not elevated on the intimal surface, containing predominately foam cells derived from monocytes and smooth muscle cells filled with minimal lipid. These lesions advance to raised fatty streaks that are characterized by lipid-filled foam cells. Raised lesions may progress to advanced fibrous plaques with lipid cores and accumulated connective matrix [26,75,99].

Lipoprotein cholesterol and atherosclerosis. Nonhuman primates provide a unique opportunity not only to understand the factors that underlie differential response to HCHF diet but the link between diet response and development of atherosclerosis in humans. In both nonhuman primates and humans, dyslipidemia is associated with atherosclerosis. High levels of non-HDL cholesterol, including LDL cholesterol, VLDL cholesterol and triglycerides, induced by HCHF diet are positively correlated with the extent and severity of atherosclerosis while HDL cholesterol is negatively correlated [75]. This implies that HCHF diets indirectly influence atherogenesis through induction of hypercholesterolemia. Another study with baboons revealed that plasma HDL1 levels are negatively correlated with extent and severity of atherosclerosis [11]. These results are consistent with results from human studies that indicate plasma lipoprotein cholesterol levels and lipoprotein subclasses are indicators of the extent of atherosclerosis [100]. Stevenson et al. [12] observed in cynomolgus monkeys that an increase in apoE correlates with extent of atherosclerosis, suggesting that apoE may represent an atherogenic feature of diet-induced hypercholesterolemia.

Arterial distribution of atherosclerosis. Atherosclerosis in nonhuman primates and humans displays a distinctive topographical distribution in the arterial system. The extent and severity of the disease is greater in the abdominal and common iliac arteries than in the thoracic and aortic arch, whereas flat lesions are more abundant in thoracic and aortic arch in nonhuman primates and humans [11,26]. It is hypothesized that the distinct localization of atherosclerotic lesions is a consequence of hemodynamic stress induced by blood flow; and anatomic, cellular, or biochemical variations in the arterial wall, particularly in the endothelium. These hypotheses are consistent with observations of more abundant lesions in branches and bifurcations of medium-sized arteries, including abdominal and common iliac arteries in nonhuman primates [101]. However, the mechanisms underlying the varied distribution of atherosclerosis in both humans and nonhuman primates are not well understood.

Variation among species and individuals in development of atherosclerosis. Nonhuman primate species display variation in susceptibility to developing atherosclerosis. Paralleling the different responses to HCHF diet, rhesus and cynomolgus monkeys are more susceptible to atherosclerosis [102] than green monkeys and baboons, which develop moderate atherosclerosis [103] as do humans [11]. Individuals within any one species also display differential susceptibility to atherosclerosis. High responders to HCHF diet develop more severe atherosclerosis than low responders, consistent with differential levels of plasma non-HDL cholesterol [26]. It is this variation that is critical for identification of genetic factors underlying variation in atherosclerosis development. This variation is heritable [104] and may correspond to genetic variation that underlies observed plasma cholesterol variation in response to HCHF diet.

5. Conclusion

ApoE deficient mice, generated by gene targeting, have a lipoprotein profile similar to humans in that most of the plasma cholesterol is carried on VLDL and IDL particles rather than HDL particles as in non-genetically modified mice. *ApoE-/-* mice have elevated levels of plasma cholesterol even on a chow diet and develop atherosclerotic lesions spontaneously. Advanced lesions with plaque rupture that resemble those in humans are frequently observed in *apoE-/-* mice fed an HCHF diet, and these mice are used for developing drugs to reduce atherosclerosis.

A nonbiliary pathway for cholesterol excretion in humans was suggested more than five decades ago based on measurement of intestinal cholesterol secretion from patients with bile duct obstruction. This finding was largely ignored because hepatobiliary secretion is believed to be the only route to dispose of cholesterol in feces. Observations from studies using several genetically modified mice (*G5G8-/-*, *Abcb4-/-* and *Npc1l1*$^{\text{-LiverTg}}$) that have severe defects in biliary cholesterol secretion, but normal or even increased fecal neutral sterol excretion, prompted several groups of researchers to investigate the TICE pathway. They reported that TICE accounts for 20%-30% of fecal neutral sterol excretion. However, mechanistic details of TICE still remain unknown. Because cholesterol excretion is an important process to eliminate cholesterol from the body, stimulation of TICE by pharmacological agents may be a novel therapeutic strategy to limit atherogenesis.

Studies using genetically modified mice have shown that they are indispensable for advancing our knowledge of the genes and pathways that govern cholesterol homeostasis, as well as for developing pharmacological agents to treat atherosclerosis. Traditional gene targeting using embryonic stem cells is a complex and time-consuming procedure to produce mutant mice and is limited to targeting one gene at a time. Mice carrying mutations in multiple genes are produced either by sequential gene targeting or intercrossing mice with a single mutation. The CRISPR (clustered regularly interspaced short palindromic repeat)-Cas9 (CRISPR-associated nuclease 9) system is a new and more efficient genome engineering technology [105]. It allows targeting multiple genes at the same time by direct co-injection of RNA encoding the Cas9 nuclease and several gene-specific guide RNA into a one-cell embryo to generate mice with multiple modified genes [106]. Application of the CRISPR/Cas system will accelerate the production of mouse models carrying multiple modified genes to study complex disease such as hypercholesterolemia.

High responding opossums have naturally occurring genetic variants that predispose them to develop hypercholesterolemia when challenged with an HCHF diet. At least two major genes control the plasma cholesterol response to dietary challenge in high responding opossums. One has been identified as the *ABCB4* gene. Mutations in *ABCB4* impair the ability of high responding opossums to secrete phospholipids into the bile. Because secretion of cholesterol into bile requires phospholipids, biliary cholesterol secretion is also impaired in high responding opossums. As a consequence, plasma V+LDL cholesterol becomes elevated in high responders, and free and esterified cholesterol accumulates in their livers. However, some opossums that are homozygous for the *ABCB4* mutations are resistant to diet-induced hypercholesterolemia. The compensatory mechanism that allows these opossums to overcome the defect in biliary cholesterol secretion is not known. In light of the finding of a nonbiliary route of cholesterol excretion that functions in normal mice as well as in mice that have very low biliary cholesterol secretion, cholesterol excretion by the nonbiliary route may compensate for the defect in biliary excretion in opossums that are homozygous for the *ABCB4* mutations.

Phylogenetic similarities between humans and nonhuman primate models are core aspects for consideration in investigations of environmental and genetic factors that contribute to complex diseases/disorders, including hypercholesterolemia and atherosclerosis. Moreover, like humans, nonhuman primates exhibit diet-induced hypercholesterolemia and naturally develop atherosclerosis, making it possible to identify phenotypic variations without altering genetic background as is required for this line of research with mice. In addition, environmental factors, including diet, can be controlled for a prolonged period of time, invasive and terminal experiments can be conducted, and tissues and organs can be easily collected. These research activities are not attainable when working with human subjects.

Recent scientific advances have led to discovery of therapeutic regimes, including statins for lowering LDL cholesterol and retarding the development of atherosclerosis [107]. However, these therapies are limited by side effects and ineffectiveness in some individuals [108,109]. Thus, there is a need for continued searching for novel therapeutic agents. Diet-induced hypercholesterolemia in nonhuman primates provides an opportunity 1) to identify lipid profiles important for the development of atherosclerosis in primates in a controlled environment, 2) to identify variation in responses to diet, and 3) to assess progression of and variation in development of atherosclerosis in response to dietary cholesterol and saturated fat. Identification of these variations is essential for genetic analysis to develop novel therapeutic agents for lowering plasma cholesterol and biomarkers for detection of early atherosclerosis, a precursor for cardiovascular disease.

Nonhuman primate genetic resources for studying complex diseases are becoming increasingly sophisticated and available at SNPRC and Texas Biomedical Research Institute. These resources enable scientific collaborations to study human diseases using multidisciplinary approaches. Significant steps have been achieved in the identification of genetic causes of hypercholesterolemia and atherosclerosis, including discovery of QTL and genes and gene variants that influence plasma LDL and HDL cholesterol levels, and triglyceride levels.

Further improvement and enhancement of unique genetic resources for research with mice, laboratory opossums, and nonhuman primates will be critical for future research aimed at understanding genetic and epigenetic factors influencing human health and disease.

Acknowledgements

This work was supported by National Institutes of Health Grants P01 HL028972, P01 HL028972-Supplement, P51 OD011133, R01 DK065058, and grants from the Robert J. Kleberg, Jr. and Helen C. Kleberg Foundation and Texas Biomedical Forum. This work was conducted in part in facilities constructed with support from Research Facilities Improvement Program Grant Numbers C06 RR013556 and C06 RR015456 from the National Center for Research Resources (now Office of Research Infrastructure Programs), National Institutes of Health.

Author details

Jeannie Chan[1*], Genesio M. Karere[1], Laura A. Cox[2] and John L. VandeBerg[2]

*Address all correspondence to: jchan@txbiomedgenetics.org

1 Department of Genetics, Texas Biomedical Research Institute, San Antonio, Texas, USA

2 Department of Genetics and Southwest National Primate Research Center, Texas Biomedical Research Institute, San Antonio, Texas, USA

References

[1] van der Wulp MY, Verkade HJ, Groen AK. Regulation of cholesterol homeostasis. Mol Cell Endocrinol 2013;368(1-2) 1-16.

[2] Executive summary of the third report of the National Cholesterol Education Program (NCEP) expert panel on detection, evaluation, and treatment of high blood cholesterol in adults (Adult Treatment Panel III). JAMA 2001;285(19) 2486-2497.

[3] Vital signs: prevalence, treatment, and control of high levels of low-density lipoprotein cholesterol--United States, 1999-2002 and 2005-2008. Morb Mortal Wkly Rep 2011;60(4) 109-114.

[4] Goldstein JL, Brown MS. The LDL receptor locus and the genetics of familial hypercholesterolemia. Annu Rev Genet 1979;13 259-289.

[5] Aliev G, Burnstock G. Watanabe rabbits with heritable hypercholesterolaemia: a model of atherosclerosis. Histol Histopathol 1998;13(3) 797-817.

[6] Yanni AE. The laboratory rabbit: an animal model of atherosclerosis research. Lab Anim 2004;38(3) 246-256.

[7] Temel RE, Rudel LL. Diet effects on atherosclerosis in mice. Curr Drug Targets 2007;8(11) 1150-1160.

[8] Fernandez ML. Guinea pigs as models for cholesterol and lipoprotein metabolism. J Nutr 2001;131(1) 10-20.

[9] Kawaguchi H, Miyoshi N, Miura N, Fujiki M, Horiuchi M, Izumi Y, Miyajima H, Nagata R, Misumi K, Takeuchi T, Tanimoto A, Yoshida H. Microminipig, a non-rodent experimental animal optimized for life science research:novel atherosclerosis model induced by high fat and cholesterol diet. J Pharmacol Sci 2011;115(2) 115-121.

[10] Rainwater DL, VandeBerg JL. Dramatic differences in lipoprotein composition among gray short-tailed opossums (*Monodelphis domestica*) fed a high cholesterol/saturated fat diet. Biochim Biophys Acta 1992;1126(2) 159-166.

[11] Kushwaha RS, McGill HC,Jr. Diet, plasma lipoproteins and experimental atherosclerosis in baboons (*Papio sp.*). Hum Reprod Update 1998;4(4) 420-429.

[12] Stevenson SC, Sawyer JK, Rudel LL. Role of apolipoprotein E on cholesteryl ester-enriched low density lipoprotein particles in coronary artery atherosclerosis of hypercholesterolemic nonhuman primates. Arterioscler Thromb 1992;12(1) 28-40.

[13] Karere GM, Glenn JP, Birnbaum S, Rainwater DL, Mahaney MC, Vanderberg JL, Cox LA. Identification of candidate genes encoding an LDL-C QTL in baboons. J Lipid Res 2013;54(7):1776-1785.

[14] Cox LA, Comuzzie AG, Havill LM, Karere GM, Spradling KD, Mahaney MC, Nathanielsz PW, Nicolella DP, Shade RE, Voruganti S, Vandeberg JL. Baboons as a model to study genetics and epigenetics of human disease. ILAR J 2013;54(2) 106-121.

[15] Shamekh R, Linden EH, Newcomb JD, Tigno XT, Jen KL, Pellizzon MA, Hansen BC. Endogenous and diet-induced hypercholesterolemia in nonhuman primates: effects

of age, adiposity, and diabetes on lipoprotein profiles. Metabolism 2011;60(8) 1165-1177.

[16] Plump AS, Smith JD, Hayek T, Aalto-Setala K, Walsh A, Verstuyft JG, Rubin EM, Breslow JL. Severe hypercholesterolemia and atherosclerosis in apolipoprotein E-deficient mice created by homologous recombination in ES cells. Cell 1992;71(2) 343-353.

[17] Zhang SH, Reddick RL, Piedrahita JA, Maeda N. Spontaneous hypercholesterolemia and arterial lesions in mice lacking apolipoprotein E. Science 1992;258(5081) 468-471.

[18] Kruit JK, Plosch T, Havinga R, Boverhof R, Groot PH, Groen AK, Kuipers F. Increased fecal neutral sterol loss upon liver X receptor activation is independent of biliary sterol secretion in mice. Gastroenterology 2005;128(1) 147-156.

[19] van der Velde AE, Vrins CL, van den Oever K, Kunne C, Oude Elferink RP, Kuipers F, Groen AK. Direct intestinal cholesterol secretion contributes significantly to total fecal neutral sterol excretion in mice. Gastroenterology 2007;133(3) 967-975.

[20] Brufau G, Groen AK, Kuipers F. Reverse cholesterol transport revisited: contribution of biliary versus intestinal cholesterol excretion. Arterioscler Thromb Vasc Biol 2011;31(8) 1726-1733.

[21] Jakulj L, Besseling J, Stroes ES, Groen AK. Intestinal cholesterol secretion: future clinical implications. Neth J Med 2013;71(9) 459-465.

[22] VandeBerg J, Cheng ML. Dyslipoproteinemia in a laboratory marsupial, *Monodelphis domestica*. Isozyme Bulletin 1985;18 66.

[23] VandeBerg JL, Chan J, VandeBerg JF, McGill HC,Jr, Kushwaha RS. Genetic Control of Lipemic Response to Dietary Cholesterol in Laboratory Opossums. In: Proceedings of the 13th International Congress on Genes and Gene Families and Isozymes (ICGGFI). Monduzzi Editore Int Proc Div Bologna; 2005. p45-56.

[24] Chan J, Mahaney MC, Kushwaha RS, VandeBerg JF, VandeBerg JL. *ABCB4* mediates diet-induced hypercholesterolemia in laboratory opossums. J Lipid Res 2010;51(10) 2922-2928.

[25] Yin W, Carballo-Jane E, McLaren DG, Mendoza VH, Gagen K, Geoghagen NS, McNamara LA, Gorski JN, Eiermann GJ, Petrov A, Wolff M, Tong X, Wilsie LC, Akiyama TE, Chen J, Thankappan A, Xue J, Ping X, Andrews G, Wickham LA, Gai CL, Trinh T, Kulick AA, Donnelly MJ, Voronin GO, Rosa R, Cumiskey AM, Bekkari K, Mitnaul LJ, Puig O, Chen F, Raubertas R, Wong PH, Hansen BC, Koblan KS, Roddy TP, Hubbard BK, Strack AM. Plasma lipid profiling across species for the identification of optimal animal models of human dyslipidemia. J Lipid Res 2012;53(1) 51-65.

[26] McGill HC,Jr, McMahan CA, Zieske AW, Sloop GD, Walcott JV, Troxclair DA, Malcom GT, Tracy RE, Oalmann MC, Strong JP. Associations of coronary heart disease risk factors with the intermediate lesion of atherosclerosis in youth. The Pathobiolog-

ical Determinants of Atherosclerosis in Youth (PDAY) Research Group. Arterioscler Thromb Vasc Biol 2000;20(8) 1998-2004.

[27] Vinson A, Mahaney MC, Cox LA, Rogers J, VandeBerg JL, Rainwater DL. A pleiotropic QTL on 2p influences serum Lp-PLA2 activity and LDL cholesterol concentration in a baboon model for the genetics of atherosclerosis risk factors. Atherosclerosis 2008;196(2) 667-673.

[28] Marotti KR, Castle CK, Murray RW, Rehberg EF, Polites HG, Melchior GW. The role of cholesteryl ester transfer protein in primate apolipoprotein A-I metabolism. Insights from studies with transgenic mice. Arterioscler Thromb 1992;12(6) 736-744.

[29] Jiang XC, Masucci-Magoulas L, Mar J, Lin M, Walsh A, Breslow JL, Tall A. Down-regulation of mRNA for the low density lipoprotein receptor in transgenic mice containing the gene for human cholesteryl ester transfer protein. Mechanism to explain accumulation of lipoprotein B particles. J Biol Chem 1993;268(36) 27406-27412.

[30] Tall AR. Plasma lipid transfer proteins. J Lipid Res 1986;27(4) 361-367.

[31] Fazio S, Linton MF, Swift LL. The cell biology and physiologic relevance of ApoE recycling. Trends Cardiovasc Med 2000;10(1) 23-30.

[32] Brown MS, Goldstein JL. A receptor-mediated pathway for cholesterol homeostasis. Science 1986;232(4746) 34-47.

[33] Hobbs HH, Brown MS, Goldstein JL. Molecular genetics of the LDL receptor gene in familial hypercholesterolemia. Hum Mutat 1992;1(6) 445-466.

[34] Watanabe Y, Ito T, Shiomi M. The effect of selective breeding on the development of coronary atherosclerosis in WHHL rabbits. An animal model for familial hypercholesterolemia. Atherosclerosis 1985;56(1) 71-79.

[35] Ishibashi S, Brown MS, Goldstein JL, Gerard RD, Hammer RE, Herz J. Hypercholesterolemia in low density lipoprotein receptor knockout mice and its reversal by adenovirus-mediated gene delivery. J Clin Invest 1993;92(2) 883-893.

[36] Chan L. Apolipoprotein B, the major protein component of triglyceride-rich and low density lipoproteins. J Biol Chem 1992;267(36) 25621-25624.

[37] Meir KS, Leitersdorf E. Atherosclerosis in the apolipoprotein-E-deficient mouse: a decade of progress. Arterioscler Thromb Vasc Biol 2004;24(6) 1006-1014.

[38] Johnson J, Carson K, Williams H, Karanam S, Newby A, Angelini G, George S, Jackson C. Plaque rupture after short periods of fat feeding in the apolipoprotein E-knockout mouse: model characterization and effects of pravastatin treatment. Circulation 2005;111(11) 1422-1430.

[39] Berge KE, Tian H, Graf GA, Yu L, Grishin NV, Schultz J, Kwiterovich P, Shan B, Barnes R, Hobbs HH. Accumulation of dietary cholesterol in sitosterolemia caused by mutations in adjacent ABC transporters. Science 2000;290(5497) 1771-1775.

[40] Jansen PL, Strautnieks SS, Jacquemin E, Hadchouel M, Sokal EM, Hooiveld GJ, Koning JH, De Jager-Krikken A, Kuipers F, Stellaard F, Bijleveld CM, Gouw A, Van Goor H, Thompson RJ, Muller M. Hepatocanalicular bile salt export pump deficiency in patients with progressive familial intrahepatic cholestasis. Gastroenterology 1999;117(6) 1370-1379.

[41] Smit JJ, Schinkel AH, Oude Elferink RP, Groen AK, Wagenaar E, van Deemter L, Mol CA, Ottenhoff R, van der Lugt NM, van Roon MA. Homozygous disruption of the murine *mdr2* P-glycoprotein gene leads to a complete absence of phospholipid from bile and to liver disease. Cell 1993;75(3) 451-462.

[42] Smith AJ, de Vree JM, Ottenhoff R, Oude Elferink RP, Schinkel AH, Borst P. Hepatocyte-specific expression of the human *MDR3* P-glycoprotein gene restores the biliary phosphatidylcholine excretion absent in *Mdr2* (-/-) mice. Hepatology 1998;28(2) 530-536.

[43] Trauner M, Boyer JL. Bile salt transporters: molecular characterization, function, and regulation. Physiol Rev 2003;83(2) 633-671.

[44] Yu L, Li-Hawkins J, Hammer RE, Berge KE, Horton JD, Cohen JC, Hobbs HH. Overexpression of ABCG5 and ABCG8 promotes biliary cholesterol secretion and reduces fractional absorption of dietary cholesterol. J Clin Invest 2002;110(5) 671-680.

[45] Yu L, Hammer RE, Li-Hawkins J, Von Bergmann K, Lutjohann D, Cohen JC, Hobbs HH. Disruption of *Abcg5* and *Abcg8* in mice reveals their crucial role in biliary cholesterol secretion. Proc Natl Acad Sci U S A 2002;99(25) 16237-16242.

[46] Langheim S, Yu L, von Bergmann K, Lutjohann D, Xu F, Hobbs HH, Cohen JC. ABCG5 and ABCG8 require MDR2 for secretion of cholesterol into bile. J Lipid Res 2005;46(8) 1732-1738.

[47] Elferink RP, Tytgat GN, Groen AK. Hepatic canalicular membrane 1: The role of mdr2 P-glycoprotein in hepatobiliary lipid transport. FASEB J 1997;11(1) 19-28.

[48] Sperry WM. Lipid excretion: IV. A study of the relationship of the bile to the fecal lipids with special reference to certain problems of sterol metabolism. J Biol Chem 1927;71 351-378.

[49] Pertsemlidis D, Kirchman EH, Ahrens EH,Jr. Regulation of cholesterol metabolism in the dog. II. Effects of complete bile diversion and of cholesterol feeding on pool sizes of tissue cholesterol measured at autopsy. J Clin Invest 1973;52(9) 2368-2378.

[50] Bandsma RH, Stellaard F, Vonk RJ, Nagel GT, Neese RA, Hellerstein MK, Kuipers F. Contribution of newly synthesized cholesterol to rat plasma and bile determined by mass isotopomer distribution analysis: bile-salt flux promotes secretion of newly synthesized cholesterol into bile. Biochem J 1998;329 (Pt 3) 699-703.

[51] van der Veen JN, van Dijk TH, Vrins CL, van Meer H, Havinga R, Bijsterveld K, Tietge UJ, Groen AK, Kuipers F. Activation of the liver X receptor stimulates trans-intestinal excretion of plasma cholesterol. J Biol Chem 2009;284(29) 19211-19219.

[52] Brown JM, Bell TA,3rd, Alger HM, Sawyer JK, Smith TL, Kelley K, Shah R, Wilson MD, Davis MA, Lee RG, Graham MJ, Crooke RM, Rudel LL. Targeted depletion of hepatic ACAT2-driven cholesterol esterification reveals a non-biliary route for fecal neutral sterol loss. J Biol Chem 2008;283(16) 10522-10534.

[53] Plosch T, Kok T, Bloks VW, Smit MJ, Havinga R, Chimini G, Groen AK, Kuipers F. Increased hepatobiliary and fecal cholesterol excretion upon activation of the liver X receptor is independent of ABCA1. J Biol Chem 2002;277(37) 33870-33877.

[54] Vrins CL, Ottenhoff R, van den Oever K, de Waart DR, Kruyt JK, Zhao Y, van Berkel TJ, Havekes LM, Aerts JM, van Eck M, Rensen PC, Groen AK. Trans-intestinal cholesterol efflux is not mediated through high density lipoprotein. J Lipid Res 2012;53(10) 2017-2023.

[55] Marshall SM, Gromovsky AD, Kelley KL, Davis MA, Wilson MD, Lee RG, Crooke RM, Graham MJ, Rudel LL, Brown JM, Temel RE. Acute sterol o-acyltransferase 2 (SOAT2) knockdown rapidly mobilizes hepatic cholesterol for fecal excretion. PLoS One 2014;9(6) e98953.

[56] Marshall SM, Kelley KL, Davis MA, Wilson MD, McDaniel AL, Lee RG, Crooke RM, Graham MJ, Rudel LL, Brown JM, Temel RE. Reduction of VLDL secretion decreases cholesterol excretion in Niemann-pick C1-like 1 hepatic transgenic mice. PLoS One 2014;9(1) e84418.

[57] Le May C, Berger JM, Lespine A, Pillot B, Prieur X, Letessier E, Hussain MM, Collet X, Cariou B, Costet P. Transintestinal cholesterol excretion is an active metabolic process modulated by PCSK9 and statin involving ABCB1. Arterioscler Thromb Vasc Biol 2013;33(7) 1484-1493.

[58] van der Velde AE, Vrins CL, van den Oever K, Seemann I, Oude Elferink RP, van Eck M, Kuipers F, Groen AK. Regulation of direct transintestinal cholesterol excretion in mice. Am J Physiol Gastrointest Liver Physiol 2008;295(1) G203-G208.

[59] Bura KS, Lord C, Marshall S, McDaniel A, Thomas G, Warrier M, Zhang J, Davis MA, Sawyer JK, Shah R, Wilson MD, Dikkers A, Tietge UJ, Collet X, Rudel LL, Temel RE, Brown JM. Intestinal SR-BI does not impact cholesterol absorption or transintestinal cholesterol efflux in mice. J Lipid Res 2013;54(6) 1567-1577.

[60] Cheng SH, Stanley MM. Secretion of cholesterol by intestinal mucosa in patients with complete common bile duct obstruction. Proc Soc Exp Biol Med 1959;101(2) 223-225.

[61] VandeBerg J, Williams-Blangero S. The Laboratory Opossum. In: Hubrecht R, Kirkwood J (eds.) The UFAW Handbook on the Care and Management of Laboratory and Other Research Animals (8th Ed.). West Sussex: Wiley-Blackwell; 2010. p246-261.

[62] Mikkelsen TS, Wakefield MJ, Aken B, Amemiya CT, Chang JL, Duke S, Garber M, Gentles AJ, Goodstadt L, Heger A, Jurka J, Kamal M, Mauceli E, Searle SM, Sharpe T, Baker ML, Batzer MA, Benos PV, Belov K, Clamp M, Cook A, Cuff J, Das R, Davidow L, Deakin JE, Fazzari MJ, Glass JL, Grabherr M, Greally JM, Gu W, Hore TA, Huttley GA, Kleber M, Jirtle RL, Koina E, Lee JT, Mahony S, Marra MA, Miller RD, Nicholls RD, Oda M, Papenfuss AT, Parra ZE, Pollock DD, Ray DA, Schein JE, Speed TP, Thompson K, VandeBerg JL, Wade CM, Walker JA, Waters PD, Webber C, Weidman JR, Xie X, Zody MC, Broad Institute Genome Sequencing Platform, Broad Institute Whole Genome Assembly Team, Graves JA, Ponting CP, Breen M, Samollow PB, Lander ES, Lindblad-Toh K. Genome of the marsupial *Monodelphis domestica* reveals innovation in non-coding sequences. Nature 2007;447(7141) 167-177.

[63] Kushwaha RS, Vandeberg JF, Rodriguez R, Vandeberg JL. Cholesterol absorption and hepatic acyl-coenzyme A:cholesterol acyltransferase activity play major roles in lipemic response to dietary cholesterol and fat in laboratory opossums. Metabolism 2004;53(6) 817-822.

[64] Chan J, Kushwaha RS, Vandeberg JF, Gluhak-Heinrich J, Vandeberg JL. Differential expression of intestinal genes in opossums with high and low responses to dietary cholesterol. J Nutr Metab 2010;2010 415075. Epub 2009 Nov 23.

[65] Russell DW. The enzymes, regulation, and genetics of bile acid synthesis. Annu Rev Biochem 2003;72 137-174.

[66] Kushwaha RS, VandeBerg JF, Jackson EM, VandeBerg JL. High and low responding strains of laboratory opossums differ in sterol 27-hydroxylase and acyl-coenzyme A:cholesterol acyltransferase activities on a high cholesterol diet. J Nutr Biochem 2001;12(12) 664-673.

[67] Temel RE, Tang W, Ma Y, Rudel LL, Willingham MC, Ioannou YA, Davies JP, Nilsson LM, Yu L. Hepatic Niemann-Pick C1-like 1 regulates biliary cholesterol concentration and is a target of ezetimibe. J Clin Invest 2007;117(7) 1968-1978.

[68] Chan J, Kushwaha RS, Vandeberg JF, Vandeberg JL. Effect of ezetimibe on plasma cholesterol levels, cholesterol absorption, and secretion of biliary cholesterol in laboratory opossums with high and low responses to dietary cholesterol. Metabolism 2008;57(12) 1645-1654.

[69] Kammerer CM, Rainwater DL, Gouin N, Jasti M, Douglas KC, Dressen AS, Ganta P, Vandeberg JL, Samollow PB. Localization of genes for V+LDL plasma cholesterol levels on two diets in the opossum *Monodelphis domestica*. J Lipid Res 2010;51(10) 2929-2939.

[70] Samollow PB, Kammerer CM, Mahaney SM, Schneider JL, Westenberger SJ, VandeBerg JL, Robinson ES. First-generation linkage map of the gray, short-tailed opossum, *Monodelphis domestica*, reveals genome-wide reduction in female recombination rates. Genetics 2004;166(1) 307-329.

[71] Gonzales E, Davit-Spraul A, Baussan C, Buffet C, Maurice M, Jacquemin E. Liver diseases related to *MDR3* (*ABCB4*) gene deficiency. Front Biosci (Landmark Ed) 2009;14 4242-4256.

[72] Mauad TH, van Nieuwkerk CM, Dingemans KP, Smit JJ, Schinkel AH, Notenboom RG, van den Bergh Weerman MA, Verkruisen RP, Groen AK, Oude Elferink RP. Mice with homozygous disruption of the *mdr2* P-glycoprotein gene. A novel animal model for studies of nonsuppurative inflammatory cholangitis and hepatocarcinogenesis. Am J Pathol 1994;145(5) 1237-1245.

[73] Fickert P, Fuchsbichler A, Wagner M, Zollner G, Kaser A, Tilg H, Krause R, Lammert F, Langner C, Zatloukal K, Marschall HU, Denk H, Trauner M. Regurgitation of bile acids from leaky bile ducts causes sclerosing cholangitis in *Mdr2* (*Abcb4*) knockout mice. Gastroenterology 2004;127(1) 261-274.

[74] Chan J, Sharkey FE, Kushwaha RS, VandeBerg JF, VandeBerg JL. Steatohepatitis in laboratory opossums exhibiting a high lipemic response to dietary cholesterol and fat. Am J Physiol Gastrointest Liver Physiol 2012;303(1) G12-G19.

[75] McGill HC,Jr, McMahan CA, Kruski AW, Mott GE. Relationship of lipoprotein cholesterol concentrations to experimental atherosclerosis in baboons. Arteriosclerosis 1981;1(1) 3-12.

[76] Sorci-Thomas M, Prack MM, Dashti N, Johnson F, Rudel LL, Williams DL. Apolipoprotein (apo) A-I production and mRNA abundance explain plasma apoA-I and high density lipoprotein differences between two nonhuman primate species with high and low susceptibilities to diet-induced hypercholesterolemia. J Biol Chem 1988;263(11) 5183-5189.

[77] Rudel LL, Parks JS, Hedrick CC, Thomas M, Williford K. Lipoprotein and cholesterol metabolism in diet-induced coronary artery atherosclerosis in primates. Role of cholesterol and fatty acids. Prog Lipid Res 1998;37(6) 353-370.

[78] Marzetta CA, Rudel LL. A species comparison of low density lipoprotein heterogeneity in nonhuman primates fed atherogenic diets. J Lipid Res 1986;27(7) 753-762.

[79] Rudel LL, Pitts LL,2nd. Male--female variability in the dietary cholesterol-induced hyperlipoproteinemia of cynomolgus monkeys (*Macaca fascicularis*). J Lipid Res 1978;19(8) 992-1003.

[80] Karere GM, Glenn JP, Vandeberg JL, Cox LA. Differential microRNA response to a high-cholesterol, high-fat diet in livers of low and high LDL-C baboons. BMC Genomics 2012;13 320.

[81] McGill HC,Jr, McMahan CA, Kruski AW, Kelley JL, Mott GE. Responses of serum lipoproteins to dietary cholesterol and type of fat in the baboon. Arteriosclerosis 1981;1(5) 337-344.

[82] McGill HC,Jr, McMahan CA, Mott GE, Marinez YN, Kuehl TJ. Effects of selective breeding on the cholesterolemic responses to dietary saturated fat and cholesterol in baboons. Arteriosclerosis 1988;8(1) 33-39.

[83] Kushwaha RS, McGill HC,Jr, Mechanisms Controlling Lipemic Responses to Dietary Lipids. In: Simopoulos AP, Nestel PJ (eds.) World Review of Nutrition and Dietetics, Vol. 80. Genetic Variation and Dietary Response. Basel: Karger; 1997. p82-125.

[84] Rogers J, Mahaney MC, Witte SM, Nair S, Newman D, Wedel S, Rodriguez LA, Rice KS, Slifer SH, Perelygin A, Slifer M, Palladino-Negro P, Newman T, Chambers K, Joslyn G, Parry P, Morin PA. A genetic linkage map of the baboon (*Papio hamadryas*) genome based on human microsatellite polymorphisms. Genomics 2000;67(3) 237-247.

[85] Cox LA, Mahaney MC, Vandeberg JL, Rogers J. A second-generation genetic linkage map of the baboon (*Papio hamadryas*) genome. Genomics 2006;88(3) 274-281.

[86] Flow BL, Cartwright TC, Kuehl TJ, Mott GE, Kraemer DC, Kruski AW, Williams JD, McGIll HC,Jr. Genetic effects on serum cholesterol concentrations in baboons. J Hered 1981;72(2) 97-103.

[87] Konigsberg LW, Blangero J, Kammerer CM, Mott GE. Mixed model segregation analysis of LDL-C concentration with genotype-covariate interaction. Genet Epidemiol 1991;8(2) 69-80.

[88] Hixson JE, Kammerer CM, Cox LA, Mott GE. Identification of LDL receptor gene marker associated with altered levels of LDL cholesterol and apolipoprotein B in baboons. Arteriosclerosis 1989;9(6) 829-835.

[89] Rainwater DL, Kammerer CM, Mahaney MC, Rogers J, Cox LA, Schneider JL, VandeBerg JL. Localization of genes that control LDL size fractions in baboons. Atherosclerosis 2003;168(1) 15-22.

[90] Rainwater DL, Cox LA, Rogers J, VandeBerg JL, Mahaney MC. Localization of multiple pleiotropic genes for lipoprotein metabolism in baboons. J Lipid Res 2009;50(7) 1420-1428.

[91] Bellacosa A, Kumar CC, Di Cristofano A, Testa JR. Activation of AKT kinases in cancer: implications for therapeutic targeting. Adv Cancer Res 2005;94 29-86.

[92] Pittet MJ, Swirski FK. Monocytes link atherosclerosis and cancer. Eur J Immunol 2011;41(9) 2519-2522.

[93] Devarajan A, Shih D, Reddy ST. Inflammation, infection, cancer and all that...the role of paraoxonases. Adv Exp Med Biol 2014;824 33-41.

[94] Ranjha R, Paul J. Micro-RNAs in inflammatory diseases and as a link between inflammation and cancer. Inflamm Res 2013;62(4) 343-355.

[95] Kleemann R, Verschuren L, van Erk MJ, Nikolsky Y, Cnubben NH, Verheij ER, Smilde AK, Hendriks HF, Zadelaar S, Smith GJ, Kaznacheev V, Nikolskaya T, Melni-

kov A, Hurt-Camejo E, van der Greef J, van Ommen B, Kooistra T. Atherosclerosis and liver inflammation induced by increased dietary cholesterol intake: a combined transcriptomics and metabolomics analysis. Genome Biol 2007;8(9) R200.

[96] Thom T, Haase N, Rosamond W, Howard VJ, Rumsfeld J, Manolio T, Zheng ZJ, Flegal K, O'Donnell C, Kittner S, Lloyd-Jones D, Goff DC,Jr, Hong Y, Adams R, Friday G, Furie K, Gorelick P, Kissela B, Marler J, Meigs J, Roger V, Sidney S, Sorlie P, Steinberger J, Wasserthiel-Smoller S, Wilson M, Wolf P, American Heart Association Statistics Committee and Stroke Statistics Subcommittee. Heart disease and stroke statistics--2006 update: a report from the American Heart Association Statistics Committee and Stroke Statistics Subcommittee. Circulation 2006;113(6) e85-151.

[97] Rosamond W, Flegal K, Furie K, Go A, Greenlund K, Haase N, Hailpern SM, Ho M, Howard V, Kissela B, Kittner S, Lloyd-Jones D, McDermott M, Meigs J, Moy C, Nichol G, O'Donnell C, Roger V, Sorlie P, Steinberger J, Thom T, Wilson M, Hong Y, American Heart Association Statistics Committee and Stroke Statistics Subcommittee. Heart disease and stroke statistics--2008 update: a report from the American Heart Association Statistics Committee and Stroke Statistics Subcommittee. Circulation 2008;117(4) e25-146.

[98] Mathers CD, Loncar D. Projections of global mortality and burden of disease from 2002 to 2030. PLoS Med 2006;3(11) e442.

[99] McGill HC,Jr, McMahan CA, Herderick EE, Tracy RE, Malcom GT, Zieske AW, Strong JP. Effects of coronary heart disease risk factors on atherosclerosis of selected regions of the aorta and right coronary artery. PDAY Research Group. Pathobiological Determinants of Atherosclerosis in Youth. Arterioscler Thromb Vasc Biol 2000;20(3) 836-845.

[100] Masulli M, Patti L, Riccardi G, Vaccaro O, Annuzzi G, Ebbesson SO, Fabsitz RR, Howard WJ, Otvos JD, Roman MJ, Wang H, Weissman NJ, Howard BV, Rivellese AA. Relation among lipoprotein subfractions and carotid atherosclerosis in Alaskan Eskimos (from the GOCADAN Study). Am J Cardiol 2009;104(11) 1516-1521.

[101] Masuda J, Ross R. Atherogenesis during low level hypercholesterolemia in the nonhuman primate. II. Fatty streak conversion to fibrous plaque. Arteriosclerosis 1990;10(2) 178-187.

[102] Masuda J, Ross R. Atherogenesis during low level hypercholesterolemia in the nonhuman primate. I. Fatty streak formation. Arteriosclerosis 1990 10(2) 164-177.

[103] Rudel LL, Bond MG, Bullock BC. LDL heterogeneity and atherosclerosis in nonhuman primates. Ann N Y Acad Sci 1985;454 248-253.

[104] Eyster KM, Appt SE, Mark-Kappeler CJ, Chalpe A, Register TC, Clarkson TB. Gene expression signatures differ with extent of atherosclerosis in monkey iliac artery. Menopause 2011;18(10) 1087-1095.

[105] Cong L, Ran FA, Cox D, Lin S, Barretto R, Habib N, Hsu PD, Wu X, Jiang W, Marraffini LA, Zhang F. Multiplex genome engineering using CRISPR/Cas systems. Science 2013;339(6121) 819-823.

[106] Yang H, Wang H, Jaenisch R. Generating genetically modified mice using CRISPR/Cas-mediated genome engineering. Nat Protoc 2014;9(8) 1956-1968.

[107] LaRosa JC, Grundy SM, Waters DD, Shear C, Barter P, Fruchart JC, Gotto AM, Greten H, Kastelein JJ, Shepherd J, Wenger NK, Treating to New Targets (TNT) Investigators. Intensive lipid lowering with atorvastatin in patients with stable coronary disease. N Engl J Med 2005;352(14) 1425-1435.

[108] Shah RV, Goldfine AB. Statins and risk of new-onset diabetes mellitus. Circulation 2012;126(18) e282-284.

[109] Goldfine AB. Statins: is it really time to reassess benefits and risks? N Engl J Med 2012;366(19) 1752-1755.

Chapter 2

Hypercholesterolemia in Childhood

Lorenzo Iughetti, Barbara Predieri and Patrizia Bruzzi

Additional information is available at the end of the chapter

http://dx.doi.org/10.5772/59760

1. Introduction

Hypercholesterolemia is a well-known risk factor for atherosclerosis in adulthood.

In the first years of life atherosclerosis is generally subclinical, but pathological studies demonstrate that, already in childhood, atherosclerotic vascular changes and their extend are associated with both the number of cardiovascular risk factors and their intensity [1, 2]. Fatty streaks and fibrous plaques at autopsy, presence of coronary artery calcium by electron-beam computed tomography, increased carotid-intima-media thickness, reduced arterial distensibility and compliance and endothelial dysfunction by ultrasound have been already associated with lipid abnormalities in youth [3]. Moreover, levels of cholesterol track strongly from childhood and adolescence over long follow-up period resulting in the progression of atherosclerosis process and increased cardiovascular disease (CVD) risk [4].

The mechanism by which hyperlipidemia contributes to atherogenesis includes several stages:

- Chronic hyperlipidemia, and especially hypercholesterolemia, might alter endothelial function, through the increased production of superoxide and other oxygen free radicals, which deactivate the nitric oxide, the main relaxing factor the endothelium
- During chronic hyperlipidemia, lipoproteins are accumulated in intima increasing endothelial permeability
- Oxidative modification of lipids, induced by free radicals, leads to the formation of oxidized low-density-lipoproteins (oxLDL), which, in their turn, are easily phagocyted by macrophages and, consequently, form foam cells. OxLDL are chemotactic for circulating monocytes, they inhibit the mobility of macrophages already in the lesion, thus, promoting their recruitment and their persistence in the plaques. They also stimulate the release of growth factors and cytokines that, in their turn, induce the production of antibodies against oxidized lipoproteins and cause a chronic inflammation [5, 6]. Such state of chronic or not-resolving inflammation facilitates lipid accumulation in the atheroma [7].

In some conditions, characterized by altered lipid assessment or other evident disorders of risk factors, premature CVD could be manifest in the first decades of life. "Vascular age" is advanced in 73% of familial dyslipidemic children, independently from the presence of others atherosclerosis-promoting risk factors [8]. The American Heart Association (AHA), endorsed by the American Academy of Pediatrics (AAP), identified 8 high-risk pediatric diagnosis and developed practical recommendations for the management of cardiovascular risk [9]. The selected diseases comprise familial hypercholesterolemia (FH), together with diabetes mellitus (type 1 and 2), chronic kidney disease, heart transplantation, Kawasaki disease, congenital heart disease, chronic inflammatory disease and childhood cancer. Subclinical endothelial dysfunction, measured through non-invasive surrogate methods such as flow-mediated dilation (FMD), occurs early in FH children indicating an increased risk for premature CVD and reflecting the need for early initiation of anticholesterolemic treatment [10]. Moreover, increasing evidences indicate that, in high-risk conditions as well as in most children with a minor degree of vascular involvement, appropriate therapy could prevent and/or reverse the progression of these cardiovascular changes [11, 12]. Therefore, the identification and the management of hypercholesterolemia in children are of great consequence.

2. Lipid concentrations in childhood and adolescence

The thresholds for defining hypercholesterolemia and elevated low density lipoprotein cholesterol (LDL-C) in childhood and adolescence are not homogeneous. One set of values were derived from the National Cholesterol Education Program (NCEP) report (Table 1) [13]. An update, published in 2011, included values of apolipoprotein B (ApoB) and apolipoprotein A-1 (ApoA-1) coming from the National Health and Nutrition Examination Survey III. NCEP cutoffs seem to accurately estimate adult values of total cholesterol (TC), LDL-C and triglycerides (TG), while high lipoprotein cholesterol (HDL-C) levels are better predicted by National Health and Nutrition Examination Survey (NHANES) cutoff points [14].

Another set of values were derived from the Lipid Research Clinics Prevalence Study [15] and revised in 2008 by the AAP [16] (Table 2).

The lack of a consensus depends on: lipid variability during infancy, childhood and adolescence, the subsequent need of using percentiles instead of cut-off values (as used in adulthood) and the lack of studies that correlate lipid values in childhood with adult cardiovascular risk.

After birth, lipids and lipoproteins gradually increase up to 2 years of life, reaching values similar to adults: therefore, before the third year of life, the determination of the lipid profile is neither recommended nor useful. An increased stability with no significant differences between genders can be observed from 5 to 10 years: until pubertal activation, the use of reference values proposed by the AAP is recommended [16]. Taking into account the changes between genders occurring during puberty, the percentiles of reference proposed by Jolliffe and Janssen for males and females from 12 to 19 years could also be used: these percentiles are based on studies that correlate the values of lipid profile with the probability of subsequent clinical cardiovascular risk [17].

Category		Acceptable < 75° p	Borderline 75-90° p	High > 90°p
TC, mg/dl		< 170	170-199	≥ 200
LDL-C, mg/dl		< 110	110-129	≥ 130
ApoB, mg/dl		< 90	90-109	≥ 110
TG, mg/dl				
	2-9 y	< 75	75-99	≥ 100
	10-19 y	< 90	90-129	≥ 130
HDL-C, mg/dl		> 45* (≥25°p)	35-45 (5-25°p)	≤ 35 (≤ 5°p)
ApoA-1, mg/dl		>120	110-120	<110

*desiderable: > 65 mg/dl, 75° p

Table 1. Plasma lipid concentration in children and adolescence modified from NCEP, 1992 [13, 14]. Legend: p, percentile

	Male			Female		
	5-9 ys	**10-14 ys**	**15-19 ys**	**5-9 ys**	**10-14 ys**	**15-19 ys**
TC, mg/dl						
50°p	153	161	152	164	159	157
75° p	168	173	168	177	171	176
90°p	183	191	183	189	191	198
95°p	186	201	191	197	205	208
TG, mg/dl						
50°p	48	58	68	57	68	64
75° p	58	74	88	74	85	85
90°p	70	94	125	103	104	112
95°p	85	111	143	120	120	126
LDL-C, mg/dl						
50°p	90	94	93	98	94	93
75° p	103	109	109	115	110	110
90°p	117	123	123	125	126	129
95°p	129	133	130	140	136	137
HDL-C, mg/dl						
5°p	38	37	30	36	37	35
10° p	43	40	34	38	40	38
25°p	49	46	39	48	45	43
50°p	55	55	46	52	52	51

Table 2. Lipid and Lipoprotein Distributions in Subjects Aged 5 to 19 Years [16]. Legend: p, percentile

Lipid concentrations vary also according to demographic variables (population specific): TC seems to be higher among Black children and adolescents than Caucasian ones [18]. Moreover, dietary habits together with current diseases and seasonality could transitionally influence cholesterol assessment.

Data from the National Health and Nutrition Examination Survey (NHANES) 1999 to 2006 for participants 6 to 17 years of age documented that 5.2%-6.6% (depending on the cut points used) and 9.6%-10.7% of them presented an elevated concentration of LDL-C and TC, respectively [19].

3. Genetic Hypercholesterolemia

Lipid abnormalities can be classified as primary disorders that encompass all genetic (monogenic) forms of dyslipidemia, as summarized in Table 3 [20], and secondary disorders.

Name	Genetic Defect	Trasmission	Clinical features
Classical Familial Hypercholesterolemia (FH)	LDLR, diminished LDL-C clearance	Autosomal dominant 1:300-1:1.000.000	Heterozygotes: TC 250-500 mg/dl (LDL-C > 135 mg/dl), xanthomas on the extensor tendons of the hands and feet, arcus cornea and premature CVD (40-60 y) Homozygotes: TC 500-1000 mg/dl, xanthomas and very premature CVD (< 10 y)
Other autosomal dominant hypercholesterolemia	PCSK9, diminished LDL-C clearance		
Autosomal recessive hypercholesterolemia (ARH)	ARH adaptor protein absent or unable to interact with the LDLR, diminished LDL-C clearance	Autosomal recessive 1:100.000 (Sardinia)	Variable, phenotype similar to homozygous FH, but generally less severe and more responsive to lipid-lowering therapy, large and bulky xanthomas from early childhood, TC > 500 mg/dl, in homozygotes: CVD < 30 y
Familial defective Apo B-100	Apo B, diminished LDL-C clearance	Autosomal dominant 1:700 (North-Centre Europe)	Heterozygotes: TC 250-500 mg/dl, xanthomas, arcus senilis and premature CVD (50-60 y) Homozygotes: TC > 500 mg/dl, premature CVD (< 30 y)
Familial combined hyperlipidemia	Polygenic		Premature CVD, Apo B elevated, TC 250-500 mg/dl, TG 250-750 mg/dl
Beta sitosterolemia	Carrier ABCG5/ABCG8	Autosomal recessive 1:1.000.000	High vegetables sterols and LDL-C

Table 3. Genetic Hypercholesterolemia [20]. Legend: LDLR, low density lipoprotein receptor; PCSK9, proprotein convertase subtilisin/kexin type 9

4. Monogenic primary Hypercholesterolemia

Monogenic hypercholesterolemias are lifelong conditions that often present during childhood and adolescence with clinically and biochemically extreme phenotypes, due to a variety of gain-of-function or loss-of-function mutations in a range of candidate genes with important roles in lipid metabolism.

FH is an autosomal dominant monogenic condition. Homozygous familial hypercholesterolemia (HoFH) is rare, with an occurrence of 1:1.000.000 individuals, but the heterozygous state (HeFH) is present in the general population with an incidence ranging from 1:300 to 1:500. On this basis we can affirm that HeFH is the most common monogenic disorder in North America and Europe. Causative FH mutation alters the function of LDL-receptor (LDLR) resulting in a reduced clearance of LDL-C particles from the circulation and consequently in an elevation of their plasma levels. In addition to LDLR defects, a similar phenotype can be caused by a number of mutations in the ApoB gene (that disrupt the binding of the LDL-C particle to the LDLR) and by gain of function mutations in the proprotein convertase subtilisin/kexin type 9 (PCSK9) gene (that increase LDLR degradation) [21]. So far, more than 1500 variants have been identified in the LDLR associated with FH, ranging from single-nucleotide substitutions to large deletions [22]. The clinical presentation of HeFH is characterized by two- to three-fold elevations in plasma LDL-C levels, by a family history positive for CVD, and, rarely in childhood, by the presence of physical symptoms of cholesterol deposits in tissues (tendon xanthomas, xanthelasma palpebrarum). Historically, left untreated, the cumulative risk of CVD in HeFH patient is greater than 50% in men by the age of 50 years and at least 30% in women by the age of 60 years. Homozygous and compound heterozygous FH subjects can experience serious cardiovascular events as early as in childhood: a six- to eight-fold increase in plasma LDL-C is found in these subjects and severe xanthomatosis and multiple types of xanthomas could occur.

Most people with FH are undiagnosed or only diagnosed after their first coronary event, but medical treatment seems to be effective and it could delay or prevent the onset of CVD. Therefore, early identification of affected individuals is crucial. Cholesterol levels alone are not sufficient to confirm a diagnosis of FH because of the extensive overlap in LDL–C levels existing between FH-causing mutation carries and non-carries (non-genetic polygenic hypercholesterolemia) and the high prevalence of modestly severe LDLR mutations that hampers the use of LDL-C cut-offs. Therefore, a diagnostic definition of FH, which supports cholesterol measurements with clinical signs and family history, has become widely used (Simon Broome Register Group definition of FH) [23]. According to this definition, a "definite" diagnosis of FH requires:

a. TC level above 260 mg/dl in children under 16 years of age

OR LDL-C levels above 160 mg/dl in children

b. PLUS tendon xanthomas in patient or relative (parent, child, sibling, grandparent, aunt, uncle)

c. OR DNA-based evidence of an LDLR mutation or familial defective Apo B.

A "possible" diagnosis of FH is suggested when (a) is present together with one of (d) or (e):

d. family history of myocardial infarction before the age of 50 years in grandparent, aunt, uncle or before age 60 in parent or siblings

e. family history of raised cholesterol in parents or siblings or levels above 290 mg/dl in grandparents, aunt or uncle.

A similar diagnostic tool has been developed by the Dutch Lipid Clinic Network. This includes similar features to the Simon Broome criteria, but adds the calculation of a numeric score [24]. These criteria differ in DNA testing and in their diagnostic effectiveness. In summary, a child with significant and isolated elevation of LDL-C (≥160 mg/dl) should be considered to have FH, particularly if there is family history of early CVD.

After diagnosis of FH, cascade screening should occur in all first degree relatives after age 2 years. Cascade screening is a term used to describe searching for affected relatives of an inherited disorder once an affected person is known. In UK guidelines, DNA-based cascade testing is recommended in affected families; however, in about 60% of patients no mutations are found [25]. This finding leads to a great concern: assigning individuals to an "uncertain" category (when mutation is not identified) is unsatisfactory and provokes confusion and ambiguity both in children and adults.

After diagnosis, an appropriate treatment should be pursued, especially after CVD risk assessment, by a lipid specialist.

5. Polygenic forms of Hypercholesterolemia

Dyslipidemia may also result from interaction of synergic environmental and genetic factors developing the group of multifactorial or polygenic hypercholesterolemia. Because of this combination of causative factors, biochemical phenotype could be variable: LDL-C and TG may be high (rarely normal), HDL-C can be normal or reduced and there is significant production of small, dense LDL-C particles. Contrary to FH, it is less likely to be diagnosed in children because LDL-C elevation may occur frequently in adolescence, but strongly tracks into adulthood (70-75% of cases).

6. Secondary Hypercholesterolemia

The prevalence of lipid abnormalities in children is increasing because of the epidemic of obesity and subsequent metabolic syndrome (MS). Data from 1999-2004 NHANES demonstrated that approximately 10% of participants aged 8-19 years had high TC, 7% had low HDL-C, 9.7% had high TG and 7.6% had high LDL-C. In addition, prevalence of adverse lipid profile in youths with high adiposity was found significantly greater than participants without it [26]. Low HDL-C, high TG and small dense LDL-C, characterizing the so called "dyslipidemia of

http://dx.doi.org/10.5772/59760

insulin resistance", are often associated with obesity and MS [27]. Promoting free-fatty acids release from visceral fat and altering the hepatic production of apolipoprotein, insulin resistance (IR) is the ethiological key of dyslipidemia in MS. Recently, the positive association demonstrated between PCSK9 activity and fasting glucose, insulin and homeostatic model assessment IR (in addition to lipid levels) suggests that PCSK9 could play a role in the development of dyslipidemia associated with the MS [28]. Moreover, the endocrine activity of adipose tissue produces inflammatory cytokines, such as adiponectin and tumor necrosis factor-alfa, influencing hepatic production of very low density lipoprotein (VLDL). All these findings highlight the importance to early counteract obesity to prevent the occurrence of dyslipidemia: the earlier the prevention begins, the better results are achieved.

Secondary dyslipidemia include also those caused by chronic disease, such as diabetes mellitus, chronic renal insufficiency, hypothyroidism, liver diseases and drugs (e.g. glucocorticoids, B-blockers, antiretroviral agents) (Table 4).

	Clinical features
Obesity	Increase TG, decreased HDL-C
Diabetes Mellitus	Increase TG and TC, decrease HDL-C
Chronic renal failure	Increase TG and TC, decrease HDL-C
HIV/AIDS wasting	Increase TG and TC, decrease HDL-C and LDL-C
HIV/AIDS (HAART)	Increase TG, TC and HDL-C
Hypothyroidism	Increase TG, TC and LDL-C
Nephrotic syndrome	Increase TC and LDL-C
Obstructive liver disease	Increase TC
Medications	Variable

Table 4. Secondary dyslipidemia.

7. Diagnosing Hypercholesterolemia in childhood

In 2011, the National Heart, Lung, and Blood Institute (NHLBI), backed by AAP, proposed an universal lipid screening to be performed with measurement of non fasting non-HDL-C (calculated by subtracting the HDL-C from the TC measurement) in all children between ages 9–11 and 17–21 years [14]. The normal variation in blood cholesterol levels within an individual over time is approximately 6%. Therefore, at least two elevated blood cholesterol measurements are required in a lapse of time between 15 days and 3 months, before a diagnosis of hypercholesterolemia can be made. In the remaining groups of age (2-8 and 12-16 years), NHLBI agrees with the use of selective screening, as proposed by the NCEP [13, 14]: lipid screening is recommended only in children with positive family history of premature CVD OR already known familial dyslipidemia OR unknown family history OR presence of multiple risk factors such as hypertension, diabetes and obesity OR overweight/obesity alone. Cholesterol screening modalities in youth have been debated for decades. The primary goal of universal screening is to identify those with FH. It has been shown that family history is incomplete in young individuals, since parents and even grandparents may be too young to have demonstrated early CVD [29]. The second goal of universal screening is to use cholesterol assessment to identify children with components of MS in an effort to highlight and prevent progression of additional components. Nevertheless, there are several critiques that comprise: the definition of risk-to-benefit ratio, especially regarding moderate dyslipidemia, the potential risk to determine anxiety in patients and families and, lastly, the financial costs [30].

8. Treatment of Hypercholesterolemia in childhood

In 2010 the AHA, while developing the 2020 Impact Goals, defined the "cardiovascular health" concept and determined the metrics needed to monitor it over time [31]. In this way the first step proposed for management of children with identified lipid abnormalities is to assess their cardiovascular risk. It includes the collection of:

- anamnestic data about familial premature cardiovascular disease (premature means before 55 years of age in males and before 65 in females)
- individual anamnestic risk factors as smoking habit, drugs and the presence of current high or moderate risk conditions such as hypercholesterolemia, diabetes, Kawasaki disease, cancer treatment survivors...
- physical examination that include blood pressure and body mass index.

In children, the definition of ideal cardiovascular health includes several goals: avoid smoking, body mass index less than 85th percentile, more than 60 minutes of moderate- or vigorous-intensity physical activity every day, health diet, TC values less than 170 mg/dl (6-19 years of age), blood pressure less than 90th percentile (8-19 years of age) and fasting plasma glucose less than 100 mg/dl (12-19 years of age) [31].

8.1. Dietary treatment and lifestyle approach

The cornerstone of lipid-lowering therapy is a healthy lifestyle [32].

Dietary recommendations emphasize the following pattern of nutrient intake:

- adequate nutrition should be achieved by eating a wide variety of foods low in saturated fat and cholesterol
- total caloric intake should be sufficient to support normal growth and development and maintain desirable body weight
- saturated fatty acids should provide <10% of total calories
- total fat should provide an average of no more than 30% and no less than 20% of total calories

- polyunsaturated fatty acids should provide up to 10% of total calories
- less than 300 mg of cholesterol should be consumed per day
- children should consume 5 or more daily serving of vegetables and fruits and 6 to 11 daily servings of whole-grain or other grain foods
- children should eat adequate amounts of dietary fiber (Age + 5 g/day).

All children with LDL-C level >130 mg/dl should receive targeted intervention and follow-up. The NCEP suggests for hypercholesterolemic patients a two level cholesterol-lowering diet [13]. In the Step 1 diet (Table 5) approximately 30% of calories derive from fat (10% from saturated fat) and the total intake of cholesterol should be limited to 300 mg/day. If the lipid values remain elevated after 6 weeks, the Step 1 diet should be reviewed to increase the compliance. If the diet for at least 3 months fails to achieve LDL-C concentrations <130 mg/dl (the ideal goal is to lower it to <110 mg/dl), a more aggressive dietary approach is needed (Step 2 diet). The two main differences between the Step 1 and Step 2 diets are that in the latter, the amount of saturated fat is reduced to 7% of total calories and the intake of cholesterol is decreased to 200 mg/day (Table 5). In order to implement this more stringent diet, advice from a nutritionist trained in dealing with children and disorders of lipids is needed. No restriction of fat or cholesterol is recommended for infants <2 years of age, when rapid growth and development require high energy intakes. Dietetic guidelines called Therapeutic Lifestyle Changes (TLC) replaced Step 1 and 2 diets. For higher risk people they recommended an adequate caloric intake, including an increased consume of whole grains, low-fat dairy products, fruits, vegetables and fish and a reduction of soft drinks and salt (Table 5) [33].

	STEP 1	STEP 2	TLC diet
Total fats (% of total calories)	30	30	25-35†
Saturated fats (% of total calories)	No more than 10	Less than 7	Less than 7
Dietary Cholesterol (mg/day)	Limited to 300	Less than 200	Less than 200
Plants stanols/sterols (grams per day)	NA	NA	2
Increased viscous soluble fiber (grams per day)	NA	NA	10-25

Legend: †The 25-35% fat recommendation allows for increased intake of unsaturated fat in place of carbohydrates in people with metabolic syndrome or diabetes.

Table 5. Characteristics and Differences between STEP 1, STEP 2 and TLC diets [33].

The improvement of dietary habits seems to be effective when hyperlipidemia is secondary to other conditions, such as obesity [34], but it is not sufficient in primary hypercholesterolemia. Nevertheless, also in the latter dietary restrictions have to be requested, in order to reduce the dose of medications and to avoid a further deterioration of the condition. No long-term (up to 10 years) adverse effects on growth and pubertal development have been documented [34-37].

In children with FH and polygenic hypercholesterolemia, additional benefit could derive from the introduction of soya protein [38] and/or plant stanols and sterol esters (2 g/day) in the diet [39]. Nevertheless, despite an improvement in TC and LDL-C levels, supplementation with stanols and sterols does not improve endothelial function, probably because they concomitantly reduce plasma carotenoids [39]. Recently, a significant reduction of small dense LDL-C has been demonstrated in 25 hypercholesterolemic children after the introduction in their diet of a yogurt-drink enriched with 2 gr/day plant sterols [40]. A large amount of sterol could also derive directly from fruits, vegetables and cereals (see table 6). Therefore, plant stanols and sterols have to be considered as beneficial, safe, tasteful, easy-accessible and low-cost lipid-lowering strategy, especially until children at risk become eligible for a more aggressive therapy.

Food	Sterol Content (mg/100 gr edible)
Fruit and vegetables	
Broccoli	44
Grean peas	25
Orange	24
Apple	13
Cucumber	6
Tomato	5
Cereals	
Wheat bran	200
Swedish knackebrot	89
Wholemeal bread	53
Rolled oats	39
Wheat Bread	29
Fats and Oils	
Corn Oil	912
Rapeseed (canola) oil	668
Liquid margarine	522
Sunflower oil	213
Spreadable butter	153
Olive oil	154

Table 6. Sterol content in food.

The efficacy of a cholesterol-lowering diet, started in childhood, upon reduction of CVD later in life, has not been firmly established yet [41].

Soluble fibers, including those from psyllium husk, have been shown to increase the cholesterol-lowering effects of a low-fat diet. In 2011 guidelines, the water soluble fiber psyllium can be added to a low fat low-saturated fat diet as cereal enriched with psyllium at a dose of 6 g/d for children 2-12 of age and 12 g/day for those ≥ 12 y of age [14]. Accordingly, it has been shown that glucomannan, a hydrosoluble fiber, may decrease TC and LDL-C levels, without changing HDL-C levels, in hypercholesterolemic children [42]. A novel pioneering approach in reducing the serum cholesterolemia could be represented by the exploitation of probiotics exerting cholesterol-lowering properties. A recent Italian randomized, double-blind, placebo-control study evaluates the effects of a probiotic formulation containing three Bifidobacterium strains on lipid profiles in 39 children affected by primary dyslipidemia: compared to placebo, probiotics reduced TC by 3.9% and LCL-C by 3.8%. Moreover, this supporting therapy seems well tolerated [43].

Lifestyle change includes: regular physical activity, screen time less than 2 hours per day, attainment of ideal body weight (body mass index ≤85th centile for age and gender) and optimization of blood pressure. In adults the combination of intensive dietary restrictions and physical exercise improves lipid metabolism, IR and cardiorespiratory fitness, thereby diminishing cardiovascular risk factors [44]. Reported trials on benefits of physical activity on lipid-profile are scarce, rarely well—performed and their results are not optimistic. However, physical activity stimulates lipoprotein lipases and the function of some enzymes like the lecithin-cholesterol acyltransferase (LCAT), improving HDL-C formation and reducing their catabolism. Moreover, exercise reduced TG levels and is effective on size and density of LDL-C particles. Finally, exercise is safe and does not require any additional cost. Therefore, children should be encouraged to undertake 60 minutes or more of vigorous aerobic activity per day. The TLC diet itself recommends expending at least 200 kcal per day [33]. The abuse of tobacco and alcohol should be avoided. An early identification and correction of eating disorders should be recommended.

8.2. Pharmacological treatment

If cholesterol does not reach acceptable levels through diet, the recourse to a pharmacological treatment is allowed and advised [45]. The NCEP recommends the administration of medications only to children > 10 years of age (better if either at pubertal Tanner stage II or higher or after onset of menses in girls) and only when an aggressive diet lasting at least 6-12 months fails [13]. A lipid specialist should be consulted. Traditionally, bile acid sequestrants (BAR) were considered the first-line therapy in hypercholesterolemic children. Since AHA statement, statins replaced BAR: their use is now recommended in children younger than 10 years of age (from 8 years of age). Surprisingly, AAP encouraged the application of this revised therapeutical approach [16] causing many controversies among experts: up to now, the efficacy of statins on adult-onset of CVD is not clearly defined and data about their long-term safety, particularly because they interfere with the production of steroid hormones and liver function, are still lacking. Nevertheless, in 2002-2005, the use of lipid-lowering drugs increased in children by

15% [46] and the American Food and Drug Administration (FDA) and the European Medicines Agency (EMEA) approved pravastatin in children > 8 years, while simvastatin, lovastatin and atorvastatin were registered by the FDA for children > 10 years of age. Ezetimibe was also approved by the FDA and EMEA for pediatric use from the age of 10 years.

8.3. 3-Hydroxy-3-MethylGlutaryl-CoA (HMG-Coa) reductase inhibitors

Statins inhibit HMG-CoA reductase, an enzyme fundamental in de novo cholesterol synthesis. Their action consequently provokes an increase in hepatic production of LDLR determining an additional decrease in LDL-C levels. Statins are commonly safe and well tolerated. However, because of the principal role of cholesterol in cellular structure and function, the use of statins is not allowed in prepubertal children. In HeFH children and adolescents, statins are effective in reducing levels of LDL-C by 20-40% and increasing HDL-C, but, because of the scarcity and the non-uniformity of trials shown by meta-analysis, no data about outcomes of different types, doses and length of therapy could be deduced [47,48]. In terms of safety, no differences in occurrence of adverse effects, alterations in sexual development and muscle or liver toxicity have been demonstrated in children treated with statins in comparison to placebo-treated ones [49]. Nevertheless, while adult guidelines do not recommend routine screening of liver and muscle enzymes during treatment, pediatric guidelines indicate to start statin at the lowest dose with baseline measurements of alanine aminotransferase (ALT), aspartate aminotransferase (AST), and creatinine kinase (CK). These levels plus a fasting lipid profile should be repeated four and eight weeks after initiation of therapy and then every 3–6 months. If liver enzymes are above 3 times the upper limit of normal and/or CK is above 10 times the upper limit of normal and/or patient complains any adverse effects, medication should be stopped to determine if there is an improvement. Some researchers have suggested hydrophilic statins, such as fluvastatin, rosuvastatin and pravastatin are less potentially toxic than lipophilic statins, such as atorvastatin, lovastatin, and simvastatin; the risk of myopathy was suggested to be lowest with pravastatin and fluvastatin, probably because they are more hydrophilic [50].

Up to now, few studies have examined vascular efficacy of statins in children, confirming an increase of impaired FMD before and a significant improvement after treatment [11, 51], long-term effects have been less studied [52]. Recently, secretory phospholipase A_2-IIA (sPLA$_2$-IIA) receives increased interest because of its role in the inflammatory process of atherosclerosis: it induce LDL-C modification, foam cell formation and activation of various immune mechanisms. Published data demonstrated no effects of 2-years-long pravastatin therapy in reducing sPLA$_2$-IIA mass or sPLA$_2$ activity levels in 91 FH children compared to placebo [53].

Statins are contraindicated during pregnancy because of potential teratogenic risk. Because of this concern, statins should be used to treat adolescent FH females only if they are aware of the risk, under a close follow-up and on contraceptive therapy when indicated.

Target LDL-C is typically below 130 mg/dl, but ideally under 100 mg/dl in high risk populations such as FH. If target levels are not achieved within 3 months, the dose of statin can be gradually increased to maximum dose. Occasionally, a second agent such as a BAR may be useful. Multiple drug therapy should be guided by a lipid specialist.

8.4. BAR

Even if FDA never approved BARs in children, they were used in the past as first-line therapy in hypercholesterolemia. Colestipol, cholestyramine and colestilan bind bile salts in the intestine preventing their re-absorption and increasing their excretion and discharge from cholesterol pool. Increased emission of bile acids causes a large conversion of cholesterol into bile salts; in liver, cholesterol pool decreases and a compensatory rise in LDLR synthesis takes place. In children with HeFH, BARs determine a decrease in TC of 10-20%. These drugs are not absorbed systematically, but local side-effects as abdominal pain and nausea could nullify compliance. Recently, a novel bile acid sequestrant, the colesevelam hydrochloride, with enhanced binding capacity for bile acids has been evaluated in HeFH children, alone or in combination with statin therapy: the therapeutical compliance has increased (about 85%) together with an effective LDL-C reduction [54].

8.5. Niacin and fibrates

Niacin, a water-soluble B complex vitamin, increases HDL-C levels and significantly reduces hepatic production and release of VLDL but it is not commonly utilized in children because of lack of information about its safety. Adverse effects consist of flushing, hepatic insufficiency, myopathy, glucose intolerance and hyperuricemia. Therefore, niacin is limited both in HoFH children and in ones with stroke and increased lipoprotein A levels.

Fibrates (gemfibrazil, fenofibrate, bezafibrate and ciprofibrate) are mainly effective in lowering TG and in increasing HDL-C, while LDL-C levels seem only partially and variably influenced. They have a complex and poorly understood way of action and, due to the lack of data on safety, their use is restricted in HeFH children with high TG levels and an increased risk for pancreatitis.

8.6. Ezetimibe

Ezetimibe is a new selective cholesterol absorption inhibitor acting at the brush border of the small intestine with no effects on the absorption of TG and fat-soluble vitamins. Target pathways may consist in the Niemann-Pick C1-like protein and the annexin-caveolin 1 complex. In 2002, FDA approved ezetimibe in FH children older than 10 years of age, but long-term effects have not been extensively evaluated yet. In HoFH, ezetimibe has a synergic effect in reducing LDL-C, if associated with statins, without increasing adverse effects. Satisfying data in term of efficacy and tolerance have also been documented in children with polygenic hypercholesterolemia, HeFH and familial combined hyperlipidemia treated with ezetimibe [55].

These positive data are partially dampened by an absolute lack of knowledge about the long-term effects of ezetimibe. In fact, the combination of statin and ezetimibe may not restore endothelial dysfunction [56]. Moreover, ezetimibe dose not influence HDL-C, an independent risk factor for CVD. Future data from the ongoing IMPROVED-IT study, enlisting 18.000 adults affected by acute coronary syndrome on simvastatin either with or without ezetimibe, may clarify the role of ezetimibe in CVD prevention [57]. In addition, systemic effects of ezetimibe, in contrast to its minimal absorption have still to be clearly defined.

In the last years, new lipid-lowering drugs are coming out. Starting from the demonstration that PCSK9 loss-of-function mutations result in a significant drop in circulating LDL-C, subsequent studies demonstrated that PCSK9 binds the epidermal growth factor precursor homology domain-A on the surface LDLR and directs LDLR and PCSK9 for lysosomal degradation. A monoclonal antibody that binds circulating PCSK9 and blocks its interactions with surface LDLR and called Alirocumab has recently demonstrated a great potentiality in reducing LDL-C in adulthood. Nevertheless, there is no data in adolescence and no evidence on its capacity in improving CVD outcome yet [58].

9. HoFH: Treatment in childhood

HoFH has to be considered an almost exclusive pediatric disease. Because of the earlier risk of CVD, HoFH patients should started pharmacological therapy as soon as possible, as recommended by AHA [45]. LDL-C apheresis and/or liver transplant have been the historical treatment in this subset, although efficacy and success are variable [59]. LDL-C apheresis is an extracorporeal plasma-perfusion method that involves selective removal of LDL-C particles. The procedure takes three or more hours and is performed at 1- to 2-week intervals. Even if it results in the regression of coronary lesions and has been found to increase life expectancy, its use is limited by its availability, higher cost and difficulties in procedures [60]. As most of the LDLR are present in the liver, liver transplantation alone or in combination with pharmacotherapy is effective in normalizing the plasma cholesterol levels. Nevertheless, the associated risks include the need of a life-long immunosuppressive therapy [61]. HoFH may also benefit from lipid-lowering drugs. However, statins require some residual LDLR function, thus they are not effective in receptor-negative HoFH. Higher risk patients will benefit from combination therapy: ezetimibe, but also niacin, fibrates, and BAR. Therapeutic efficacy, safety, medication adherence, and compliance should be monitored closely. Novel medical therapies for adults with HoFH have recently been approved in the US. These include inhibitors of PCSK9, microsomal triglyceride transfer protein and cholesteryl ester transfer protein (CETP), as well as mipomersen, an apolipoprotein B synthesis inhibitor [62, 63].

10. Conclusions

The role of pediatrician in the prevention of chronic and disabling diseases in adulthood is reinforced by the extensive scientific evidence that proves the beginning of causative processes, such as atherosclerosis, in childhood. Therefore, the identification of patients at risk of premature CVD has become, today, one of the primary aims of pediatricians. The evaluation of hypercholesterolemic children should not be based exclusively on lipid assessment: it is essential to quantify the overall cardiovascular risk through the collection of a full medical history (including familial history), the performance of an accurate physical examination, the assessment of eating habits and the identification of concomitant risk factors. Moreover, in

http://dx.doi.org/10.5772/59760

hypercholesterolemic children, the monitoring over time of cardiovascular function through non-invasive methods can be useful.

Childhood could be considered as the best period of life to acquire a proper lifestyle and healthy eating habits, especially in patients at risk of premature CVD. The diet, low in saturated fat and cholesterol, should be the first therapeutic approach to be proposed in children with hypercholesterolemia. Early pharmacological treatment could be planned in cases of genetic hypercholesterolemia or when diet alone persistently fails. Several studies have demonstrated the short-term efficacy and safety of statins in childhood.

The definition of pediatric population-specific percentiles for lipid values, the achievement of a shared screening strategy and the demonstration of long-term safety and efficacy of statin therapy have to be considered the current priorities for improving the approach to childhood hypercholesterolemia.

Nomenclature

AHA; American Heart Association

AIDS; Acquired Immune Deficiency Syndrome

ALT; Alanine aminotransferase

Apo; Apolipoprotein

AAP; American Academy of Pediatrics

AST; Aspartate aminotransferase

BAR; Bile acid sequestrants

CK; Creatine phosphokinase

CVD; Cardiovascular disease

EMEA; European Medicines Agency

FDA; Food and Drugs Administration

FH; Familial Hypercholesterolemia

FMD; Flow-mediated dilation

HAART; Hightly active antiretroviral therapy

HDL; High-density lipoprotein

HDL-C; High-density lipoprotein cholesterol

HeFH; Heterozygous familial hypercholesterolemia

HIV; Human immunodeficiency virus

HMG-CoA; 3-Hydroxy-3-MethylGlutaryl-CoA

HoFH; Homozygous familial hypercholesterolemia

IR; insulin resistance

LCAT; Lecithin-cholesterol acyltransferase

LDL; Low-density lipoprotein

LDL-C; Low-density lipoprotein cholesterol

LDLR; Low-density lipoprotein receptor

MS; Metabolic syndrome

NCEP; National Cholesterol Education Program

NHANES; National Health and Nutrition Examination Survey

NHLBI; National Heart, Lung, and Blood Institute

oxLDL; oxidized low-density lipoprotein

PCSK9; Proprotein convertase subtilisin/kexin type 9

$sPLA_2$-AII; Secretory phospholipase A_2-IIA

TC; Total cholesterol

TG; Triglycerides

TLC; Therapeutic lifestyle change

VLDL; Very low density lipoprotein

Author details

Lorenzo Iughetti*, Barbara Predieri and Patrizia Bruzzi

*Address all correspondence to: iughetti.lorenzo@unimore.it

Department of Medical and Surgical Sciences of Mothers, Children and Adults, University of Modena & Reggio Emilia, Pediatric Unit, Modena, Italy

References

[1] Relationship of atherosclerosis in young men to serum lipoprotein cholesterol and smoking: a preliminary report from the Pathobiological Determinants of Atherosclerosis in Youth (PDAY) Research Group. JAMA 1990; 264: 3018-3024.

[2] Berenson GS, Srinivasan SR, Bao W, Newman WP III, Tracy RE, Wattigney WA. Association between multiple cardiovascular risk factors and atherosclerosis in children and young adults: the Bogalusa Heart Study. N Engl J Med 1998; 338: 1650-1656.

[3] Davis PH, Dawson JD, Riley WA, Lauer RM. Carotid intimal-medial thickness is related to cardiovascular risk factors measured from childhood through middle age: the Muscatine Study. Circulation 2001;104: 2815-2819.

[4] Miettinen TA, Hallikainen M, Raitakari OT, et al. Twenty-one year tracking of serum non-cholesterol sterol. The Cardiovascular Risk in Young Finns study. Nutrition, Metabolism & Cardiovascular Disease 2009; 19:525-531.

[5] Tabas I. Consequences of cellular cholesterol accumulation: basis concepts and physiological implications. J Clin Invest 2002;110:905-911.

[6] Libby P, Ridker PM, Hansson GK. Inflammation in atherosclerosis. J Am Coll Cardiol 2009;54:2129-38.

[7] Narverud I, Rettestol K, Iversen PO, Halvorsen B, Ueland T, Ulven SM et al. Markers of atherosclerotic development in children with familial hypercholesterolemia: a literature review. Atherosclerosis 2014;235:299-309.

[8] Le J, Zhang D, Chen J, Raghuveer G. "Vascular age" is advanced in children with atherosclerosis promoting risk. Circ Cardiovasc Imaging 2010:3(1):8-14.

[9] Kavey REW, Allada V, Daniels SR, Hayman LL, McCrindle BW, Newburger JW, Parekh RS, Steinberger J. Cardiovascular Risk Reduction in High-Risk Pediatric Patients. Circulation 2006; 114:2710-2738.

[10] Vlahos AP, Naka KK, Bechlioulis A, Theoharis P, Vakalis K, Moutzouri E et al. endothelial dysfunction, but not structural atherosclerosis, is evident early in children with heterozygous familial hypercholesterolemia. Pediatr Cardiol. 2014;35(1):63-70.

[11] DeJongh S, Lilien MR, op't Roodt J, Stroes ES, Bakker HD, Kastelein JJ. Early statin therapy restores endothelial function in children with familial hypercholesterolemia. J Am Coll Cardiol 2002; 40: 2117-2121.

[12] Wiegman A, Hutten BA, deGroot E, Rodenburg J, Bakker HD, Buller HR, Sijbrands EJ, Kastelein JJ. Efficacy and safety of statin therapy in children with familial hypercholesterolemia: a randomized controlled trial. JAMA 2004;292:331-337.

[13] National Cholesterol Education Program. Report of the Expert Panel on Blood Cholesterol Levels in Children and Adolescents. Pediatrics 1992; 89(S):525–584.

[14] Expert Panel on Integrated Guidelines for Cardiovascular Health and Risk Reduction in Children and Adolescents. Expert panel on integrated guidelines for cardiovascular health and risk reduction in children and adolescents: summary report. Pediatrics 2011 S128; 5:S213-256.

[15] Lipid Research Clinics Population Studies data Book, Vol 1. The Prevalence Study. NIH Publication n°80-1527. Washington, DC, National Institutes of Health, 1980

[16] Daniels SR, Greer FR et al. American Academy of Pediatrics Committee on Nutrition. Lipid screening and cardiovascular Health in Childhood. Pediatrics 2008; 122: 198-208.

[17] Jolliffe CJ and Janssen I. Distribution of lipoproteins by age and gender. Circulation 2006; 114:1056-1062.

[18] Hickman TB, Briefel RR, Carroll MD, Rifkind BM, Cleeman JI, Maurer KR, Johnson CL. Distributions and trends of serum lipid levels among United States children and adolescents ages 4-19 years: data from the Third National health and Nutrition Examination Survey. Prev Med 1998;27:879-890.

[19] Ford ES, Li C, Zhao G, Mokdad AH. Concentrations of low-density lipoprotein cholesterol and total cholesterol among children and adolescents in the United States. Circulation 2009;119:1108-1115.

[20] Rahalkar AR, Hegele RA. Monogenic pediatric dyslipidemias: classification, genetics and clinical spectrum. Molecular genetics and Metabolism 2008;93:282-294.

[21] Braamskamp MJ1, Hutten BA, Wiegman A, Kastelein JJ. Management of hypercholesterolemia in children. Paediatr Drugs. 2014;16(2):105-14.

[22] Usifo E, Leigh SE, Whittall RA, Lench N, Taylor A, Yeats C, Orengo CA, Martin AC, Celli J, Humphries SE. Low-density lipoprotein receptor gene familial hypercholesterolemia variant database: update and pathological assessment. Ann Hum Genet. 2012;76(5):387-401.

[23] Scientific Steering Committee on behalf of the Simon Broome Register Group. Risk of fatal coronary heart disease in familial hypercholesterolemia. BMJ 1991;303:893-6.

[24] WHO-Human Genetics. Familial Hypercholesterolemia. Report of a second WHO Consultation. Ed. WHO. 1999, Geneva.

[25] Wald D. Commentary: Controversies in NICE guidance on familial hypercholesterolemia. BMJ 2008; 337:a1304.

[26] Lamb MM, Ogden CL, Carroll MD, Lacher DA, Flegal KM. Association of body fat percentage with lipid concentrations in children and adolescents: United States, 1999-2004. Am J Clin Nutr 2011;94:877-83.

[27] Korsten-Reck U, Kromeyer-Hauschild K, Korsten K, et al. Frequency of secondary dyslipidemia in obese children. Vascular Health and Risk Management 2008;4(5): 1089-1094.

[28] Baass A, Dubuc G, Tremblay M, et al. Plasma PCSK9 is associated with age, sex, and multiple metabolic markers in a population-based sample of children and adolescents. Clin Chem 2009;55(9):1637-1645.

[29] Ritchie SK, Murphy EC, Ice C, Cottrell LA, Minor V, Elliott E, Neal W. Universal versus targeted blood cholesterol screening among youth: The CARDIAC project. Pediatrics 2010;126:260–265.

[30] Bamba V, Update on screening, etiology and treatment of dyslipidemia in children. J Clin Endocrinol Metab 2014; 99: 3093-3102.

[31] Lloyd-Jones DM, Hong Y, Labarthe D, Mozaffarian D, Appel LJ, Van Horn L, Greenlund K, Daniels S, Nichol G, Tomaselli GF, Arnett DK, Fonarow GC, Ho PM, Lauer MS, Masoudi FA, Robertson RM, Roger V, Schwamm LH, Sorlie P, Yancy CW, Rosamond WD; American Heart Association Strategic Planning Task Force and Statistics Committee. Defining and setting national goals for cardiovascular health promotion and disease reduction: the American Heart Association's strategic Impact Goal through 2020 and beyond. Circulation. 2010;121(4):586-613.

[32] Gidding SS, Dennison BA, Birch LL, et al. Dietary recommendations for children and adolescents. A guide for practitioners. Consensus statement from the American Heart Association. Circulation 2005; 112: 2061-2075.

[33] National Cholesterol Education Program ATP III : httw://www.americanheart.org/presenter.jhtml?identifier=4764.

[34] Nemet D, Barkan S, Epstein Y, et al. Short- and long-term beneficial effects of a combined dietary-behavioral-physical activity intervention for the treatment of childhood obesity. Pediatrics 2005; 115:e443-e449.

[35] Iughetti L, Predieri B, Balli F, Calandra S. Rational approach to the treatment for heterozygous familial hypercholesterolemia in childhood and adolescence: a review. J Endocrinol Invest 2007; 30(8): 700-719.

[36] Obarzanek E, Kimm SY, Barton BA, for DISC Collaborative Research Group et al. Long-term safety and effects of a cholesterol lowering lipoprotein cholesterol: seven year result of the Dietary Intervention Study in Children (DISC). Pediatrics 2001; 104: 256-264.

[37] Talvia S, Lagstrom H, Rasanen M, et al. A randomized intervention since infancy to reduce intake of saturated fat; calories (energy) and nutrient intakes up to 10 years in the Special Turku Coronary Risk Factor Intervention Project. Arch Pediatr Adolesc Med 2004; 158: 41-47.

[38] Weghuber D, Widhalm K. Effect of 3-month treatment of children and adolescents with familial and polygenic hypercholesterolemia with a soya-substituted diet. Br J Nutr 2008; 99(2): 281-286.

[39] Jakuli L, Vissers MN, Rodenburg J, et al. Plant stanols do not restore endothelial function in prepubertal children with familial hypercholesterolemia despite reduction of low-density lipoprotein cholesterol levels. J Pediatr 2006;148: 495-500.

[40] Garoufi A, Vorre S, Soldatou A, Tsentidis C, Kossiva L, Drakatos A, Marmarinos A, Gourgiotis D. Plant sterols-enriched diet decreases small, dense LDL-cholesterol levels in children with hypercholesterolemia: a prospective study. Ital J Pediatr 2014;40:42.

[41] Malhotra A, Shafiq N, Arora A, Singh M, Kumar R, Malhotra S. Dietary interventions (plant sterols, stanols, omega-3 fatty acid, soy protein and dietary fibers) for familial hypercholesterolaemia. Cochrane Database Syst Rev 2014;6: CD001918.

[42] Martino F, Martino E, Morrone F, Carnevali E, Forcone R, Niglio T. Effect of dietary supplementation with glucomannan on plasma total cholesterol and low density lipoprotein cholesterol in hypercholesterolemic children. Nutr Metab Cardiovasc Dis 2005;15(3):174-80.

[43] Guardamagna O, Amaretti A, Puddu PE, Raimondi S, Abello F, Cagliero P, Rossi M. Bifidobacteria supplementation: effects on plasma lipid profiles in dyslipidemic children. Nutrition. 2014;30(7-8):831-6.

[44] Kelley GA, Kelley KS. Effects of aerobic exercise on NON-HDL-C in children and adolescents: a meta-analysis of randomized controlled trials. Prog Cardiovasc Nurs 2008;23(3):128-132).

[45] McCrindle BW, Urbina EM, Dennison BA, et al. American Heart Association Atherosclerosis, Hypertension, and Obesity in Youth Committee; American Heart Association Council of Cardiovascular Disease in the Young, American Heart Association Council on Cardiovascular Nursing. Drug therapy of high-risk lipid abnormalities in children and adolescents: a scientific statement from the American Heart Association Atherosclerosis, Hypertension, and Obesity in Youth Committee, Council of Cardiovascular Disease in the Young, with the Council on Cardiovascular Nursing. Circulation 2007;115:1948-1967

[46] Cox ER, Halloran DR, Homan SM et al. Trends in the prevalence of chronic medication use in children: 2002-2005. Pediatrics 2008;122:e1053-e1061.

[47] Vuorio A, Kuoppala J, Kovanen PT, Humphries SE, Tonstad S, Wiegman A, Drogari E. Statins for children with familial hypercholesterolemia. Cochrane Database Syst Rev 2014;7:CD006401.

[48] O'Gorman CS, Higgins MF, O'Neil MB. Systematic review and meta-analysis of statins for heterozygous familial hypercholesterolemia in children: evaluation of cholesterol changes and side effects. Pediatr Cardiol 2009; 30: 482-489.

[49] Arambepola C, Farmer AJ, Perera R, Neil HAW. Statin treatment for children and adolescents with heterozygous familial hypercholesterolaemia: A systematic review and meta-analysis. Atherosclerosis 2007;195: 339-347.

[50] Hanai J, Cao P, Tanksale P, Imamura S, Koshimizu E, Zhao J, Kishi S, Yamashita M, Phillips PS, Sukhatme VP, Lecker SH. The muscle-specific ubiquitin ligase atrogin-1/MAFbx mediates statin-induced muscle toxicity. J Clin Invest 2007; 117 (12): 3940–51.

[51] Ferreira WP, Bertolami MC, Santos SN, et al. One-month therapy with simvastatin restores endothelial function in hypercholesterolemic children and adolescents. Pediatr Cardiol 2007; 28: 8-13.

[52] Kusters DM, Avis HJ, de Groot E, Wijburg FA, Kastelein JJ, Wiegman A, Hutten BA. Ten-year follow-up after initiation of statin therapy in children with familial hypercholesterolemia. JAMA 2014;312(10):1055-7.

[53] Braamskamp MJAM, Tsimikas S, Wiegman A, Kastelein JJP, Hutten BA. Statin therapy and secretory phopholipase A2 in children with heterozygous familial hypercholesterolemia. Atherosclerosis 2013; 229:404-407.

[54] Stein EA, Marais AD, Szamosi T, et al. Colesevelam hydrochloride: efficacy and safety in pediatric subjects with heterozygous familial hypercholesterolemia. J Pediatr 2010;156(2): 231-6.

[55] Yeste D, Chacon P, Clemente M, et al. Ezetimibe as monotherapy in the treatment of hypercholesterolemia in children and adolescents. J Pediatr Endo Metab 2009; 22:487-492.

[56] Kastelein JJP, Akdim F, Stroes ESG, et al. Simvastatin with or without ezetimibe in familial hypercholesterolemia. N Engl J Med 2008; 385: 1431-1443.

[57] Blazing MA, Giugliano RP, Cannon CP, Musliner TA, Tershakovec AM, White JA, Reist C, McCagg A, Braunwald E, Califf RM. Evaluating cardiovascular event reduction with ezetimibe as an adjunct to simvastatin in 18,144 patients after acute coronary syndromes: final baseline characteristics of the IMPROVE-IT study population. Am Heart J 2014;168(2):205-12.

[58] Tavori H, Melone M, Rashid S. Alirocumab: PCSK9 inhibitor for LDL cholesterol reduction. Expert Rev cardiovasc Ther 2014; 12(10):1137-44.

[59] Marais AD, Firth JC, Blom DJ. Homozygous familial hypercholesterolemia and its management. Semin Vasc Med 2004;4:43-50.

[60] Page MM, Bell DA, Hooper AJ, Watts GF, Burnett JR. Lipoprotein apheresis and new therapies for severe familial hypercholesterolemia in adults and children. Best Pract Res Clin Endocrinol Metab 2014;28(3):387-403.

[61] Malatack JJ. Liver transplantation as treatment for familial homozygous hypercholesterolemia: too early or too late. Pediatr Transplant 2011;15(2):123-5.

[62] Cuchel M, Meagher EA, du Toit Theron H, Blom DJ, Marais AD, Hegele RA, Averna MR, Sirtori CR, Shah PK, Gaudet D et al. Efficacy and safety of a microsomal triglyceride transfer protein inhibitor in patients with homozygous familial hypercholesterolaemia: a single-arm, open-label, phase 3 study. Lancet 2013; 381:40–46.

[63] Thomas GS, Cromwell WC, Ali S, Chin W, Flaim JD, Davidson M. Mipomersen, an Apolipoprotein B Synthesis Inhibitor, Reduces Atherogenic Lipoproteins in Patients with Severe Hypercholesterolemia at High Cardiovascular Risk: A Randomized, Double-Blind, Placebo-Controlled Trial. J Am Coll Cardiol 2013;62(23):2178-84.

Chapter 3

Role of Oxidized LDL in Atherosclerosis

E. Leiva, S. Wehinger, L. Guzmán and R. Orrego

Additional information is available at the end of the chapter

http://dx.doi.org/10.5772/59375

1. Introduction

Nowadays, Atherosclerosis is the most important source of morbidity and mortality in the world, and is detected by the accumulation of lipids deposits (mainly cholesterol) in macrophages located not only in large but also in medium sized arteries. Currently, the association between atherosclerosis and heightened oxidative stress is widely accepted. Nevertheless, despite numerous efforts the role of oxidative stress in the progression of Atherosclerosis is still not clear.

Oxidation is a biochemical process of loss of electrons, which is essential for life due to its involvement in the production of cellular energy. However, when oxidation is excessive causing cellular damage is when Oxidative Stress appears. This process is complex; therefore, it cannot be measured or defined by a single parameter. For this reason, currently the interest lies on developing antioxidant therapies and diets enriched with antioxidants that prevent or at least decrease cellular damage and atheromatous plaque formation originated by the excess of oxidative stress.

Aim. The aim of this review is to analyze the state of the art on oxidized LDL role within the pathogenesis of atherosclerosis.

This chapter will be developed according to the following titles,

1. Oxidative stress and atherosclerosis.
2. LDL Oxidation
3. OxLDL in atheromatous plaque formation
4. Study Models
5. OXIDATIVE STRESS AND ATHEROSCLEROSIS

The word “Atherosclerosis” comes from the ancient Greeks where "sclerosis” means hardening and “athere” is gruel or accumulation of lipid. The physiopathological process is characterized by the aggregation of cholesterol, infiltration of macrophages and the proliferation of smooth muscle cells (SMCs) as accumulation of connective tissues and thrombus creation. In early stages of the disease, the growth of the lesion starts in the sub endothelial space and its progress may even cause total cessation in blood flow with intermittent periods of quiescence. The accumulation of lipids and other organic molecules lead to a proliferation of certain cell types within the arterial wall that gradually impinge the vessel lumen and block up the blood flow in large and medium sized arteries. Furthermore, this disease tends to be more common in white than black men [1]. The magnitude of this problem is deep, because atherosclerosis claims more lives than all types of combined cancer and economic costs are considerably high[2]. Currently, the idea that atherosclerosis constitutes a state of high levels of oxidative stress is widely accepted and this phenomenon is associated with lipid and protein oxidation in the vascular wall[3, 4].

Despite the countless efforts made to explain the role of oxidative stress in progression of atherosclerosis, its predictive role is still not clear. Goldstein and Brown discovered the LDL incorporation process in peripheral cells as fibroblasts, macrophages and others -which meant for them the Nobel Prize- has been the basis for a series of subsequent discoveries, from 1979 up to now, which have intended to explain the development of the atherosclerosis' process [5-8]. The hypothesis of oxidative modification in atherosclerosis, reviewed by Steinberg and others in several opportunities argues that the oxidation of low-density lipoprotein (LDL) is an early stage of the disease and that oxidized LDL (OxLDL) would contribute to atherogenesis [9-12].

Until 1991, the strength of the scientific evidence regarding the role of the oxidation of LDL in the phenomenon of atherosclerosis was such that the National Heart, Lung and Blood Institute recommended the initiation of clinical trials [8, 13-17]. In relationship to this hypothesis, based on *in vitro* assays, the evidence showed the following relevant aspects: 1) the LDL oxidation is the first event in the foam cell formations [18, 19] the LDL lipids in human arterial lesions are extensively oxidized and 3) the presence of Ox LDL is evident *in vivo*[20]. On the other hand, the existence of several structurally unrelated compounds such as probucol and vit E that inhibit atherosclerosis in animals, prevent the initiation of the disease due to a reduction of the oxidization of LDL [21]. In relationship to probucol, It seems to be a more effective protection against lesion formation on an early-stage of the disease than the statin-mediated lipid-lowering effects [22].

The events involving the process of atherosclerosis begin with LDL oxidation in the vascular wall. This happens due to the production of reactive oxygen species (ROS) and nitrogen species (NOS) by endothelial cells, therefore, oxidative modifications would be crucial in the clinical aspect of coronary artery disease such as endothelial dysfunction and plaque disruption [23].

Although it is known by scientific evidence that LDL oxidation plays a central role in the pathophysiology of atherosclerosis, up to now there is no convincing proofs related to the protective effect of antioxidant therapy as a way to prevent the damage caused by that process on vital macromolecules such as lipids, proteins and DNA.This may be due to the discrepancies

http://dx.doi.org/10.5772/59375

between human and animal studies that use antioxidant therapies either to try or to limit the atherosclerotic process and cardiovascular events. It is not clear if oxidative stress is cause or consequence of the atherogenic process. In this sense, it has been proposed that inflammation could be considered as a primary process and oxidative stress as a secondary event of atherosclerosis [24].

2. LDL oxidation

Oxidation is a biochemical process of loss of electrons, which is essential for life due to its involvement in the production of cellular energy. Oxidative stress appears when oxidation is excessive. This apparently simple process is actually complex in all biological levels, and cannot be measured or defined by a single parameter.

The oxidation process of lipids and proteins is the result of an excess of free radical and other oxidant species derived from oxygen, nitrogen and other chemical elements in the body. Chemically, the oxidative stress is associated with an increased production of oxidizing species or a significant decrease in the effectiveness of antioxidants defenses such as reduced glutathione, catalase, peroxidases and others. The cell proliferation and death are key processes in the progression of atherosclerosis and severe oxidative stress can cause cell death and even mild oxidation can trigger cellular stress and apoptosis, while more intense stress may cause necrosis [25].

There is a constant production of ROS and other oxidative species derived from the normal and xenobiotic metabolism, ionizing radiation and smoke snuff exposure, among others. Oxidative molecules can exert positive or negative effects over cells and tissues, depending on their concentration. ROS plays an important role in several physiological cell processes, such as signaling and regulation cascades, however excesses can induce chemical and structural modifications which has been proven that alter the function of cellular components, inhibit protein function, induce DNA damage, viral activation and lipid peroxidation which can promote cell death (Figure 1).

In addition, redox systems such as gluthation peroxidase, thioredoxine reductase and pyridine nucleotide redox status can change their physiological function when modified by ROS and others reactive species, affecting the normal cell signaling including apoptotic cell death [26].

Today there are clear proofs that LDL oxidation plays a significant role in atherogenesis. In fact, this has been demonstrated throughout time. So, between 1985 and 1989, 62 papers about OxLDL were published; between 1992 and January 1997, the number of publications related to OxLDL went up to 727, and up to day only considering PubMed entry, it is possible to find over 7000 publications associated with the key words Oxidized LDL. This growing interest is supported by the large amount of evidence which confirms that oxidative modification of LDL plays a pivotal role in atherosclerosis and hence, makes it an obvious target for therapeutic approaches [10, 27].

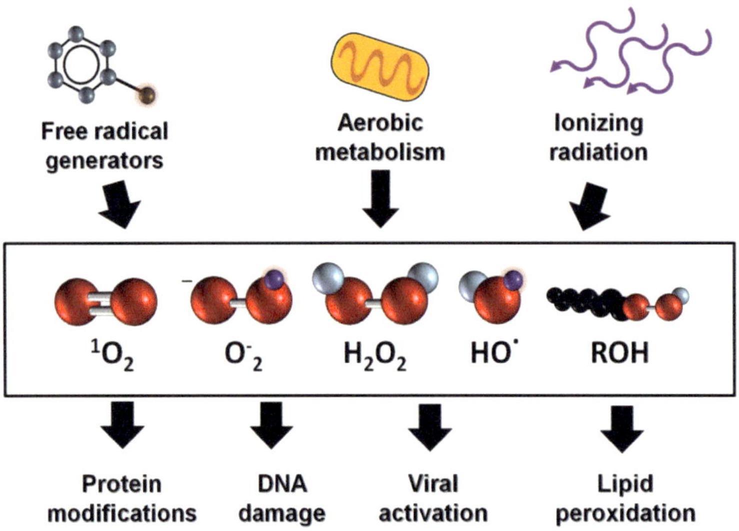

Figure 1. The figure shows some sources and consequences of oxidative stress.

In 2002, Friedman et al. showed that the oxidized lipids from OxLDL are biologically active. Specifically, polyunsaturated fatty acids (PUFA) either free or bound to an ester from phospholipid are converted into hydroperoxides, which break down to form highly reactive molecules, such as malondialdehyde and 4-hydroxynonenal among other metabolic products. These reactive aldehydes can then form Schiff-bases, covalent Michael-type adducts with lysine residues of apolipoprotein B in LDL molecules. Besides, the sn-2 oxidized fatty acid fragments which can remain attached via ester bridges may also contain terminal reactive aldehydes. However, this reactive phospholipid also called "aldehyde phospholipid core" may also form adducts with Schiff-base lysine residues of apolipoprotein B and presumably also with other proteins and amines-containing phospholipids, such as phosphatidylethanolamine and phosphatidylserine (Figure 2).Finally, the authors proved that when LDL presents substantial oxidative modifications, a great number of neoepitopes are generated transforming it in a highly immunogenic LDL. Indeed, there are a variety of autoantibodies directed to epitopes of OxLDL derived from specific oxidation in animals and human, that appear to increase in individuals with clinical and morphological signs of atherosclerosis [28].

On the contrary, OxLDL is thought to promote atherosclerosis through complex inflammatory and immunologic mechanisms that lead to lipid dysregulation and foam cell formation. Matsuura et al (2006) proposed that in the intima of atherosclerotic lesions, the OxLDL forms complex with the Beta 2 glycoprotein I (beta2GPI) and / or C-reactive protein (CRP). In patients with systemic lupus erythematosus (SLE) and/or antiphospholipid syndrome (APS), anti-OxLDL/beta2GPI complex autoantibodies have been found which has been significantly related to arterial thrombosis. In a non-immunized animal model of APS (NZWxBXSB F1 mice), it was demonstrated that anti-OxLDL/beta2GPI complex IgG autoantibodies can emerge spontaneously. Moreover, a monoclonal autoantibody (WB-CAL-1; IgG2a) against a complex beta-2-GPI was derived from the same mice. WB-CAL-1 significantly increased the

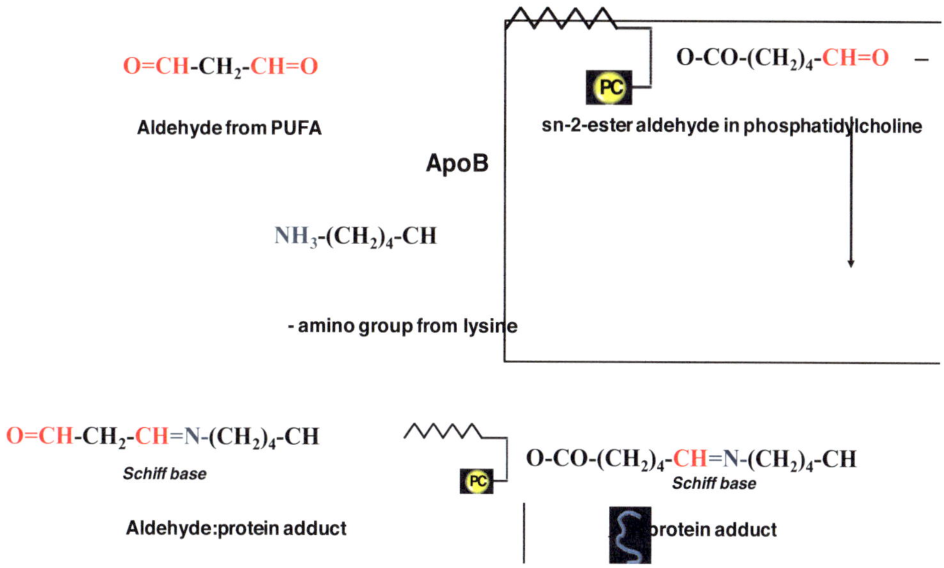

Figure 2. Oxidative modifications in ApoB present in lipoproteins.

in vitro uptake of OxLDL/beta-2-GPI complex by macrophages, suggesting that these IgG auto antibodies are pro-atherogenic. As opposed, IgM antibodies to OxLDL found in pro- atherogenic mice ApoE (-/-) and LDL -R (-/-) seemed to be protective. In human beings it has been widely reported the presence of IgG anti-Ox - LDL antibodies, but their clinical significance is not clear yet [29].

In the beginning, OxLDL was characterized by its biological properties, specifically for being a ligand for acetyl LDL receptor instead of a native LDL receptor. The Acetyl LDL receptor, present in macrophages, uptakes the OxLDL much faster than the native receptors, favoring the excessive intracellular accumulation of cholesterol. LDL oxidation and its uptake can be accomplished *in vitro* by an overnight incubation with macrophages cultured on an appropriate medium with 5 - 10 μM Cu^{2+} (oxidant) for 8-16 h allowing the study of the mechanism and kinetics of OxLDL.[30]

LDL oxidative modification, produces numerous structural changes, resulting in an increment of electrophoretic mobility, higher density, a polipoprotein B degradation, hydrolysis of phosphatidylcholine, changes on the amino groups of lysine residues and generation of fluorescent adducts caused by the covalent binding of lipid oxidation products to Apo B[31].

In vitro assays have shown that oxidative modification of LDL can be mutated by cultured endothelial cells or by cupric ions, which results in an increase of the lipoprotein uptake into macrophages [32, 33]. Therefore, it seems to be obvious that LDL oxidation is a crucial step for macrophage-derived foam cells formation in early stages of an atherosclerotic lesion. Moreover, LDL can be oxidized by specific enzymes such as lipooxygenase and phopholipase A2, even when these modifications are not necessarily identical to the endothelial cells-dependent modifications, they are still useful for studying oxidative alterations of LDL. In fact, in 1998, it was demonstrated that the oxidative modification of LDL by specific enzymes leads to an increased recognition by macrophages [32]. In conclusion, it is possible to say that oxidation of LDL in cells depends on at least three possibilities: (a) lipid oxidation by the action of lipoxygenase within the cells followed by the LDL exchange on its medium; (b) direct lipoxygenase-dependent lipid oxidation during cell contact with LDL and (c) both possibilities mentioned above [34].

It is has been reported that the *in vitro* addition of acetyl groups to LDL (acetylation), generates a modified LDL which can induce cholesterol accumulation in macrophages. Indeed, acetylated LDL is incorporated by "scavenger receptors" (SRA), which in contrast to the normal LDL receptor, are not "down regulated", so they induce a great intracellular lipid accumulation. Thus, acetylated LDL increases the formation of foam cells [35].

Another process that needs to be taken into account is the autoxidation of glucose or the early glycation products (carbonyl compounds) generated by oxygen free radicals (superoxide and hydroxyl) and hydrogen peroxide that can cause oxidative damage. Baynes et al in 1991 introduced the "glycoxidation hypothesis", which proposes that oxidative stress concomitant to glycation plays an important role in the stage of advanced glycation of proteins. Modifications of lipoproteins by glycation and oxidation alter their structure to make them sufficiently immunogenic. In type 2 diabetes, high titles of antibodies have been found against glicosylated-LDL and glicosylated-OxLDL. Immunogenic properties of glycosilated-OxLDL induce immune complex formation. It has been shown that glycosilated-OxLDL is trapped in the artery wall *in situ* [36-40].

Various pathologies can be originated by oxidative stress-induced apoptotic signaling which is a consequence of an increase of ROS and a decrease of other oxidative species and/or antioxidants, disruption of intracellular redox homeostasis and irreversible oxidative modifications of lipids, proteins or DNA. A better understanding of redox control over the development of apoptotic process in the cell, could better guide the course of the therapeutic strategies associated with disorders related to oxidative stress [25].

A great number of diseases have been related to oxidative stress and generation of free radicals, for this reason, antioxidant therapies and diets (such as Mediterranean diet) rich or enriched with antioxidants are thought to be a promising way to prevent or at least to attenuate the organic deterioration originated by the excessive oxidative stress.

3. OxLDL in atheromatous plaque formation

Atherosclerosis is a chronic inflammatory disease of the arterial wall that culminates with the atheromatous plaque formation. At present, there is a consensus that oxidation of LDL in the endothelial wall is an early event in atherosclerosis, according to the oxidative hypothesis [24]. First, the circulating LDL particles are transported from the vascular space into the arterial wall, mainly across trancytosis[41]. LDL is retained in the extracellular matrix of subendothelial space, through the binding of basic aminoacids in a polipoprotein B100 to negatively charged sulphate groups of proteoglycans in the extracellular matrix (ECM) [42, 43], where it is prone to be oxidized by oxidative stress, generating OxLDL[21], as we previously mentioned in this article.

It is known that OxLDL participates actively in atheromatous plaque formation, where it is retained. Multiple studies provide evidence suggesting OxLDL contribute in atherosclerotic plaque formation in several ways. In fact, at least four mechanisms have been proposed, being they complementary to each other: a) endothelial dysfunction, b) foam cell formation, c) SMCs migration and proliferation and c) induction of platelet adhesion and aggregation.

3.1. Endothelial dysfunction

The Endothelial dysfunction is a pathological condition in which the endothelium presents an impairment of anti-inflammatory, anti-coagulant and vascular regulatory properties. Nowadays, it is considered a key event in the atherosclerosis development. OxLDL formed and retained in the sub-entothelial space, activates endothelial cells (ECs) through the induction of the cell surface adhesion molecules which in turn, induce the rolling and adhesion of blood monocytes and T cells. It is reported that OxLDL induces the expression of intercellular adhesion molecule-1 (ICAM-1) and vascular-cell adhesion molecule-1 (VCAM-1), increasing the adhesive properties of endothelium in a similar manner to the effects of pro-inflammatory cytokines as interleukin 1 beta [44].

The blood leukocytes recruited migrate into the tunica intima, guided by chemokines. Indeed, OxLDL stimulates ECs and SMCs to secrete monocyte chemotactic protein-1 (MCP-1) and monocyte colony stimulating factor (mCSF) that induce the recruitment of monocytes into the endothelial wall [45-47]. On another hand, OxLDL can be chemotactic itself for monocytes and T lymphocytes (since it possesses lyso-phosphatidylcholine) and also for macrophages [48].

Nitric oxide (NO), is recognized as an important cardiovascular protective molecule, because exerts vasodilator properties and inhibits the adhesion of leucocytes and platelets to endothelium. This is generated in the vasculature by endothelial NO sythase (eNOS); the impairment of NO production and secretion by ECs is considered one of the most important characteristic of endothelial dysfunction [49].

The NO production from ECs is inhibited by OxLDL, given that the OxLDL is able to induce cholesterol depletion in the plasma membrane invaginations called caveolae, which causes the translocation of the protein caveolin and eNOS from the membrane domains, inhibiting eNOS activity in ECs [50]. Besides, another mechanisms to explain the inhibitory effect of OxLDL over NO production in ECs, has been proposed. It has been reported that OxLDL leads to an increased oxidative stress in ECs, producing significant amounts of superoxide, which chemically inactivates NO, forming peroxynitrite [51].

Lectin-like oxidized LDL receptor-1 (LOX-1), identified as the mayor OxLDL receptor in ECs, is expressed in several pro-inflammatory conditions and seems to play a crucial role in endothelial dysfunction induced by OxLDL[52]. Indeed, in human atherosclerotic lesions, LOX-1 overexpression in ECs has been reported, especially in the early stage of plaque formation [53]. It has been observed that the knockdown of LOX-1, inhibits the MCP-1 expression in human ECs stimulated with OxLDL and mitogen-activated protein kinase (MAPK) pathway would play a critical role [54]. Also, up-regulation of endothelial adhesion molecules as ICAM-1 and VCAM-1, can be induced by OxLDL in a LOX-1-dependent manner and this is mediated by the nuclear factor κB (NF-κB) [55]. Furthermore, the inhibitory effects of OxLDL over endothelial NO productions has been associated with LOX-1 function [51, 56]. Finally, it has been proposed that OxLDL can induce endothelial cell death through the activation of NF-κB and AP-1 pathways [57], worsening endothelial dysfunction and promoting the progression of the atherosclerotic plaque.

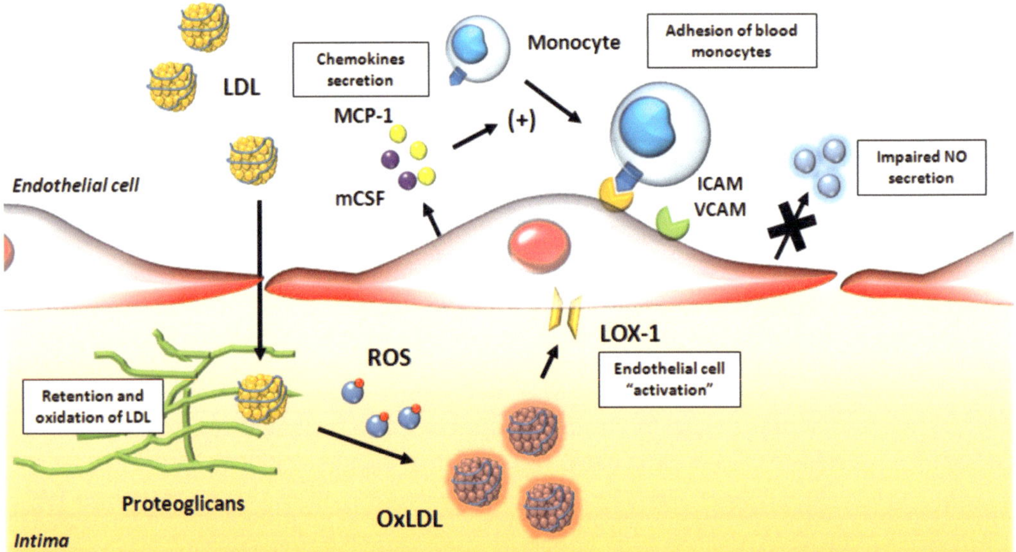

Figure 3. Role of OxLDL in endothelial dysfunction.

3.2. Foam cell formation

Once inside the sub-endothelial ECM, monocytes differentiate into macrophages that express several scavenger receptors (SRs) such as SR-AI/II, SR-BI, cluster of differentiation 36 (CD36) and LOX-1, and toll-like receptors (TLRs). It is important to remark that this phenotypic change, since the internalization of native LDL, occurs at a very low rate to account for foam cells formation and this process is prone to suffer down regulation of LDL receptor. In contrast, scavenger receptors have high affinity for OxLDL and they are not down regulated, leading to a massive intracellular lipid accumulation [20], which results in the foam cells formation [58, 59]. This differentiation into macrophages that promotes pro-inflammatory milieu, is part of a "macrophage trapping", a vicious circle that involves cell retention, oxidation of new LDL and the recruitment of more monocytes [18].

http://dx.doi.org/10.5772/59375

OxLDL also induce the expression of a number of genes associated to inflammation in macrophages: MCP-1, serum amyloid A, ceruloplasmin and hemeoxigenase-1 [60]. Moreover, macrophage activation induces the release of pro-inflammatory cytokines (interleukin 1-β, tumor necrosis factor), reactive oxygen species (ROS) and metalloproteases, which are associated with progression of inflammation [58].

Internalized OxLDL provides oxidized lipids as ligands for PPAR-γ pathway, upregulating CD36 expression, facilitating in turn, the internalization of more OxLDL[61, 62]. This internalization activates the macrophage, inducing the secretion of cytokines that recruits immune cells to intima and the secretion of the enzymes myeloperoxidase and 12/15-lipoxigenase, which are thought to participate in the oxidization of new LDL, increasing the local pool of OxLDL[63, 64]. Also, the internalization of OxLDL by CD36 seems to induce the inhibition of macrophage migration, favoring cell spreading and the activation of focal adhesion kinase, in a process mediated by src-kinases and oxidative stress [65]. Besides, OxLDL-CD36 interaction induces the loss of cell polarization in macrophages, an essential process to cell migration [66]. Thus, the evidence suggests that OxLDL not only participates in monocyte differentiation and macrophage activation, but also macrophage retention.

As mentioned, LOX-1 is one of the SRs expressed in macrophages and when it occurs by the influence of pro inflammatory cytokines, OxLDL or other stimuli, the OxLDL uptake increases significantly favoring the foam cells formation [67, 68]. The accumulation of OxLDL can lead to foam cell apoptosis or necrosis, forming cellular debris deposited in the core of the atherosclerotic plaque and contributing to inflammatory progression.

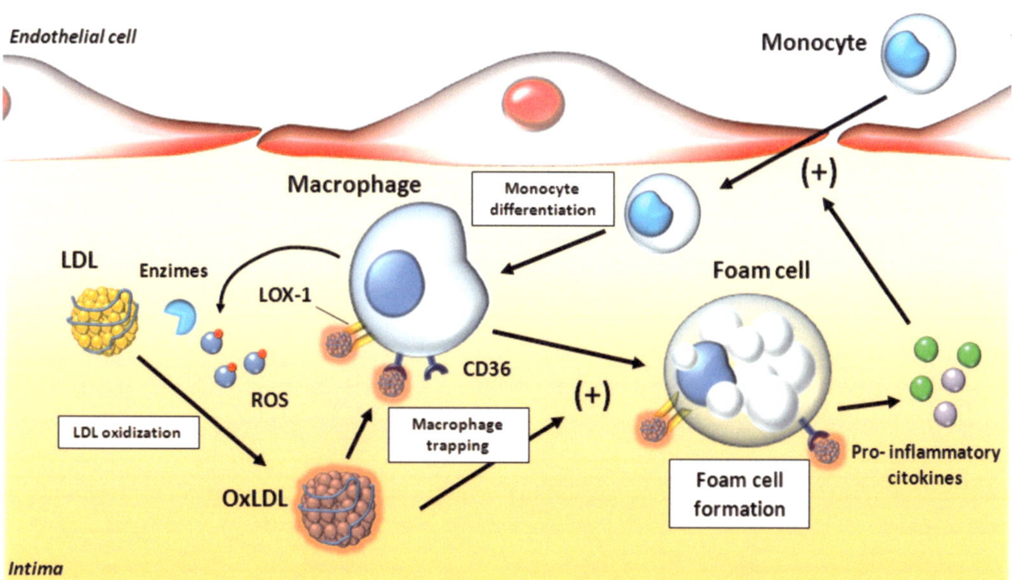

Figure 4. Role of OxLDL in foam cell formation.

3.3. Smooth muscle cell migration and proliferation

The migration and subsequent focal proliferation of SMCs in tunica intima are some of the hallmarks of the atheromatous phenomenon and they play a critical role on it. The SMCs migrate from tunica media to the subendothelial space, where they proliferate in response to growth factors. The proliferation of SMCs can be stimulated by OxLDL, since these particles enhance platelet-derived growth factor (PDGF) and basic fibroblast growth factor (bFGF) expression and secretion [69, 70] by ECs and macrophages. On the other hand, OxLDL also induces the secretion of a variety of other growth factors and their receptors: insulin-like growth factor-1(IGF-1) and epidermal growth factor (EGF), all with mitogenic effects inducing SMCs proliferation [71].

OxLDL has also been shown to induce changes directly in SMCs. OxLDL increases migration and leads to changes in SMCs phenotype making them to produce large amounts of ECM [72]. The production of interstitial collagen and elastin leads to the building of a fibrous cap that covers the developing atherosclerotic plaque, forming a "necrotic core" containing foam cells, cellular debris, extracellular lipids and lysosomal enzymes [73]. Thus, OxLDL participate in the expansion of the atherosclerotic lesion size.

OxLDL also induce LOX-1 expression in SMCs and recently, it has been proposed that many of the named effects of OxLDL are mediated by LOX-1[71]. Another important effect mediated by LOX-1 is the increment of ROS generation induced by OxLDL in SMCs, which can induce the cell death, contributing to plaque instability and rupture in the final stage of atherosclerosis [74]. Taken together, the evidence suggests that OxLDL has a crucial role in the plaque instability and hence, in the development of its complications.

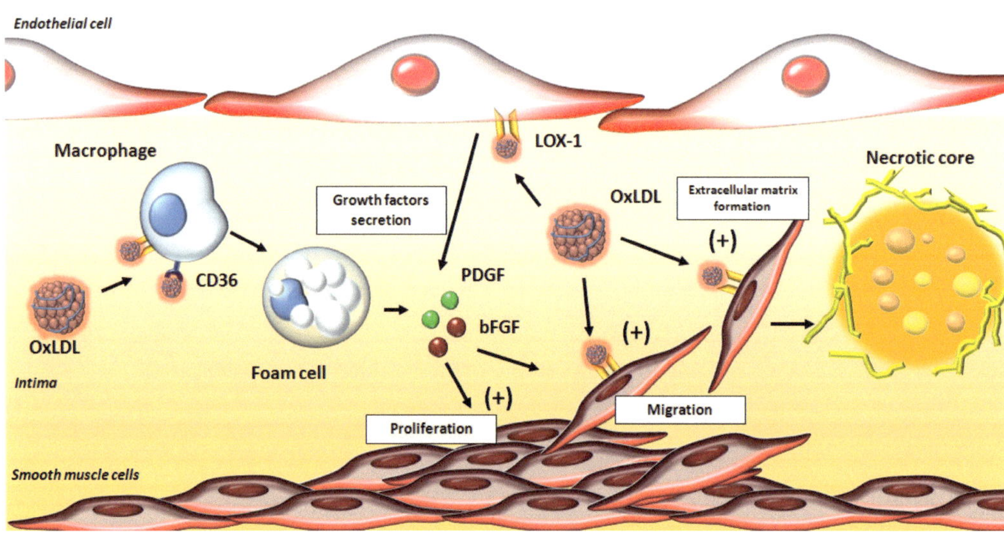

Figure 5. Role of OxLDL in smooth muscle cells proliferation and migration.

3.4. Induction of platelet adhesion and aggregation

Platelets are important players in atherosclerosis plaque development, especially after the plaque rupture, where they promote thrombus formation. In this process, OxLDL also is implicated. The impairment of endothelial NO production by OxLDL has been associated with an increase in prostaglandin secretion and thus, platelet aggregation [73]. CD36 is expressed in resting platelets and its interaction with OxLDL has been implicated with platelet activation, evidenced by P-selectin expression and the activation of integrin $\alpha_{IIb}\beta_3$[75].

OxLDL seems to induce a hyperactive state in platelets, since when they are cultured with OxLDL, they show more sensitivity to the classic platelet-activator ADP, in a process mediated by JNK and Vav family members [76, 77]. OxLDL is able to promote shape change and fast platelet activation through the action of Src kinases and Rho kinase-signaling pathways [78]. The effects of OxLDL over platelets could account also for additional pro-atherogenic phenomena. Platelets exposed to OxLDL release chemokines that favors atherosclerotic development [79] and promote endothelial dysfunction and foam cells formation [80, 81].

LOX-1 is expressed in platelets once they are activated [82], where it contributes to OxLDL internalization together with CD36. Since LOX-1 is able to binds anionic phospholipids as the present in the surface of activated platelets, has been proposed that endothelial LOX-1 mediates platelet adhesion to ECs [68]. Indeed, platelet binding to LOX-1 enhances endothelin-1 (ET-1) release from ECs [83] and induces oxidative inactivation of NO in ECs [56], suggesting that LOX-1 participates in endothelial dysfunction also through activated platelets. Thus, OxLDL seems to play a pivotal role in the pro-atherosclerotic behavior of activated platelets.

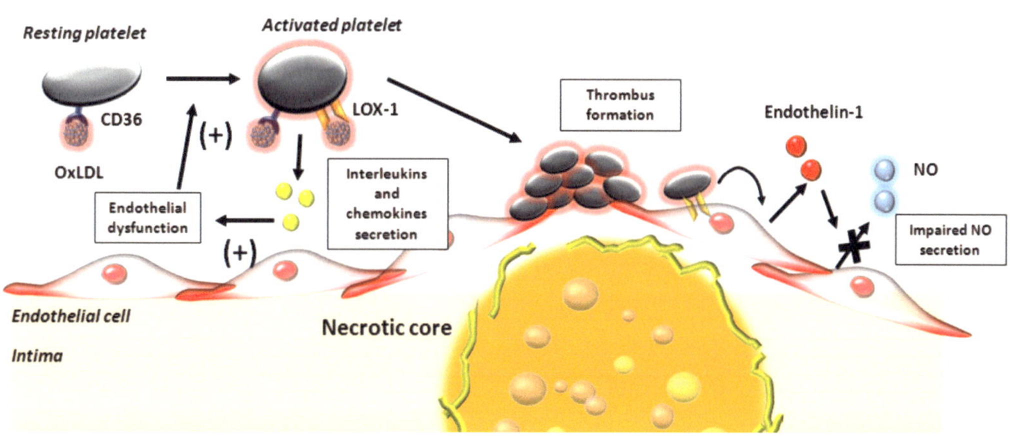

Figure 6. Role of OxLDL in pro-atherosclerotic function of platelets.

4. Mouse models for atherosclerosis

Given the importance of knowing the role of oxidized LDL in the process of atherosclerotic plaque formation, the study of animal models has been an important tool, where the examination of genetically modified mice has significantly contributed towards a better understanding of the mechanisms involved in this pathology.

It is worth noting that the use of small animals in research benefits from easy availability and low cost compared to large animals like primates. In addition, working with small animals reduces ethical concerns and limits the quantity of new agents needed for *in vivo* studies.

Transgenic and knockout mouse models for atherosclerosis have also been instrumental in evaluating existing, finding and testing new atherosclerotic drugs [84]. Small-animal models have the advantage of a well-defined genetic characterization which opens the possibility to transform them into transgenic and gene knockout animals [85].

Atherosclerosis is it not developed by wild-type mice; in fact they have high levels of anti-atherogenic high-density lipoprotein (HDL) and low levels of pro-atherogenic LDL and very-low-density lipoprotein (VLDL). Furthermore, mice do not express cholesteryl ester transfer protein (CETP), a plasma protein known to transfer cholesteryl ester from HDL particles and other lipoprotein fractions to pro-atherogenic apolipoprotein-B-containing lipoproteins LDL, VLDL and intermediate low-density lipoproteins (ILDL).

The current mouse models of atherosclerosis are based on disorders on the metabolism of lipoproteins through diets or genetic manipulations [84]. These perturbations have been made thanks to the current availability of genetic information, a variety of inbred strains and the development of molecular biology technics [86]. Atherosclerotic mice were first reported by Thompson et al., 1969, [87] using C57BL/6 inbred mice fed for five weeks with a diet containing a 50% of fat, whereas control mice were fed with a regular diet of 5% of fat. Nevertheless, this diet had a high percentage of mortality [86]. Paigen et al. modified the diet proposed by Thompson supplementing it with a regular diet containing 1.25% of cholesterol, 0.5% of cholic acid and 15% of fat. Nowadays, this diet is named the "Paiged diet" [88]. However, Ignatowski et al., [89] reported in 1980 the first evidence of atherosclerosis in the aorta of a rabbit model fed with a diet containing animal proteins like meat, eggs and milk.

Nowadays, the most used model of atherosclerosis in mice is based on the alteration of genes that codify the low-density lipoprotein receptor (LDLr) and the apolipoprotein E (ApoE), being both key elements for the lipid metabolism.

5. Apolipoprotein E-deficient (*Apo E* $^{-/-}$) mice

The ApoE, is a glycoprotein found in almost every lipoprotein with the exception of LDL. The purpose of this glycoprotein mainly synthesized in the brain and liver is to serve as a ligand for receptors that removes the VLDL and chylomicrons remnants. Since the ApoE can also be synthesized by macrophages and monocytes in the atherosclerotic vessels, is thought to have an important role on inflammatory processes and on the cholesterol homeostasis [90]. Moreover, it has been reported that ApoE may function in the biliary excretion and in dietary absorption of cholesterol [91].

Plump et al., [92] in 1992, produced the first mice models deficient in apolipoprotein E (*ApoE*$^{-/-}$). These animals were fed with a diet of 4.5% fat to develop a strong atherosclerosis model. This became an important tool in the research of atherosclerosis.

To inactivate the mice's *ApoE* gene, a homologous recombination of genes was made in embryonic stem cells. Two plasmids (pNMC109 and pJPB63) with a neomycin-resistance gene were used to disrupt the structure of the *ApoE* gene. Chimeric mice were generated by blastocyst injection with targeted lines [93]. The fact that homozygous animals were born at the expected frequency and that they appeared to be healthy, was of significant importance.

Currently, the *ApoE*$^{-/-}$mice are available on Jackson Laboratories which are direct descendants of the original *ApoE*$^{-/-}$ mouse created by the Maeda group (002052 B6.129P2-Apoe^{tm1Unc}).

Under a normal chow-fed diet, the mice developed a fatty streak observed in the aorta as early as a 3-month-old [93]. Foam cells at 10 weeks of age under the same diet were observed using a light microscopy. At 15 weeks of age, lesions containing SMCs and foam cells were observed, and at 20 weeks of age, fibrous plaques could be seen. It is worth mentioning that when a Western diet is used, the process is accelerated [94].

Although it is known that this model of *ApoE*$^{-/-}$ has considerable limitations, it has been used widely, because of the rapid development of atherosclerosis. A major drawback of the complete absence of ApoE protein is that most plasma cholesterol is confined to VLDL and not to LDL particles as in humans.

6. LDL receptor-deficient (*LDLr*$^{-/-}$) mice

In humans, mutations in the *LDLr* gene cause familial hypercholesterolemia. The *LDLr*$^{-/-}$mouse has a milder lipoprotein alteration than *ApoE*$^{-/-}$mice when fed standard low-fat chow, with plasma cholesterol levels around 250 mg/dL due mainly to the accumulation of LDL [95].

In 1993, *LDLr*$^{-/-}$ mice were created by gene targeting of embryonic stem cells [96]. By feeding them with a 10% fat diet, an increase of total cholesterol level (2-fold) was observed on these mice, due mainly to the high levels of VLDL and LDL. When fed on a high-fat/high-cholesterol diet, *LDLr*$^{-/-}$ mice showed a rapid increase in the severity of hypercholesterolemia and atherosclerotic lesion development throughout the coronary arteries, aortic root, and aorta [85, 97]. The plasma lipoprotein profile of *LDLr*$^{-/-}$ mice resembled the one of humans, with the cholesterol being confined mainly to the LDL fraction. Nevertheless, this mice model of atherosclerosis is very responsive to the diet. In fact, their cholesterol levels rose up to 1500 mg/dL when they were under the Paigen diet [98]. The lesions produced in *LDLr-/-* mice were similar to the lesions produced in the *ApoE-/-* mice, in terms of their development of plaques in a time-dependent manner. On the contrary, the *LDLr-/-* mouse produced a more moderate murine model of atherosclerosis than the *ApoE-/-* mouse. This characteristic is produced mainly due to a milder degree of hyperlipidemia [99].

In 1998, a mouse model deficient in the Apo B mRNA editing activity (*Apobec1*$^{-/-}$) and LDL receptor (*LDLr*$^{-/-}$) were generated by Powell-Braxton et al [100]. The lipoprotein profile of this animal model resembles the human familial hypercholesterolemia and when fed with a chow diet, exhibited atherosclerosis at its 8-month of age. The characteristics of this animal model provided an advantage to study the interactions between the environment (high fat diet) and the gene response in the onset of atherosclerosis [101].

7. ApoE3-leiden transgenic mice

Mutations in the gene encoding ApoE can lead to a binding-defective ApoE, which mediates the binding of lipoproteins to LDL receptor and is an essential ligand for the receptor-mediated uptake of chylomicron and VLDL remnants by hepatic lipoprotein receptors. This results in a disturbed receptor-mediated clearance of lipoprotein remnants by the liver, as has been described for patients with familial dysbetalipoproteinemia[102]. Premature atherosclerosis is produced by a genetic disorder named familial dysbetalipoproteinemia, which presents high levels of plasmatic triglycerides and cholesterol, mainly due to the increase in the VLDL remnants and chylomicron. The ApoE3-Leiden, a genetic variant of ApoE, is related with an inherited familial dysbetalipoproteinemia [103].

The ApoE3-Leiden mutation it is characterized by a rare dominant-negative tandem duplication of codons 120 to 126 in human *ApoE3* gene. Introducing a human ApoE3-Leiden gene construct into C57BL/6 mice has generated the ApoE3-Leiden transgenic mice. The ApoE3-Leiden gene consists of a construct with the *ApoC1*and *ApoE* genes with a promoter element to regulate the expression. While, this mice model of atherosclerosis still expresses ApoE protein, the clearance of lipoproteins containing ApoE is impaired, being less dramatic than the *ApoE*$^{-/-}$ mice model of atherosclerosis. The introduction of the *ApoC1* gene in transgenic mice has exhibited elevated levels of cholesterol and triglycerides owing to an accumulation of VLDL-size particles in the circulation, increasing plasma lipid levels by diminished lipolysis and VLDL uptake through both the LDLr and low density lipoprotein receptor-related protein (LRP) [84, 104].The ApoE3-Leiden mice have a hyperlipidemic phenotype, develop atherosclerosis on being fed cholesterol, and are more sensitive to lipid-lowering drugs than *ApoE*$^{-/-}$ and *LDLr*$^{-/-}$ mice [105]. The ApoE3-Leiden mice model is very responsive to diets containing sugar, fat and cholesterol, developing high levels of plasma triglycerides and cholesterol, with a prominent increase in LDL and VLDL lipoproteins.

Compared with *ApoE*$^{-/-}$ and *LDLr*$^{-/-}$ mice, ApoE3-Leiden mice represent a moderate mouse model for hyperlipidemia. Therefore, diets and drugs that influence the production of VLDL and chylomicron also show parallel effects on plasma levels of triglycerides and cholesterol. In this sense, the ApoE3-Leiden mice are more responsive to hypolipidemic compounds than the *LDLr*$^{-/-}$ and *ApoE*$^{-/-}$ mice [84, 106].

8. Double knockout mice models

A model that develops severe hyperlipidaemia and atherosclerosis was obtained with an *ApoE* and *LDLr* double knockout (*ApoE*$^{-/-}$/ *LDLr*$^{-/-}$ / DKO) [98]. It has been observed that, even on a regular chow diet, the atherosclerosis progression is generally more considerable than in mice only deficient in ApoE [107, 108]. Hence, the *ApoE*$^{-/-}$/, *LDLr*$^{-/-}$/, DKO mouse is appropriate to study the effect of compounds with anti-atherosclerotic activity without the need of atherogenic diets.

Besides, the role of the ApoE and the LDLr in the development of the atherosclerosis and dysregulation of the NOS system leading to impairment of NO bioavailability, has been documented for some time in atherosclerotic vessels of both experimental animals and humans [109]. To study the contribution of endothelial eNOS to lesion formation, Kuhlencordt et al. [110] created *ApoE*$^{-/-}$/ *eNOS*$^{-/-}$/double knockout mice (*ApoE*$^{-/-}$/ *eNOS*$^{-/-}$ / DKO), which presents a more pronounced atherosclerosis than ApoE-/- mouse model. Besides, eNOS absence favors the development of peripheral coronary disease, chronic myocardial ischemia, heart failure and an array of other vascular complications not detected in *ApoE*$^{-/-}$ mice [111].

Additionally, key structural proteins like apoB100 and apoB48, are needed to assemble lipoproteins rich in triacylglycerol; moreover, these proteins are part of all classes of atherogenic lipoproteins [112]. Veniant et al., 1998, characterized *LDLr*$^{-/-}$ and *ApoE*$^{-/-}$ mice which were homozygous to the ApoB-100 allele, founding that the *LDLr*$^{-/-}$/ApoB$^{100/100}$ mice model develop an extensive atherosclerosis, even when were fed with a normal chow diet, [113]

In summary, the experimental evidences show that the oxidative stress plays a pivotal role in atherogenesis, having OxLDL as a crucial player. Nevertheless, the clinical trials that used antioxidants strategies have shown poor results in relationship to the development of atherosclerosis, besides strong discrepancies between the different studies to establish the correlation between oxidative stress and atherogenic process. Therefore, the achievement of a successful therapy in humans based on the oxidative modification hypothesis is still a major challenge.

Author details

E. Leiva*, S. Wehinger, L. Guzmán and R. Orrego

*Address all correspondence to: eleivam@utalca.cl

Interdisciplinary Excellence Research Program on Healthy Aging (PIEI-ES), Universidad de Talca, Talca, Chile

References

[1] Hegele, R. A. The genetic basis of atherosclerosis. *Int J Clin Lab Res* 27:2-13; 1997.

[2] Mathers, C. D.; Loncar, D. Projections of global mortality and burden of disease from 2002 to 2030. *PLoS Med* 3:e442; 2006.

[3] Napoli, C.; D'Armiento, F. P.; Corso, G.; Ambrosio, G.; Palumbo, G.; Zuliani, P.; Malorni, A.; Gallotta, G.; Somma, P.; Postiglione, A.; Chiariello, M. Occurrence of the same peroxidative compounds in low density lipoprotein and in atherosclerotic lesions from a homozygous familial hypercholesterolemic patient: a case report. *Int J Cardiol* 62:77-85; 1997.

[4] Uppal, N.; Uppal, V.; Uppal, P. Progression of Coronary Artery Disease (CAD) from Stable Angina (SA) Towards Myocardial Infarction (MI): Role of Oxidative Stress. *J Clin Diagn Res* 8:40-43; 2014.

[5] Henriksen, T.; Evensen, S. A.; Carlander, B. Injury to human endothelial cells in culture induced by low density lipoproteins. *Scand J Clin Lab Invest* 39:361-368; 1979.

[6] Hessler, J. R.; Robertson, A. L., Jr.; Chisolm, G. M., 3rd. LDL-induced cytotoxicity and its inhibition by HDL in human vascular smooth muscle and endothelial cells in culture. *Atherosclerosis* 32:213-229; 1979.

[7] Goldstein, J. L.; Ho, Y. K.; Basu, S. K.; Brown, M. S. Binding site on macrophages that mediates uptake and degradation of acetylated low density lipoprotein, producing massive cholesterol deposition. *Proc Natl Acad Sci U S A* 76:333-337; 1979.

[8] Brown, M. S.; Goldstein, J. L. Lipoprotein metabolism in the macrophage: implications for cholesterol deposition in atherosclerosis. *Annu Rev Biochem* 52:223-261; 1983.

[9] Morel, D. W.; Hessler, J. R.; Chisolm, G. M. Low density lipoprotein cytotoxicity induced by free radical peroxidation of lipid. *J Lipid Res* 24:1070-1076; 1983.

[10] Steinberg, D. Low density lipoprotein oxidation and its pathobiological significance. *J Biol Chem* 272:20963-20966; 1997.

[11] Steinberg, D. The LDL modification hypothesis of atherogenesis: an update. *J Lipid Res* 50 Suppl:S376-381; 2009.

[12] Steinberg, D.; Witztum, J. L. Oxidized low-density lipoprotein and atherosclerosis. *Arterioscler Thromb Vasc Biol* 30:2311-2316; 2010.

[13] Parthasarathy, S.; Khan-Merchant, N.; Penumetcha, M.; Khan, B. V.; Santanam, N. Did the antioxidant trials fail to validate the oxidation hypothesis? *Curr Atheroscler Rep* 3:392-398; 2001.

[14] Stocker, R. Dietary and pharmacological antioxidants in atherosclerosis. *Curr Opin Lipidol* 10:589-597; 1999.

[15] Navab, M.; Berliner, J. A.; Watson, A. D.; Hama, S. Y.; Territo, M. C.; Lusis, A. J.; Shih, D. M.; Van Lenten, B. J.; Frank, J. S.; Demer, L. L.; Edwards, P. A.; Fogelman, A. M. The Yin and Yang of oxidation in the development of the fatty streak. A review

based on the 1994 George Lyman Duff Memorial Lecture. *Arterioscler Thromb Vasc Biol* 16:831-842; 1996.

[16] Sevanian, A.; Asatryan, L.; Ziouzenkova, O. Low density lipoprotein (LDL) modification: basic concepts and relationship to atherosclerosis. *Blood Purif* 17:66-78; 1999.

[17] McCall, M. R.; Frei, B. Can antioxidant vitamins materially reduce oxidative damage in humans? *Free Radic Biol Med* 26:1034-1053; 1999.

[18] Park, Y. M. CD36, a scavenger receptor implicated in atherosclerosis. *Exp Mol Med* 46:e99; 2014.

[19] Apostolov, E. O.; Ok, E.; Burns, S.; Nawaz, S.; Savenka, A.; Shah, S.; Basnakian, A. G. Carbamylated-oxidized LDL: proatherosclerotic effects on endothelial cells and macrophages. *J Atheroscler Thromb* 20:878-892; 2013.

[20] Barbieri, S. S.; Cavalca, V.; Eligini, S.; Brambilla, M.; Caiani, A.; Tremoli, E.; Colli, S. Apocynin prevents cyclooxygenase 2 expression in human monocytes through NADPH oxidase and glutathione redox-dependent mechanisms. *Free Radic Biol Med* 37:156-165; 2004.

[21] Steinberg, D.; Parthasarathy, S.; Carew, T. E.; Khoo, J. C.; Witztum, J. L. Beyond cholesterol. Modifications of low-density lipoprotein that increase its atherogenicity. *N Engl J Med* 320:915-924; 1989.

[22] Niimi, M.; Keyamura, Y.; Nozako, M.; Koyama, T.; Kohashi, M.; Yasufuku, R.; Yoshikawa, T.; Fan, J. Probucol inhibits the initiation of atherosclerosis in cholesterol-fed rabbits. *Lipids Health Dis* 12:166; 2013.

[23] Karimi, S.; Dadvar, M.; Modarress, H.; Dabir, B. Kinetic modeling of low density lipoprotein oxidation in arterial wall and its application in atherosclerotic lesions prediction. *Chem Phys Lipids* 175-176:1-8; 2013.

[24] Stocker, R.; Keaney, J. F., Jr. Role of oxidative modifications in atherosclerosis. *Physiol Rev* 84:1381-1478; 2004.

[25] Circu, M. L.; Aw, T. Y. Reactive oxygen species, cellular redox systems, and apoptosis. *Free Radic Biol Med* 48:749-762; 2010.

[26] Zhang, Y.; Chen, N.; Zhang, J.; Tong, Y. Hsa-let-7g miRNA targets caspase-3 and inhibits the apoptosis induced by ox-LDL in endothelial cells. *Int J Mol Sci* 14:22708-22720; 2013.

[27] Actis Dato, S. M.; Rebolledo, O. R. [Lipoprotein glycation and glycoxidation: their importance in diabetes mellitus]. *Medicina (B Aires)* 60:645-656; 2000.

[28] Friedman, P.; Horkko, S.; Steinberg, D.; Witztum, J. L.; Dennis, E. A. Correlation of antiphospholipid antibody recognition with the structure of synthetic oxidized phospholipids. Importance of Schiff base formation and aldol condensation. *J Biol Chem* 277:7010-7020; 2002.

[29] Matsuura, E.; Kobayashi, K.; Tabuchi, M.; Lopez, L. R. Oxidative modification of low-density lipoprotein and immune regulation of atherosclerosis. *Prog Lipid Res* 45:466-486; 2006.

[30] Esterbauer, H.; Gebicki, J.; Puhl, H.; Jurgens, G. The role of lipid peroxidation and antioxidants in oxidative modification of LDL. *Free Radic Biol Med* 13:341-390; 1992.

[31] Steinbrecher, U. P.; Zhang, H. F.; Lougheed, M. Role of oxidatively modified LDL in atherosclerosis. *Free Radic Biol Med* 9:155-168; 1990.

[32] Sparrow, C. P.; Parthasarathy, S.; Steinberg, D. Enzymatic modification of low density lipoprotein by purified lipoxygenase plus phospholipase A2 mimics cell-mediated oxidative modification. *J Lipid Res* 29:745-753; 1988.

[33] Jayaraman, S.; Gantz, D. L.; Gursky, O. Effects of oxidation on the structure and stability of human low-density lipoprotein. *Biochemistry* 46:5790-5797; 2007.

[34] Parthasarathy, S.; Wieland, E.; Steinberg, D. A role for endothelial cell lipoxygenase in the oxidative modification of low density lipoprotein. *Proc Natl Acad Sci U S A* 86:1046-1050; 1989.

[35] Kodama, T.; Freeman, M.; Rohrer, L.; Zabrecky, J.; Matsudaira, P.; Krieger, M. Type I macrophage scavenger receptor contains alpha-helical and collagen-like coiled coils. *Nature* 343:531-535; 1990.

[36] Gillotte, K. L.; Horkko, S.; Witztum, J. L.; Steinberg, D. Oxidized phospholipids, linked to apolipoprotein B of oxidized LDL, are ligands for macrophage scavenger receptors. *J Lipid Res* 41:824-833; 2000.

[37] Horkko, S.; Miller, E.; Dudl, E.; Reaven, P.; Curtiss, L. K.; Zvaifler, N. J.; Terkeltaub, R.; Pierangeli, S. S.; Branch, D. W.; Palinski, W.; Witztum, J. L. Antiphospholipid antibodies are directed against epitopes of oxidized phospholipids. Recognition of cardiolipin by monoclonal antibodies to epitopes of oxidized low density lipoprotein. *J Clin Invest* 98:815-825; 1996.

[38] Steinberg, D.; Witztum, J. L. Is the oxidative modification hypothesis relevant to human atherosclerosis? Do the antioxidant trials conducted to date refute the hypothesis? *Circulation* 105:2107-2111; 2002.

[39] Hulthe, J.; Wiklund, O.; Hurt-Camejo, E.; Bondjers, G. Antibodies to oxidized LDL in relation to carotid atherosclerosis, cell adhesion molecules, and phospholipase A(2). *Arterioscler Thromb Vasc Biol* 21:269-274; 2001.

[40] Crawford, R. S.; Mudaliar, S. R.; Henry, R. R.; Chait, A. Inhibition of LDL oxidation in vitro but not ex vivo by troglitazone. *Diabetes* 48:783-790; 1999.

[41] Simionescu, M.; Simionescu, N. Proatherosclerotic events: pathobiochemical changes occurring in the arterial wall before monocyte migration. *FASEB J* 7:1359-1366; 1993.

[42] Tabas, I.; Williams, K. J.; Boren, J. Subendothelial lipoprotein retention as the initiating process in atherosclerosis: update and therapeutic implications. *Circulation* 116:1832-1844; 2007.

[43] Skalen, K.; Gustafsson, M.; Rydberg, E. K.; Hulten, L. M.; Wiklund, O.; Innerarity, T. L.; Boren, J. Subendothelial retention of atherogenic lipoproteins in early atherosclerosis. *Nature* 417:750-754; 2002.

[44] Frostegard, J.; Haegerstrand, A.; Gidlund, M.; Nilsson, J. Biologically modified LDL increases the adhesive properties of endothelial cells. *Atherosclerosis* 90:119-126; 1991.

[45] Rajavashisth, T. B.; Andalibi, A.; Territo, M. C.; Berliner, J. A.; Navab, M.; Fogelman, A. M.; Lusis, A. J. Induction of endothelial cell expression of granulocyte and macrophage colony-stimulating factors by modified low-density lipoproteins. *Nature* 344:254-257; 1990.

[46] Yla-Herttuala, S.; Lipton, B. A.; Rosenfeld, M. E.; Sarkioja, T.; Yoshimura, T.; Leonard, E. J.; Witztum, J. L.; Steinberg, D. Expression of monocyte chemoattractant protein 1 in macrophage-rich areas of human and rabbit atherosclerotic lesions. *Proc Natl Acad Sci U S A* 88:5252-5256; 1991.

[47] Catapano, A. L.; Maggi, F. M.; Tragni, E. Low density lipoprotein oxidation, antioxidants, and atherosclerosis. *Curr Opin Cardiol* 15:355-363; 2000.

[48] Quinn, M. T.; Parthasarathy, S.; Fong, L. G.; Steinberg, D. Oxidatively modified low density lipoproteins: a potential role in recruitment and retention of monocyte/macrophages during atherogenesis. *Proc Natl Acad Sci U S A* 84:2995-2998; 1987.

[49] Forstermann, U.; Sessa, W. C. Nitric oxide synthases: regulation and function. *Eur Heart J* 33:829-837, 837a-837d; 2012.

[50] Blair, A.; Shaul, P. W.; Yuhanna, I. S.; Conrad, P. A.; Smart, E. J. Oxidized low density lipoprotein displaces endothelial nitric-oxide synthase (eNOS) from plasmalemmal caveolae and impairs eNOS activation. *J Biol Chem* 274:32512-32519; 1999.

[51] Cominacini, L.; Rigoni, A.; Pasini, A. F.; Garbin, U.; Davoli, A.; Campagnola, M.; Pastorino, A. M.; Lo Cascio, V.; Sawamura, T. The binding of oxidized low density lipoprotein (ox-LDL) to ox-LDL receptor-1 reduces the intracellular concentration of nitric oxide in endothelial cells through an increased production of superoxide. *J Biol Chem* 276:13750-13755; 2001.

[52] Chen, M.; Masaki, T.; Sawamura, T. LOX-1, the receptor for oxidized low-density lipoprotein identified from endothelial cells: implications in endothelial dysfunction and atherosclerosis. *Pharmacol Ther* 95:89-100; 2002.

[53] Kataoka, H.; Kume, N.; Miyamoto, S.; Minami, M.; Moriwaki, H.; Murase, T.; Sawamura, T.; Masaki, T.; Hashimoto, N.; Kita, T. Expression of lectinlike oxidized low-density lipoprotein receptor-1 in human atherosclerotic lesions. *Circulation* 99:3110-3117; 1999.

[54] Li, D.; Mehta, J. L. Antisense to LOX-1 inhibits oxidized LDL-mediated upregulation of monocyte chemoattractant protein-1 and monocyte adhesion to human coronary artery endothelial cells. *Circulation* 101:2889-2895; 2000.

[55] Li, D.; Chen, H.; Romeo, F.; Sawamura, T.; Saldeen, T.; Mehta, J. L. Statins modulate oxidized low-density lipoprotein-mediated adhesion molecule expression in human coronary artery endothelial cells: role of LOX-1. *J Pharmacol Exp Ther* 302:601-605; 2002.

[56] Cominacini, L.; Fratta Pasini, A.; Garbin, U.; Pastorino, A.; Rigoni, A.; Nava, C.; Davoli, A.; Lo Cascio, V.; Sawamura, T. The platelet-endothelium interaction mediated by lectin-like oxidized low-density lipoprotein receptor-1 reduces the intracellular concentration of nitric oxide in endothelial cells. *J Am Coll Cardiol* 41:499-507; 2003.

[57] Valente, A. J.; Irimpen, A. M.; Siebenlist, U.; Chandrasekar, B. OxLDL induces endothelial dysfunction and death via TRAF3IP2: Inhibition by HDL3 and AMPK activators. *Free Radic Biol Med* 70C:117-128; 2014.

[58] Hansson, G. K.; Robertson, A. K.; Soderberg-Naucler, C. Inflammation and atherosclerosis. *Annu Rev Pathol* 1:297-329; 2006.

[59] Mietus-Snyder, M.; Friera, A.; Glass, C. K.; Pitas, R. E. Regulation of scavenger receptor expression in smooth muscle cells by protein kinase C: a role for oxidative stress. *Arterioscler Thromb Vasc Biol* 17:969-978; 1997.

[60] Liao, F.; Andalibi, A.; deBeer, F. C.; Fogelman, A. M.; Lusis, A. J. Genetic control of inflammatory gene induction and NF-kappa B-like transcription factor activation in response to an atherogenic diet in mice. *J Clin Invest* 91:2572-2579; 1993.

[61] Nagy, L.; Tontonoz, P.; Alvarez, J. G.; Chen, H.; Evans, R. M. Oxidized LDL regulates macrophage gene expression through ligand activation of PPARgamma. *Cell* 93:229-240; 1998.

[62] Tontonoz, P.; Nagy, L.; Alvarez, J. G.; Thomazy, V. A.; Evans, R. M. PPARgamma promotes monocyte/macrophage differentiation and uptake of oxidized LDL. *Cell* 93:241-252; 1998.

[63] Carr, A. C.; McCall, M. R.; Frei, B. Oxidation of LDL by myeloperoxidase and reactive nitrogen species: reaction pathways and antioxidant protection. *Arterioscler Thromb Vasc Biol* 20:1716-1723; 2000.

[64] Cyrus, T.; Witztum, J. L.; Rader, D. J.; Tangirala, R.; Fazio, S.; Linton, M. F.; Funk, C. D. Disruption of the 12/15-lipoxygenase gene diminishes atherosclerosis in apo E-deficient mice. *J Clin Invest* 103:1597-1604; 1999.

[65] Park, Y. M.; Febbraio, M.; Silverstein, R. L. CD36 modulates migration of mouse and human macrophages in response to oxidized LDL and may contribute to macrophage trapping in the arterial intima. *J Clin Invest* 119:136-145; 2009.

[66] Park, Y. M.; Drazba, J. A.; Vasanji, A.; Egelhoff, T.; Febbraio, M.; Silverstein, R. L. Oxidized LDL/CD36 interaction induces loss of cell polarity and inhibits macrophage locomotion. *Mol Biol Cell* 23:3057-3068; 2012.

[67] Schaeffer, D. F.; Riazy, M.; Parhar, K. S.; Chen, J. H.; Duronio, V.; Sawamura, T.; Steinbrecher, U. P. LOX-1 augments oxLDL uptake by lysoPC-stimulated murine macrophages but is not required for oxLDL clearance from plasma. *J Lipid Res* 50:1676-1684; 2009.

[68] Pirillo, A.; Norata, G. D.; Catapano, A. L. LOX-1, OxLDL, and atherosclerosis. *Mediators Inflamm* 2013:152786; 2013.

[69] Stiko-Rahm, A.; Hultgardh-Nilsson, A.; Regnstrom, J.; Hamsten, A.; Nilsson, J. Native and oxidized LDL enhances production of PDGF AA and the surface expression of PDGF receptors in cultured human smooth muscle cells. *Arterioscler Thromb* 12:1099-1109; 1992.

[70] Kohno, M.; Yokokawa, K.; Yasunari, K.; Minami, M.; Kano, H.; Hanehira, T.; Yoshikawa, J. Induction by lysophosphatidylcholine, a major phospholipid component of atherogenic lipoproteins, of human coronary artery smooth muscle cell migration. *Circulation* 98:353-359; 1998.

[71] Mitra, S.; Goyal, T.; Mehta, J. L. Oxidized LDL, LOX-1 and atherosclerosis. *Cardiovasc Drugs Ther* 25:419-429; 2011.

[72] Shen, C. M.; Mao, S. J.; Huang, G. S.; Yang, P. C.; Chu, R. M. Stimulation of smooth muscle cell proliferation by ox-LDL- and acetyl LDL-induced macrophage-derived foam cells. *Life Sci* 70:443-452; 2001.

[73] Maiolino, G.; Rossitto, G.; Caielli, P.; Bisogni, V.; Rossi, G. P.; Calo, L. A. The role of oxidized low-density lipoproteins in atherosclerosis: the myths and the facts. *Mediators Inflamm* 2013:714653; 2013.

[74] Hsieh, C. C.; Yen, M. H.; Yen, C. H.; Lau, Y. T. Oxidized low density lipoprotein induces apoptosis via generation of reactive oxygen species in vascular smooth muscle cells. *Cardiovasc Res* 49:135-145; 2001.

[75] Podrez, E. A.; Byzova, T. V.; Febbraio, M.; Salomon, R. G.; Ma, Y.; Valiyaveettil, M.; Poliakov, E.; Sun, M.; Finton, P. J.; Curtis, B. R.; Chen, J.; Zhang, R.; Silverstein, R. L.; Hazen, S. L. Platelet CD36 links hyperlipidemia, oxidant stress and a prothrombotic phenotype. *Nat Med* 13:1086-1095; 2007.

[76] Chen, K.; Febbraio, M.; Li, W.; Silverstein, R. L. A specific CD36-dependent signaling pathway is required for platelet activation by oxidized low-density lipoprotein. *Circ Res* 102:1512-1519; 2008.

[77] Chen, K.; Li, W.; Major, J.; Rahaman, S. O.; Febbraio, M.; Silverstein, R. L. Vav guanine nucleotide exchange factors link hyperlipidemia and a prothrombotic state. *Blood* 117:5744-5750; 2011.

[78] Wraith, K. S.; Magwenzi, S.; Aburima, A.; Wen, Y.; Leake, D.; Naseem, K. M. Oxidized low-density lipoproteins induce rapid platelet activation and shape change through tyrosine kinase and Rho kinase-signaling pathways. *Blood* 122:580-589; 2013.

[79] Siegel-Axel, D.; Daub, K.; Seizer, P.; Lindemann, S.; Gawaz, M. Platelet lipoprotein interplay: trigger of foam cell formation and driver of atherosclerosis. *Cardiovasc Res* 78:8-17; 2008.

[80] Daub, K.; Seizer, P.; Stellos, K.; Kramer, B. F.; Bigalke, B.; Schaller, M.; Fateh-Moghadam, S.; Gawaz, M.; Lindemann, S. Oxidized LDL-activated platelets induce vascular inflammation. *Semin Thromb Hemost* 36:146-156; 2010.

[81] Curtiss, L. K.; Black, A. S.; Takagi, Y.; Plow, E. F. New mechanism for foam cell generation in atherosclerotic lesions. *J Clin Invest* 80:367-373; 1987.

[82] Chen, M.; Kakutani, M.; Naruko, T.; Ueda, M.; Narumiya, S.; Masaki, T.; Sawamura, T. Activation-dependent surface expression of LOX-1 in human platelets. *Biochem Biophys Res Commun* 282:153-158; 2001.

[83] Kakutani, M.; Masaki, T.; Sawamura, T. A platelet-endothelium interaction mediated by lectin-like oxidized low-density lipoprotein receptor-1. *Proc Natl Acad Sci U S A* 97:360-364; 2000.

[84] Zadelaar, S.; Kleemann, R.; Verschuren, L.; de Vries-Van der Weij, J.; van der Hoorn, J.; Princen, H. M.; Kooistra, T. Mouse models for atherosclerosis and pharmaceutical modifiers. *Arterioscler Thromb Vasc Biol* 27:1706-1721; 2007.

[85] Badimon, L.; Casani, L.; Vilahur, G. Chapter 10 - Models for the Study of Atherosclerosis and Thrombosis. In: Conn, P. M., ed. *Animal Models for the Study of Human Disease*. Boston: Academic Press; 2013: 221-239.

[86] Ohashi, R.; Mu, H.; Yao, Q.; Chen, C. Cellular and molecular mechanisms of atherosclerosis with mouse models. *Trends Cardiovasc Med* 14:187-190; 2004.

[87] Thompson, J. S. Atheromata in an inbred strain of mice. *J Atheroscler Res* 10:113-122; 1969.

[88] Paigen, B.; Morrow, A.; Brandon, C.; Mitchell, D.; Holmes, P. Variation in susceptibility to atherosclerosis among inbred strains of mice. *Atherosclerosis* 57:65-73; 1985.

[89] Ignatowski A.C. Influence of animal food on the organism of rabbits. *S Peterb Izviest Imp Voyenno-Med. Akad* 16:154-173; 1908.

[90] Curtiss, L. K.; Boisvert, W. A. Apolipoprotein E and atherosclerosis. *Curr Opin Lipidol* 11:243-251; 2000.

[91] Sehayek, E.; Shefer, S.; Nguyen, L. B.; Ono, J. G.; Merkel, M.; Breslow, J. L. Apolipoprotein E regulates dietary cholesterol absorption and biliary cholesterol excretion: studies in C57BL/6 apolipoprotein E knockout mice. *Proc Natl Acad Sci U S A* 97:3433-3437; 2000.

[92] Plump, A. S.; Smith, J. D.; Hayek, T.; Aalto-Setala, K.; Walsh, A.; Verstuyft, J. G.; Rubin, E. M.; Breslow, J. L. Severe hypercholesterolemia and atherosclerosis in apolipoprotein E-deficient mice created by homologous recombination in ES cells. *Cell* 71:343-353; 1992.

[93] Piedrahita, J. A.; Zhang, S. H.; Hagaman, J. R.; Oliver, P. M.; Maeda, N. Generation of mice carrying a mutant apolipoprotein E gene inactivated by gene targeting in embryonic stem cells. *Proc Natl Acad Sci U S A* 89:4471-4475; 1992.

[94] Reddick, R. L.; Zhang, S. H.; Maeda, N. Atherosclerosis in mice lacking apo E. Evaluation of lesional development and progression. *Arterioscler Thromb* 14:141-147; 1994.

[95] Ishibashi, S.; Goldstein, J. L.; Brown, M. S.; Herz, J.; Burns, D. K. Massive xanthomatosis and atherosclerosis in cholesterol-fed low density lipoprotein receptor-negative mice. *J Clin Invest* 93:1885-1893; 1994.

[96] Ishibashi, S.; Brown, M. S.; Goldstein, J. L.; Gerard, R. D.; Hammer, R. E.; Herz, J. Hypercholesterolemia in low density lipoprotein receptor knockout mice and its reversal by adenovirus-mediated gene delivery. *J Clin Invest* 92:883-893; 1993.

[97] Knowles, J. W.; Maeda, N. Genetic modifiers of atherosclerosis in mice. *Arterioscler Thromb Vasc Biol* 20:2336-2345; 2000.

[98] Ishibashi, S.; Herz, J.; Maeda, N.; Goldstein, J. L.; Brown, M. S. The two-receptor model of lipoprotein clearance: tests of the hypothesis in "knockout" mice lacking the low density lipoprotein receptor, apolipoprotein E, or both proteins. *Proc Natl Acad Sci U S A* 91:4431-4435; 1994.

[99] Sjoland, H.; Eitzman, D. T.; Gordon, D.; Westrick, R.; Nabel, E. G.; Ginsburg, D. Atherosclerosis progression in LDL receptor-deficient and apolipoprotein E-deficient mice is independent of genetic alterations in plasminogen activator inhibitor-1. *Arterioscler Thromb Vasc Biol* 20:846-852; 2000.

[100] Powell-Braxton, L.; Veniant, M.; Latvala, R. D.; Hirano, K. I.; Won, W. B.; Ross, J.; Dybdal, N.; Zlot, C. H.; Young, S. G.; Davidson, N. O. A mouse model of human familial hypercholesterolemia: markedly elevated low density lipoprotein cholesterol levels and severe atherosclerosis on a low-fat chow diet. *Nat Med* 4:934-938; 1998.

[101] Dutta, R.; Singh, U.; Li, T. B.; Fornage, M.; Teng, B. B. Hepatic gene expression profiling reveals perturbed calcium signaling in a mouse model lacking both LDL receptor and Apobec1 genes. *Atherosclerosis* 169:51-62; 2003.

[102] Marais, A. D.; Solomon, G. A.; Blom, D. J. Dysbetalipoproteinaemia: a mixed hyperlipidaemia of remnant lipoproteins due to mutations in apolipoprotein E. *Crit Rev Clin Lab Sci* 51:46-62; 2014.

[103] Murase, T.; Ebara, T.; Okubo, M. Hepatic lipase activity is decreased in Japanese patients with type III hyperlipoproteinemia. *Clin Chim Acta* 414:185-187; 2012.

[104] Jong, M. C.; Hofker, M. H.; Havekes, L. M. Role of ApoCs in lipoprotein metabolism: functional differences between ApoC1, ApoC2, and ApoC3. *Arterioscler Thromb Vasc Biol* 19:472-484; 1999.

[105] van Vlijmen, B. J.; van den Maagdenberg, A. M.; Gijbels, M. J.; van der Boom, H.; HogenEsch, H.; Frants, R. R.; Hofker, M. H.; Havekes, L. M. Diet-induced hyperlipoproteinemia and atherosclerosis in apolipoprotein E3-Leiden transgenic mice. *J Clin Invest* 93:1403-1410; 1994.

[106] Vainer, B.; Nielsen, O. H. Correlation between circulating soluble ICAM-1 and prednisolone-induced amelioration of ulcerative colitis. *Scand J Gastroenterol* 38:283-287; 2003.

[107] Witting, P. K.; Pettersson, K.; Ostlund-Lindqvist, A. M.; Westerlund, C.; Eriksson, A. W.; Stocker, R. Inhibition by a coantioxidant of aortic lipoprotein lipid peroxidation and atherosclerosis in apolipoprotein E and low density lipoprotein receptor gene double knockout mice. *FASEB J* 13:667-675; 1999.

[108] Kostogrys, R. B.; Franczyk-Zarow, M.; Maslak, E.; Gajda, M.; Mateuszuk, L.; Jackson, C. L.; Chlopicki, S. Low carbohydrate, high protein diet promotes atherosclerosis in apolipoprotein E/low-density lipoprotein receptor double knockout mice (apoE/LDLR(-/-)). *Atherosclerosis* 223:327-331; 2012.

[109] Perrotta, I.; Brunelli, E.; Sciangula, A.; Zuccala, V.; Donato, G.; Tripepi, S.; Martinelli, G. L.; Cassese, M. Inducible and endothelial nitric oxide synthase expression in human atherogenesis: an immunohistochemical and ultrastructural study. *Cardiovasc Pathol* 18:361-368; 2009.

[110] Kuhlencordt, P. J.; Gyurko, R.; Han, F.; Scherrer-Crosbie, M.; Aretz, T. H.; Hajjar, R.; Picard, M. H.; Huang, P. L. Accelerated atherosclerosis, aortic aneurysm formation, and ischemic heart disease in apolipoprotein E/endothelial nitric oxide synthase double-knockout mice. *Circulation* 104:448-454; 2001.

[111] Wang, Y. X. Cardiovascular functional phenotypes and pharmacological responses in apolipoprotein E deficient mice. *Neurobiol Aging* 26:309-316; 2005.

[112] Veniant, M. M.; Kim, E.; McCormick, S.; Boren, J.; Nielsen, L. B.; Raabe, M.; Young, S. G. Insights into apolipoprotein B biology from transgenic and gene-targeted mice. *J Nutr* 129:451S-455S; 1999.

[113] Veniant, M. M.; Zlot, C. H.; Walzem, R. L.; Pierotti, V.; Driscoll, R.; Dichek, D.; Herz, J.; Young, S. G. Lipoprotein clearance mechanisms in LDL receptor-deficient "Apo-B48-only" and "Apo-B100-only" mice. J Clin Invest 102:1559-1568; 1998.

Chapter 4

A Practical Case-Based Approach to Dyslipidaemia in Light of the European Guidelines

Olivier S. Descamps , Lale Tokgozoglu and Eric Bruckert

Additional information is available at the end of the chapter

http://dx.doi.org/10.5772/59481

1. Introduction

The European Atherosclerosis Society and the European Society of Cardiology have made new recommendations regarding the treatment of dyslipidaemia (1). Such recommendations build upon the "Joint European Societies' Task Force Guidelines on the Prevention of CVD in Clinical Practice" of 2007 [1, 2]. The most important changes include the redefinition of the risk categories and the addition of a 'very high-risk' category. For these new risk categories, the LDL-C targets have been redefined. In the highest risk individuals, the lowering of LDL to 70 mg/dl is recommended. Furthermore, HDL-c has been added to the new SCORE risk chart and non-HDL cholesterol is now considered to be a secondary target.

In this study, we illustrate how these guidelines can be used in clinical practice. We also give some tips on how to make them more user-friendly for clinicians (Figure 1). The discussed case (Clinical Case 1) was developed to combine a series of difficulties in therapeutic decision-making. We accepted the principle that any correctable secondary causes of dyslipidaemia had been excluded and that the patient had already received all the care to improve the other risk factors but without real (enough) success. These risk factors included smoking cessation, weight loss and/or blood pressure reduction. Unfortunately, this case is far from an exception. The reality is that it is often more difficult to quantitatively reduce risk factors, than it is to reduce cholesterol levels.

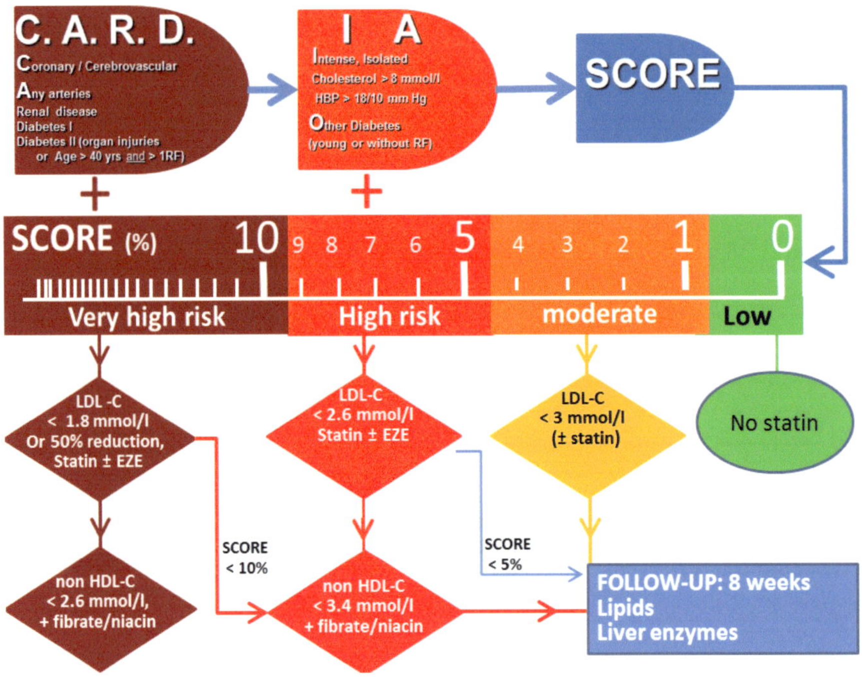

Figure 1. Algorithm of dyslipidaemia management in cardiovascular prevention.

Clinical Case 1. Presentation.

The patient,a woman of 59 years of age, has come to visit her doctor because she has reached the same age as when her sister suffered from a heart attack (two years ago).

Personal history:*Without particularity.*

Family history:*Her mother is obese and has been treated for diabetes since the age of 60 years. Her sister has undertaken a coronary bypass surgery following a heart attack at 59 years of age.*

Lifestyle-dietary habits.*Smokes (15 cigarettes per day), sedentary (works in an office, does not practice sport and only engages in interior recreation).*

Clinical examination.*Weight: 92 kg; height: 1,74 m (Body mass index – BMI : 30,5 kg/m²); waist circumference: 99 cm ; blood pressure: 145 / 85 mm Hg, no xanthoma, no corneal arcus.*

Biology:*Total cholesterol: 5.8 mmol/l; HDL cholesterol(HDL-C) : 1.0 mmol/l; triglycerides (TG): 3.5 mmol/l: cholesterol LDL (LDL-C) : 3.2 mmol/l (tableau 1); glycaemia : 112 mg/dl ; hs-CRP= 1,2 mg/dL; normal levels of creatinin, hepatic enzymes and thyroid hormones.*

---

http://dx.doi.org/10.5772/59481

Clinical Case 2. What is the Cardiovascular Risk of this Patient?

Our patient has no cardiovascular history, diabetes or any severe risk factors. Thus, we should calculate the risk SCORE, i.e., the risk of cardiovascular mortality in 10 years (we should take into consideration that we are a country with a high-risk population).

- Based on the classical risk factors (gender, age, systolic blood pressure and total cholesterol levels) and according to the classical SCORE table, the risk SCORE is 4% (Figure 2).

- Based on the new way to calculate the risk, the risk of our patient is quite high. After adjusting the HDL-C (near 1 mmol/l), using the four tables or using multipliers plus the reference chart, the SCORE reached should be 6 -6,4%. Given her family history (her sister, a woman of 60 years), this must be multiplied by 1.7 (Figure 2). Thus, the calculation is 10-11%. In addition, the presence of other risk factors (high levels of triglycerides, obesity, sedentariness and high hs-CRP) justifies the multiplication by 1.5 (~1.46=1.1 x 1.1 x 1. 1 x 1.1). This gives us 15-16% (let us take 15% as a base to facilitate later calculations). Thus, in total, we estimate that the risk of the patient dying of cardiovascular disease in 10 years is likely to be 15 % (Table 1). The patient is, therefore, in the category of risk labelled very high. The global risk (fatal and non-fatal) can be calculated by multiplying this by three (as the patient is a woman of nearly 60 years of age), giving a value of ~ 45%, which is very high.

2. First question: What is the cardiovascular risk of this patient?

To determine whether the patient is in the highest/high-risk category, we propose the acronym "C.A.R.D.I.A.SCORE". This will make it easy to remember (Figure 1).

2.1. Acronym « C.A.R.D.I.A. SCORE »

If there is an history of **c**ardiovascular **(« C »)** disease, **c**oronary**, c**erebrovascular or any **ar**tery injuries **(« A ») in** general (peripheral arteries, aneurism, etc.); if there is **r**enal insufficiency **(« R »)** defined by a glomerular filtration below 60 ml/min/1,73 m^2; if there is **d**iabetes **(« D »)**, either type I or II complicated of organ injuries (microalbuminuria) or type II without complications; if the patient is older than 40 years of age and displaying other risk factors (notice that, in diabetes, the three conditions of « **c**omplication, **a**ge and **r**isk factor give the acronym « CAR »), the patient should be considered as « very high-risk ».

For patients who show an isolated, yet severe, risk factor **(« I »),** like diabetes, without any other risk factor, severe hypercholesterolemia (cholesterol > 7.5 mmol/l and/or familial hypercholesterolemia) or severe hypertension (>180 mm Hg), they should be considered as « **high-risk** ». Furthermore, patients who have been diabetic since a young age **(« I »)** should also be considered as **« high-risk** ».

All other individuals who do not present one of the above characteristics should be examined using SCORE (6).

2.2. SCORE with two novelties

First novelty. It is now possible to qualify the risk SCORE quantitatively, according to the presence of a family history of early cardiovascular disease and the level of HDL cholesterol (1, 3and 4).We can do this by using either the four specific tables (one for each of the four HDL-C levels) (1) or the HDL-C specific multipliers to adjust the SCORE risk based on one reference table (the table for HDL-C = 0.8 mmol/l)(6) (Figure 2). In addition, we should consider the patient as higher risk if other risk factors are present (high levels of triglycerides, obesity, sedentariness, etc.). For these factors, the guidelines do not provide any multipliers but, as a rule of thumb, we should accept a minimum value of 1.1 as a multiplier for each additional factor. Indeed, in epidemiological studies, it is rare that a parameter can be identified as statistically independent and a clinically meaningful risk factor if it does not increase the risk to a minimum of 10%, after adjusting for other risk factors.

Second novelty. Patients should not be categorized according to a single "frontier of risk" (below or above 5%). Instead, they should be categorized based on the three "frontiers of risk": 1%, 5% and 10%. Thus, the risk SCORE should be defined as “**low**” if it is less than 1%,"**moderate**" if it is between 1% and 5%, "**high**" if it is between 5% and 10% and "**very high**" if it is over 10% (Figure 1).

Our case (Clinical Case 2) illustrates how a "moderate" 4% risk can be significantly enhanced in refining the other risk factors such as HDL-C, family history and so on. It is possible to calculate the global risk (fatal and non-fatal) simply by multiplying by three for men, by four for women and by a little less for older people. Taking this into consideration, for our female patient of 59 years, we should multiply by three. Thus, the overall risk is 45%. This is another way of expressing the CVD risk (with a higher number!). It should be used to increase our patient’s awareness of CVD and encourage her to be more motivated to follow the regime and take her medication.

3. Second question, how do we treat this patient?

The LDL-C remains the primary target, as in the previous guidelines. The target LDL-C is determined as a function of the patient’s risk.For each risk category, there is a different LDL GOAL. There is also a simplified chart to calculate the LDL reduction percentage to reach that goal. The evidence to decrease LDL-C to such low levels is supported by previous studies that indicate a possible regression of atherosclerotic plaques (i.e., a "rejuvenation" of the arteries) in this condition.

What if the level of LDL-C is unavailable because it is non-computable by the Friedewald formula (when TG levels are above 4.5 mmol/l)? In this case, we should use another target. The alternative target is not the level of total cholesterol, as proposed in the previous guidelines. Instead, it is the level of non HDL-C that will become, in this case, the primary target (see §4).

http://dx.doi.org/10.5772/59481

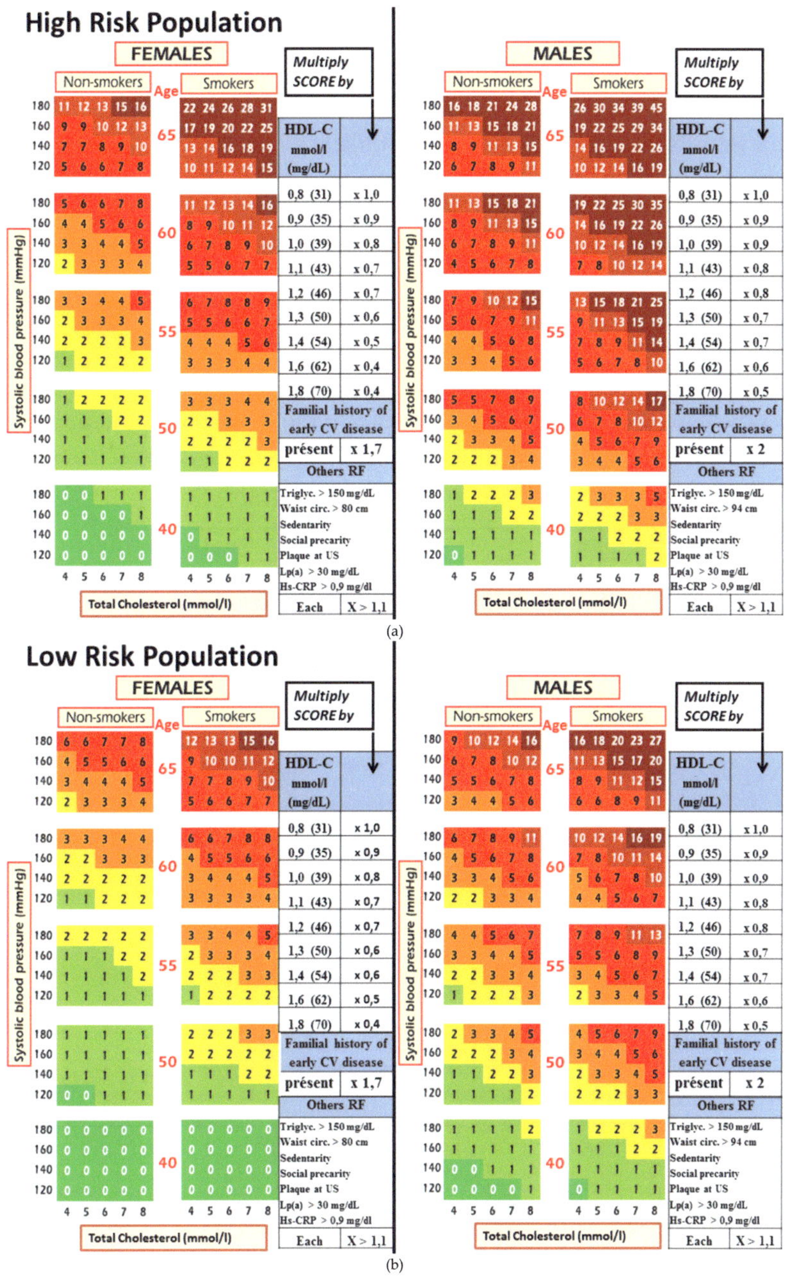

Figure 2. Table of risk SCORE, (the risk of cardiovascular death at 10 years) and the adjustments according to the level of HDL-C (8) as well as any family history of early cardiovascular disease (before 50 years of age in men and before 60 years of age in women). The table should be used as a reference chart; the table of SCORE at 0.8 mmol/l HDL-C, which contains the highest risk values. This allows the multipliers for the other HDL levels to be between 0 and 1 (which facilitates multiplication, e.g., to multiply by 0.4, multiply by 4 and divide by 10). Figure 2a. displays the SCORE in the high-risk population and Figure 2.b, in the low risk population.

3.1. Which Statin, What Dose and How Fast

Statin should always be the first line treatment (even for dyslipidaemia mixed with elevations of cholesterol and triglycerides, as we will demonstrate below (§4)). We should begin by prescribing a statin at a dosage that is the most likely to be effective in obtaining the correct reduction target. The rationale to choose the statin type and dosage is quite mathematical and is based on the baseline level, the LDL-C target and knowledge of the different statins' power (Figure 3). In terms of power (for a same dosage), these are fluvastatin < pravastatin < simvastatin <pitavastatin< atorvastatin < rosuvastatin [5]. Another rule is that, on average, doubling each of the statin dosage leads to a further decline in the rate of LDL-C of 4% to 6%. Another way to intensify the treatment is to associate the statin with one of the other anti-dyslipidaemia drugs (Figure 3). Among these, ezetimibe has the largest (20% to 25%) additional reduction of LDL-C. When the risk is high and the target is not reached, it is important to adjust the treatment as quickly as possible. The compliance and satisfaction of the patient, as well as the physician, depends on it.

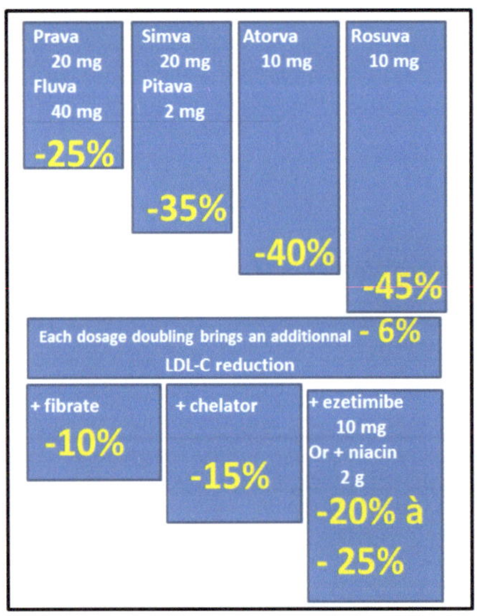

Figure 3. The choice and the statin dose should be based on a near mathematical criterion: the target reduction of LDL-C. The necessary reduction is easily estimated by the difference between the baseline LDL-C level and its target (according to the risk level) divided by the baseline LDL-C. The figure displays the power of different treatments in reducing LDL-C. For better precision of atorvastatin, we should use the following rule (dosage→ % LDL-C reduction): 10 mg → 38%, 20 mg → 45%, 40 mg → 49%, 80 mg → 52%). Other drugs also influence the HDL-C and TG levels. Statins have a small effect on the levels of HDL-C (slight ↑) and triglycerides (slight ↓). Fluva: fluvastatin; prava: pravastatin; pita: pitavasatin; simva: simvastatin; rosuva:rosuvastatin; atorva: atorvastatin.

3.2. Before prescribing a statin, we will check

Before the initiation of treatment, it is important to ensure that the CK (creatine phosphokinase) levels are not too high. If they are very high (> 5 times the upper limit of normal), it is better to delay and to check again six weeks later. Furthermore, it is important to determine the cause of these levels (intense physical exercise, trauma or recent intramuscular injection). To reduce

http://dx.doi.org/10.5772/59481

the risk of muscle side effects, we have to be more vigilant in elderly patients or in cases where the simultaneous use of treatment is interfering (via cytochrome P 450) with the metabolism of the proposed statin. We also have to be particularly careful if the patient has previously suffered from hepatic or renal insufficiencies.

For our patient in the very high-risk category, the LDL-C target is below 1.8 mmol/l. To achieve this target, we should reduce the patient's LDL-C by 40% (Clinical Case 3).

Clinical Case 3. How do we Treat Cholesterol in this Patient?

For our patient with a very high-risk,

- The target is < 1.8 mmol/l

- The necessary LDL-C reduction is: 3.0 mmol/l - 1.8 mmol/l = 1.2 mmol/l, which requires a reduction of 40% of the LDL-C (1.2 / 3.0 = 40%).

- The statins that are able to achieve a 40% reduction (Figure 3) are, for example, 40 mg simvastatin or 20 mg atorvastatin (there is very little chance of achieving such a reduction with pravastatin, even with 20 mg simvastatin).

- Prior to prescribing the drug, we should first verify the levels of CPK and liver enzymes, if this has not already been achieved.

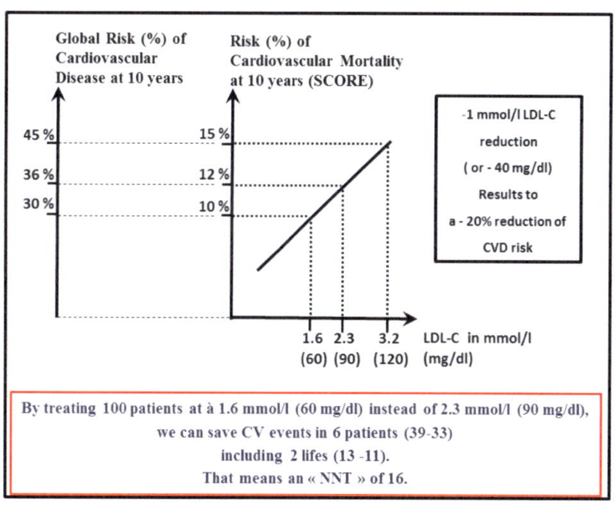

Figure 4. Shows how various LDL reductions decrease the risk of cardiovascular mortality up to 10 years (SCORE) and the risk of global cardiovascular risk (fatal and non-fatal) up to 10 years (this is calculated by multiplying the risk SCORE by three). (1) The current 0.9 mmol/l reduction of LDL-C relatively reduces CV events by 18%. Hence, the absolute risk of mortality CV decreases from 15% to 12%. Similarly, the global CV risk (multiplied by 3, see above) decreases from 45% to 36%. (2) A greater reduction below the target of 1.8 mmol/l allows a relative reduction in the amount of CV events by 32%. Hence, the absolute risk of mortality CV decreases from 15% to 10% and the CV global risk decreases from 45% to 30%.

4. Third question, how to follow up the patient?

In order to verify the effectiveness and safety of the patient's prescription, the improved guidelines recommend a patient follow up eight weeks later. Once the lipid levels have reached the target levels (according to the risk of the patient) and a safe level is maintained, an annual follow up will suffice.

4.1. Tolerance monitoring

Throughout the therapy, the monitoring of liver enzymes (Figure 5) is required. In subjects complaining of muscle pain, the muscle enzymes should be analysed. As long as the enzymes are not too high (< 3 x the upper limit of normal or ULN), we should continue the statin. However, if the enzymes exceed by 3 x ULN for liver enzymes or 5 X ULN for muscle enzymes (Figure 5), the statins should be stopped. Furthermore, the enzymes should be checked four to six weeks later (or two weeks later if the CK is very high). For high elevation of the CK, we should check the renal function. When the enzymes return to a normal value, treatment (or an alternative treatment) should be carefully reintroduced. In all cases, other common causes of the elevation of these enzymes should be excluded. In the instance of high CK, this means intensive muscle efforts and injuries (including intramuscular injections, etc.). For cases of high ALT, this means weight gain, excess of sugar, fat or alcohol, steatosis, hepatitis, lithiasis migration and other medications, etc.

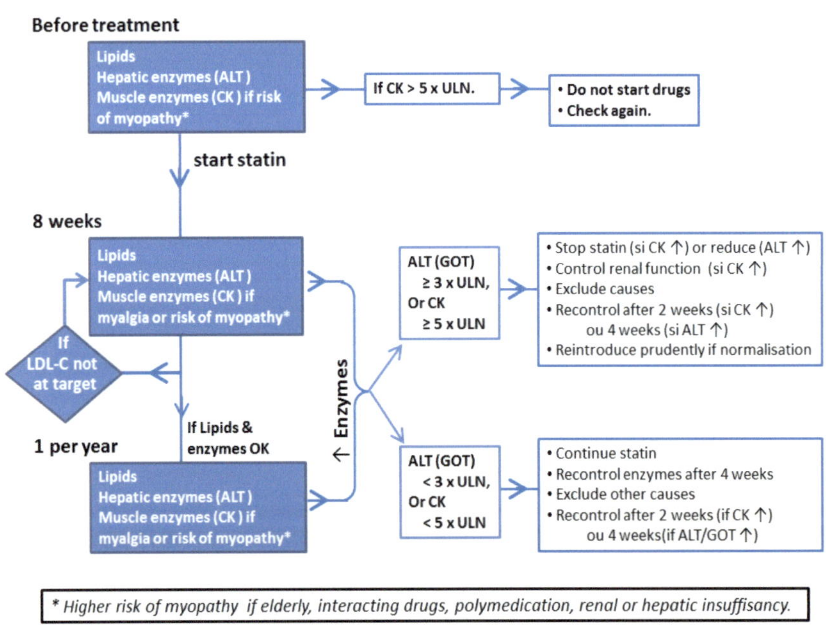

Figure 5. Biological monitoring of liver and muscle enzymes. CK: Creatine kinase. ALT. Alanine aminotransferase (also called SGPT).

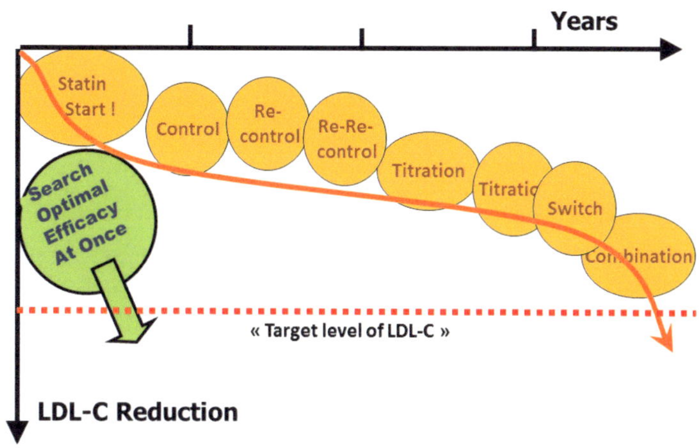

Figure 6. In the intensity of treatment, a rapid escalation is more beneficial than a slow progression.

4.2. Efficacy monitoring

If the target is not achieved and, especially, if the observed reduction is lower than expected, as is the case here (Clinical Case 4), we should first check whether the patient has been compliant. We know that, after one year, approximately half of patients do not correctly take their medication [6]. If the patient has been compliant with her medication, it is possible that the inadequate response is due to a resistance to the statin. This occurs in 10% of patients. If this is the case, we should adapt the treatment.

Clinical Case 4. How do we Follow up the Patient?

Eight weeks after the prescription of 40 mg simvastatin, the patient is not complaining of myalgia. CPK levels have not been controlled and the GOT rates are normal. However, we are slightly disappointed with the lipid profile of the patient, which has become (Table 1):

Total cholesterol: 4.8 mmol/l; LDL-C: 2, 3 mmol/l; HDL-C: 1.1 mmol/l; Triglycerides: 3.1 mmol/l

The treatment appears to be well tolerated but the target has not been reached. Curiously, the reduction has not achieved the expected 40% (but only 28%!).

4.2.1. Why is it important that the target is reached?

In a recent meta-analysis of the results of 118,000 subjects from 26 intervention trials with statins, there was evidence of a relationship between the reduction of LDL-C and the reduction of the incidence of CV disease in 4-5 years. Every decrease of 1 mmol/l for LDL - C by a statin (Figure 4) was associated with a relative reduction in about 20% coronary events, stroke and heart deaths [7]. This relationship was universal (regardless of age, sex and other risk factors). Furthermore, it was almost linear over the range of studied LDL-C levels.

The absolute benefit produced by statins not only depends on their capacity to lower LDL-C but also, on the initial CV risk. Thus, the greater the initial CV risk, the greater the reduction of absolute risk. In such cases, it is crucial to ensure the reduction of LDL-C. For our patient (Clinical Case 4 and Figure 4), we calculated that a reduction ofLDL-C to 1.6 mmol/l (below the target of 1.8 mmol/l), instead of the current reached level of 2.3 mmol/l (Clinical Case 4), should reduce the risk of mortality from 12% to 10% CV. This should also reduce the CV global risk (multiplied by three) from 36% to 30% (Figure 4). This means that if this target was not achieved in 100 patients, six (30-36%) patients would experience a CV event and two patients would die (10%-12%). This highlights the importance of achieving values below the target, even if it sometimes seems difficult.

4.2.2. What to do if the target is not reached?

In our patient's case (Clinical Case 5), we should try to obtain her compliance by reassuring her. If, in spite of this, the target is still not reached, we should adapt the treatment. This can be achieved by increasing the dosage of the statin (doubling each = 6% further LDL reduction) or replacing it with a more powerful statin. Another option is to combine the treatment with Ezetimibe (with an additional reduction of 20-25%) (Figure 3). The latter option is particularly useful when the observed reduction appears lower than expected, despite the patient's compliance with the treatment. Indeed, this suggests that the patient has a resistance to the statins. This usually affects all statins at all doses (the effect of each doubling statin dose does not allow the patient to achieve more than 4% or even 3%).

Clinical Case 5. What do we do if the Target is not Reached?

Due to the disappointing result at the second visit, we ask the patient about her resistance to comply. The patient says that she is scared of the side effects of the medication and thus, she only takes half a pill and tends to forget to take her medication. We answer all of her questions. We put the patient's mind at ease and encourage her to correctly take her medicine. Thus, the patient finally complies. This is confirmed at her third visit. However, at this visit, the patient's LDL-C still remained above 1.8 mmol/l. This means that we should adapt the statin (Table 1).

Eight weeks later (visit 4, Table 1), the lipid profile of the patient becomes (Table 1):

Total cholesterol: 4.0 mmol/l; LDL-C : 1.6 mmol/l; HDL-C : 1.2 mmol/l; Triglycerides: 2.8 mmol/l.

The target of LDL - C (less than 1.8 mmol/l) has now been reached. However, elevated levels of triglycerides and low level of HDL – C still remain! Should we be concerned about them?

4.2.3. Reach the target« ASAP[2] ».

As mentioned above, the benefit of the LDL-C reduction can be seen within the first year treatment. The goal of "as quickly as possible" is all the more important in patients that are considered as high-risk. In a patient such as ours, there is a 15% risk of her dying from CVD in the next 10 years. Furthermore, there is a 45% (almost a "chance" on 2) risk of her having a global (fatal and non-fatal) CV event in the next 10 years. This means that there is a respective 1.5% risk and 4.5% (almost a "chance" on 20) risk of CV mortality and global CV risk per year. Although this may seem like a relatively small number, the delay in the necessary reduction of LDL-C for a year in 100 individuals (like our patient) would result in at least four to five CV events (including one death). However, in our practice, we should take note of the excuses given by the patient or by ourselves (anniversary cake, Christmas or Easter celebration, carnivals, holidays in all-inclusive hotels, etc., are a few days before blood sampling!). Such legions delay treatment adaption and obtaining satisfactory results. Taking this into consideration, it is clear that a more honest escalation in treatment would be more beneficial for the patient (Figure 6).

5. Fourth question: Should we go beyond LDL?

This leads us to three questions: (1) under statin therapy, does the patient still have a residual CV risk? (2) Is it necessary to target HDL-C and triglycerides? (3) Finally, is there scientific evidence that suggests further intervention would be beneficial? To answer these three questions, the guidelines respond affirmatively. Even after the reduction of LDL–C under the correct value target, a residual risk persists (between 60 and 80% of the initial risk). Part of this residual risk is attributed to the persistence of other alterations in a lipid profile.

Thus, if after the LDL-C correction, the patient still displays a high or very high-risk and has combined dyslipidaemia (triglycerides [TG] high > 1.7 mmol/l and HDL cholesterol [HDL - C] too low < 1.2 mmol/l for men or < 1.4 mmol/l for women), she may benefit from further improvement in her lipid profile.

The next question is: at this stage, how should a therapeutic target be set? Should we correct these levels of HDL-C and triglycerides or should we seek another target? In practice, it is often impossible to completely correct TG and HDL-C levels to achieve levels of 1.7 mmol/l for TG or 1.2 mmol/l in men and1.4 mmol/l in women for HDL-C. On the one hand, TG levels vary too much from one day to the next. On the other hand, HDL-C levels are difficult to increase. For example, a baseline HDL-C at 0.8 mmol/l gives a rise of 20%, equivalent to 0.16 mmol/l. This only allows the HDLL-C levels to reach 1 mmol/l - a difference barely perceptible, given the limited accuracy of laboratory measurements. Thus, the new guidelines recommend a more realistic target: the level of **non-HDL cholesterol** (non-HDL-C). This level is measured by a simple calculation:

$$Non-HDL-C \ = \ total\ cholesterol \ - \ HDL-C$$

In fact, as we can understand from the formula of Friedewald, this non-HDL-C is the sum [LDL-C + VLDL cholesterol]. The originality of this parameter is that it integrates all the potentially atherogenic lipoproteins, namely LDL and VLDL. These have a particularly high presence of low HDL-C and high TG (e.g., in the metabolic syndrome) [8].

The conditions and level of non-HDL-C targets are easy to deduct from the target levels of LDL–C. This is because they integrate the target value of LDL-C (< 1.8 or <2.5 mmol/l) plus the ideal value of VLDL-C (< 0.8 mmol/l; 0.8 is obtained by dividing the ideal 1.7 mmol/l level of TG by 2.2, see the Friedewald formula). Consequently, the level of non-HDL-C should be less than 2.5 mmol/l or 3.3 mmol/l as the risk is very high or high, respectively (Clinical Case 6).

Clinical Case 6. Should we go Further in Correcting the Dyslipidaemia?

The presence of high levels of triglycerides and low levels of HDL –C signal the calculation of the level of **cholesterol non-HDL** *and the examination of the patient's residual risk.*

At this stage, the calculated risk SCORE (with a total cholesterol of 4 mmol/l) is still very high. The SCORE is equal to 10.4%, taking into account the SCORE, HDL-C and family history, as well as the other risk factors such as TG, obesity, sedentariness and high hs-CRP (Table 1). Another way to calculate this risk is by considering the initial risk SCORE of 15% and removing the CV risk reduction produced by the LDL - C reduction (Figure 4). This leads to the same result.

Non-HDL cholesterol, which is equal to 2,8 mmol/l (tot chol – HDL-C = 4.0 – 1.2), should certainly be reduced below 2.5 mmol/l (= target for very high-risk). To do so, we can either strengthen the power of the statin or add ezetimibe to further reduce LDL–C. Another option is to add a fibrate or niacin to reduce TG (and LDL for niacin). Although these alternatives result in approximately the same reduction of the non - HDL cholesterol, they lead to different final lipid patterns (Table 1).

	Visit 1	**Visit 2**	**Visit 4**	**Visit 5 (2 alternatives)**	
Time line	0	2 months	6 months	10 months	
Therapeutic target(s)		LDL-C < 1,.8 mmol/l < 70 mg/dl	Second attempt to correct LDL-C	Non HDL-C < 2.5 mmol/l (↓ LDL-C)	Alternative to ↓ non HDL-C < 2,5 mmol/l (↓ VLDL-C)
Current treatment	Baseline	Simva 40 mg	- Better compliance - Atorva 40 mg or rosuva 20 mg	Same as visit 4 + ezetimibe 10 mg	Same as visit 4 +fenofibrate 145 mg
Total cholesterol	5,8 mmol/l (224 mg/dl)	4,8 mmol/l (185 mg/dl)	4,0 mmol/l (156 mg/dl)	3,6 mmol/l (140 mg/dl)	3,7 mmol/l (141 mg/dl)

	Visit 1	Visit 2	Visit 4	Visit 5 (2 alternatives)	
HDL-C	1,0 mmol/l (39 mg/dl)	1,1 mmol/l (42 mg/dl)	1,2 mmol/l (45 mg/dl)	1,2 mmol/l (47 mg/dl)	1,3 mmol/l (49 mg/dl)
Triglycerides	3,5 mmol/l (308 mg/dl)	3,1 mmol/l (271 mg/dl)	2,8 mmol/l (246 mg/dl)	2,6 mmol/l (232 mg/dl)	2,0 mmol/l (172 mg/dl)
LDL-C	3,2 mmol/l (124 mg/dl)	2,3 mmol/l (89 mg/dl)	1,6 mmol/l (62 mg/dl)	1,2 mmol/l (46 mg/dl)	1,5 mmol/l (58 mg/dl)
Non HDL-C	5,8-1,0=4,8 mmol/l (224-39=185 mg/dl)	4,8-1,1=3,7 mmol/l (185-42=143 mg/dl)	4,0-1,2=2,9 mmol/l (156-45=111 mg/dl)	3,6-1,2=2,4 mmol/l (140-47=93 mg/dl)	3,7-1,3=2,4 mmol/l (141-49=92 mg/dl)
LDL reduction (from baseline level)		-0,9 mmol/l (-28%) (- 35 mg/dl)	-1,6 mmol/l (-50%) (- 62 mg/dl)	-2,0 mmol/l (-63%) (- 77 mg/dl)	-1,7 mmol/l (-53%) (- 66 mg/dl)
Relative risk reduction (Absolute risk reduction or ARR)		- 18% (- 2,7%)	- 32% (- 4,8%)	- 40% (- 6,0%)	> - 34%* (>- 5,1%)*
SCORE evolution calculated from the initial SCORE and the subsequent ARR	15,0%	12,3%	10,2%	9,0%	<9,9%
SCORE evolution estimated from SCORE Chart (see Figure 2).	15,9%	12,2%	10,4%	10,4%	8,1%

The relative risk reduction (RRR) is calculated from the CTT regression (every LDL-C reduction of 1 mmol/l LDL-C leads to a 20% CVD risk reduction). * The effect associated with the combination of statin and fibrate is expected to be greater than the effect of the LDL reduction. According to a recent study of diabetes (ACCORD), the addition of fibrate to statin in patients (including non-diabetic patients) with high TG and low HDL-C brings an additional 30% reduction in the risk of CVD. In our SCORE calculation, the smaller risk (8-9%) is due to the increase in HDL-C (the multiplier is 0.6 instead of 0.7) and the suppression of TG amongst the "other risk factors" (only obesity, sedentariness and hs-CRP remain, therefore, the multiplier for the other risk factor is 1.1 x 1.1 x 1.1 = 1.3 instead of 1.5). Simva: simvastatin; rosuva: rosuvastatin; atorva: atorvastatin.

Table 1. The evolution of the lipid profiles and CV risk in relation to our patient's increased treatment.

The reduction in the level of non-HDL-C should be achieved by an additional lowering of the LDL-C level. There are a number of ways to do this, including the prescription of a higher statin dosage, a stronger statin, a combination with ezetimibe (if intolerant) or by lowering the level of TG (and therefore, VLDL-C) via the association of the statin with fibrate or niacin (Clinical Case 6).

6. Conclusions

The new recommendations offer a practical approach. They are more precise in supporting the lipid profile of CV prevention. The four levels of risk and the possible adjustment of the new targets (non-HDL-C or apoB) next to the traditional targets of the LDL–C and HDL-C rate will allow better prescriptions of appropriate therapeutic drugs.

The present case illustrates step by step (visit by visit) the rationale for escalating treatment in order to achieve the best cardiovascular prevention. We hope that such an example can help give a better understanding of the EAS/ESC guidelines. The rigorous mathematical reasoning is, of course, only displayed here to better quantify the benefit of the various therapeutic choices. It is unlikely that it would be used in clinical practice. It is important to note that the practical implementation of guidelines requires the intuitive clinical skill of the practitioner, as well as open discussions with the patient. We would also like to highlight that, if the correction of the lipid profile is accepted as the cornerstone of CV prevention, the importance of lifestyle change (smoking, diet and physical activity) and the need to correct other risk factors should not be forgotten.

Author details

Olivier S. Descamps [1*], Lale Tokgozoglu[2] and Eric Bruckert[3]

*Address all correspondence to: olivierdescamps@hotmail.com

1 Département de Médecine Interne, Centre de Recherche Médicale de Jolimont, Hôpital de Jolimont, Haine Saint-Paul, Belgium

2 Cardiology, Hacettepe University, Ankara, Turkey

3 Service d'endocrinologie-métabolisme, Hôpital de La Pitié Salpêtrière, Paris, France

References

[1] Graham I, Atar D, Borch-Johnsen K, Boysen G, Burell G, Cifkova R et al. 'European Guidelines on Cardiovascular Disease Prevention in Clinical Practice. Fourth Joint Task Force of the European Society on Cardiovascular Disease Prevention in Clinical Practice'. Eur J CardiovascPrevRehabil 2007; 14 (Suppl 2): S1-S112.

[2] www.escardio.org/guidelines.

[3] Cooney MT, Dudina A, De Bacquer D, Fitzgerald A et al. 'How Much Does HDL Cholesterol Add to Risk Estimation? A report from the SCORE Investigators'. Eur J Cardiovasc Prev Rehabil 2009; 16: 304-314.

[4] Descamps OS, et al. 'A Simple Multiplier to Calculate the Impact of HDL Cholesterol on Cardiovascular Risk Estimation Using SCORE'. Atherosclerosis (2012), http://dx.doi.org/10.1016/j.atherosclerosis.2012.03.035.

[5] Weng TC, Yang YH, Lin SJ, Tai SH. 'A Systematic Review and Meta-analysis on the Therapeutic Equivalence of Statins'.J Clin Pharm Ther. 2010;35(2):139-51.

[6] Choudhry NK, Avorn J, Glynn RJ, Antman EM, Schneeweiss S, Toscano M, Reisman L, Fernandes J, Spettell C, Lee JL, Levin R, Brennan T, Shrank WH.'Post-Myocardial Infarction Free Rx Event and Economic Evaluation (MI FREEE) Trial. Full Coverage for Preventive Medications after Myocardial Infarction'. N Engl J Med. 2011;365:2088-97. Epub 2011 Nov 14.

[7] Nicholls SJ, Brandrup-Wognsen G, Palmer M, Barter PJ. 'Meta-analysis of Comparative Efficacy of Increasing Dose of Atorvastatin Versus RosuvastatinVersus Simvastatin on Lowering Levels of AtherogenicLipids (from VOYAGER). Am J Cardiol 2010; 105: 69-76.

[8] Chapman MJ, Ginsberg HN, Amarenco P, Andreotti F, Borén J, Catapano AL, Descamps OS, Fisher E, Kovanen PT, Kuivenhoven JA, Lesnik P, Masana L, Nordestgaard BG, Ray KK, Reiner Z, Taskinen MR, Tokgözoglu L, Tybjærg-Hansen A, Watts GF.'European Atherosclerosis Society Consensus Panel. Triglyceride-rich Lipoproteins and High-Density Lipoprotein Cholesterol in Patients at High Risk of Cardiovascular Disease: Evidence and Guidance for Management. Eur Heart J. 2011 Jun; 32(11):1345-61.

Chapter 5

Hypercholesterolemia Effect on Potassium Channels

Anna N. Bukiya and Avia Rosenhouse-Dantsker

Additional information is available at the end of the chapter

http://dx.doi.org/10.5772/59761

1. Introduction

Cholesterol is a major lipid component of the plasma membrane in mammalian cells constituting up to 45 mol % with respect to other lipids [1, 2]. Yet, even a limited increase in blood and/or tissue cholesterol of up to 2-3 fold above the physiological level is cytotoxic [1-3] and is associated with the development of cardiovascular disease [4-6]. The underlying source for the effect of cholesterol on cellular functions is its ability to alter the function of multiple membrane proteins including ion channels (see, for example, reviews [7-9]).

In recent years, high cholesterol diet has been shown to affect the function of multiple ion channels. In this chapter we focus on the effect of dietary-induced increase in blood and tissue cholesterol levels on potassium channels. Potassium channels are among the largest and most complex types of ion channels. They are widely expressed in human tissues and are involved in many aspects of cell function including membrane excitability, regulation of heart rate, neuronal signaling, vascular tone, insulin release and salt flow across epithelia (see, for example, reviews [10-17]). In addition, they also play a critical role in the protection of neurons and muscle under metabolic stress. As a result, mutations in potassium channels lead to a wide range of disease in the brain (epilepsy, episodic ataxia), ear (deafness), heart (arrhythmia), muscle (myokymia, periodic paralysis), kidney (hypertension), pancreas (hyperinsulinemic hypoglycemia, neonatal diabetes). Therefore, the effect of hypercholesterolemia on potassium channel function has important pathophysiological implications.

The most common effect of a high-cholesterol diet on ion channels in general and potassium channels in particular is a decrease in channel activity. Yet, the activity of some channels is increased following a high cholesterol diet. For example, hypercholesterolemia suppressed the function of the Kir2 subfamily of inwardly rectifying potassium (Kir) channels in different cell types by ~2 fold [18-19]. However, atrial G-protein gated inwardly rectifying potassium channels (GIRK or Kir3) that underlie K_{ACh} currents in the heart are enhanced by a high-cholesterol diet [19]. Several types of voltage gated (Kv) channels were sensitive to changes in the level of cellular membrane and dietary cholesterol [20-26]. The majority of the reports described suppression of channel function by high-cholesterol diet. Moreover, large conductance calcium-activated potassium (BK) channels were often suppressed following a high-cholesterol diet [27-31].

In this chapter, we will describe the implications of high-cholesterol dietary intake on members of three major families of potassium channels: voltage gated potassium (K_v) channels, calcium-activated potassium (K_{Ca}) channels of large conductance (BK) and inwardly rectifying potassium (Kir) channels. We will demonstrate that not only does high-cholesterol diet increase the levels of blood cholesterol but it also increases the level of cholesterol in tissues in which these types of channels are expressed. We will show that this cholesterol accumulation *in-vivo* is reflected in the function of potassium channels. Lastly, we will discuss the importance of the observed effects to organ function.

2. High-cholesterol diet model

Cholesterol-rich diet that is characteristic of Western societies critically controls blood lipid levels in several species, including humans [32-33]. Regression models have been reported for serum total cholesterol, triacylglycerol, and low-density-, high-density-, and very-low-density-lipoprotein cholesterol. In particular, correlations between increased levels of dietary cholesterol and these plasma lipids and lipoproteins were found to be 0.74, 0.65, 0.41, 0.14, and 0.34, respectively [32]. It has been predicted that compliance with the dietary recommendation to consume <300 mg cholesterol per day (with 30% of energy from fat, < 10% from saturated fat) will reduce plasma total and low-density-lipoprotein-cholesterol (LDL) concentrations by approximately 5% compared with amounts associated with the average American diet [32]. Restriction of dietary cholesterol intake represents a widely used preventative measure against numerous pathological conditions since increased total cholesterol and LDL levels are well-recognized risk factors for several largely prevalent pathologies, including stroke [34-37], coronary heart disease [38-39], vascular dementia [40], and atherosclerosis [41]. Therefore, it is not surprising that a cholesterol-rich diet has been recreated in a research laboratory setting to study the deleterious effects of cholesterol-rich food intake.

High-cholesterol diet-induced hypercholesterolemia is widely used for studies on monkeys [42], hamsters [43], guinea pigs [44], rabbits [20, 27, 29, 45, 46], rats [19, 47-49] and mice [50]. The dietary-induced hypercholesterolemia model has several advantages. First, it mimics the high-cholesterol food intake that is characteristic to the US population, and which impacts cholesterol levels in the blood of human individuals [32-33]. Second, it does not require alteration of the genetic background of the animal. These advantages make high-cholesterol diet a useful tool to manipulate cholesterol levels in species in which genetic alterations to achieve hypercholesterolemia are challenging. For example, diet-induced changes in blood cholesterol level have been detected in primates besides humans, such as baboons *Papiospp* (reviewed by [51]) and Japanese monkeys *Macacafuscata* [42].

It should be noted that earlier studies have documented the existence of "hyper-" and "hyporesponders" to a cholesterol-rich diet in the human population. Trials with the same subjects demonstrated that the human population includes people with a consistently low or high response to increased dietary intake of cholesterol (reviewed by [52]). Similarly to humans, other primates also vary in their blood lipid responses to dietary lipid composition. Selective breeding of primates based on their individual responses to the composition of the diet resulted in lines that are characterized by low versus high responses to changes in dietary lipids. Thus, similarly to humans, changes in lipoprotein patterns in response to dietary cholesterol seem to be heritable in primates (reviewed by [51]). Further studies have shown that the differential response to cholesterol consumption in smaller laboratory animals also results in inbred strains of rabbits, rats, and mice that differ in their sensitivity to high-cholesterol diet. Their responsiveness to high-cholesterol diet is largely influenced by the genetic background [52]. Compared to humans, changes in blood cholesterol and LDL levels induced by high-cholesterol diet in lab animals are robust and of high magnitude. Therefore, a high-cholesterol diet represents a useful and practical tool to induce an increase in blood cholesterol levels that ultimately leads to hypercholesterolemia in animal models.

In a typical protocol for a high-cholesterol diet in animal models, the animal would be fed (*ad libitum* of via gavage) cholesterol-rich food. The ability of a high-cholesterol diet to increase blood cholesterol and LDL levels is well documented in various animal models. For instance, consumption of food containing 2% cholesterol for 20 months leads to up to a 2-fold increase in total cholesterol and LDL levels in the blood of a macaque [42]. An even more drastic increase was documented multiple times in rabbits: feeding animals with dietary cholesterol supplementation in the amount of 1 g per day for 4 weeks resulted in ~20-fold increase in total serum cholesterol concentration in rabbits [29], 1% cholesterol food for 8 weeks resulted in a nearly 30-fold increase in total serum cholesterol level [20], and 0.5% cholesterol for 12 weeks raised blood cholesterol level by nearly 33-fold [45]. Another study reported a 10-fold increase in plasma cholesterol concentration in rabbits fed by 0.5% cholesterol food for 16 weeks [27]. Mice and rats usually respond with a lower magnitude of increase in blood cholesterol and LDL levels in response to diet, yet these changes are still easily detected. In mice, consumption of 1, 000 mg/kg cholesterol per day for 8 weeks increased blood cholesterol and LDL levels by 2-3 times [50]. Significant increase in blood cholesterol and LDL levels have been documented following feeding with 4% cholesterol food for 4 weeks in Sprague-Dawley rats [48], 2% cholesterol diet for 20-24 weeks in the same strain [19], and 5% cholesterol diet for 3 weeks led to a significant increase in the plasma cholesterol level in Wistar rats [47].

In our rat model of a high-cholesterol diet, male Sprague-Dawley rats (50 g) were subjected to an *ab libitum* high-cholesterol diet (2% cholesterol). The total cholesterol plasma level remained unchanged for 11-12 weeks of diet, but significantly increased during weeks 18-23 and was increased even further during weeks 27-28 of the high-cholesterol diet compared to the control group (Figure 1A). After receiving a high-cholesterol diet for 11-12 weeks, the rats displayed a significant increase in the LDL plasma level, with the increase becoming more pronounced during weeks 18-23 on a high-cholesterol diet and reaching a nearly 5-fold increase during weeks 27-28 on a high-cholesterol diet when compared to the control group (Figure 1B). High-density-lipoproteins (HDL), however, seemed to be less sensitive to high-cholesterol diet intake, as HDL level increased significantly only during weeks 27-28 on a high-cholesterol diet (Figure 1C). Triglycerides followed the pattern of response of cholesterol and LDL: triglyceride level increased significantly during weeks 18-23 and became even higher during weeks 27-28 of the high-cholesterol diet (Figure 1D). Overall, changes in the blood lipid profile correlated with the duration of the high-cholesterol diet. Therefore, a high-cholesterol diet constitutes a valuable tool when the degree of change in the blood lipid profile needs to be controlled tightly.

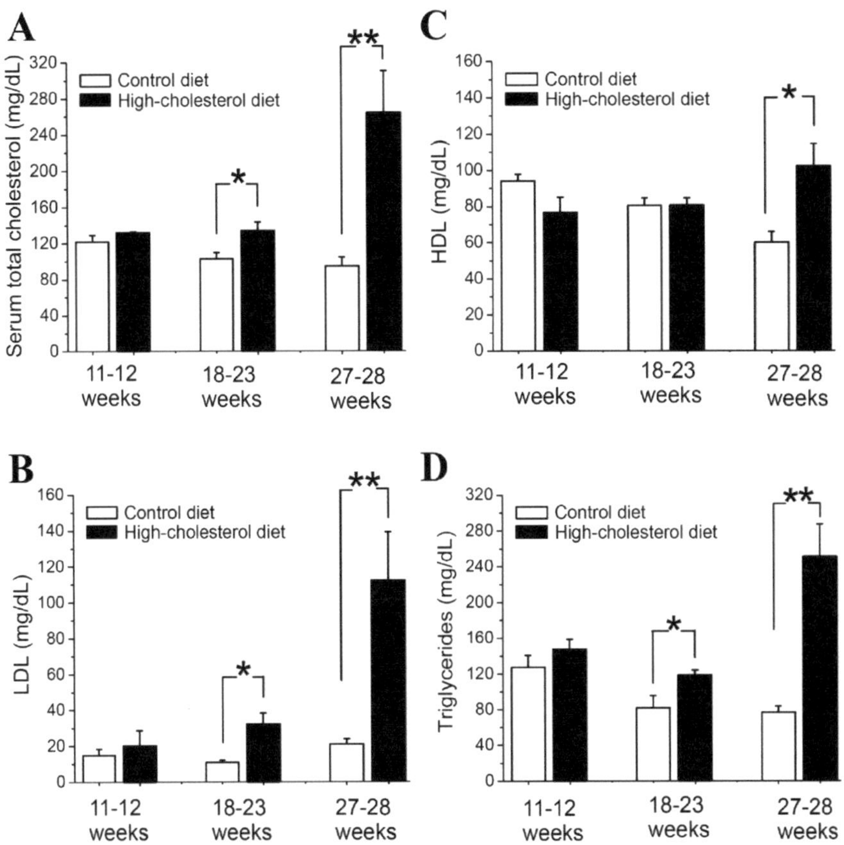

Figure 1. Blood lipid profile in Sprague-Dawley rats fed high-cholesterol diet. (A) Serum total cholesterol. (B) Low-density-lipoprotein-cholesterol. (C) High-density-lipoprotein. (D) Triglycerides. Here and in all figures: significantly different from control is indicated by an asterisk (*, $p<0.05$; **, $p<0.01$).

3. Effect of high-cholesterol diet on potassium channels.

In view of the advantages of a high cholesterol diet described above and its ability to adequately represent the characteristics of high cholesterol food intake in the US, it is widely used for studies on ion channel function during dyslipidemia and hypercholesterolemia. For instance, dietary-induced hypercholesterolemia was shown to up-regulate the function of L-type Ca^{2+}-channels in detrusor smooth muscle [48], transient receptor potential channels 5 and 6 (TRPC5 and TRPC6) in aortic endothelial cells [53], cardiac G protein gated inwardly rectifying potassium channels [19], and epithelial Na^{+} channels (eNaC) [54].

In this chapter, we will focus on high-cholesterol diet-driven changes in the function of potassium channels. In particular, we will discuss the effect of an increase in the dietary intake of cholesterol on voltage gated (Kv) channels, calcium activated potassium channels (K_{Ca}) and inwardly rectifying potassium channels (Kir).

Voltage-gated potassium (K_V) channels. Several reports describing the effect of a high-cholesterol diet on potassium channel function came from studies on voltage-gated potassium channels (K_V) [21]. These channels are transmembrane proteins that are located on the plasma membrane and sensitive to changes in the transmembrane potential [55]. Upon membrane depolarization, voltage-gated potassium channels conduct outward potassium currents as these channels exhibit the highest selectivity for K^{+} ions compared to other monovalent cations. Activation of K_V channels usually results in decreased depolarization and the return of the plasma membrane potential to the resting level. Vertebrate K_V channels are tetramers of four pore-forming subunits, each contributing to the wall of the K^{+} conducting pore. Each pore-forming subunit is composed of six transmembrane α-helices with intracellular N- and C-termini (Figure 2A). Helices S1-S4 contribute to voltage-sensing and S5-S6 form the pore region. Voltage-gated potassium channels play a key role in cellular excitability including vascular smooth muscle [55]. The effect of a high-cholesterol diet on K_V channel function has been extensively studied in the cardiovascular system.

High-cholesterol diet failed to modulate K_V channel function after a brief placement of an Ossabaw miniature swine model on a high-fat/high-cholesterol/high-fructose diet [26]. The animals were fed by the diet for 9 weeks. The authors considered the duration of diet administration to be relatively short. As a result, only an early stage of a complex metabolic syndrome developed. The diet caused ~4-fold increase in blood cholesterol level in the group on diet compared to the control group on standard chow. Coronary arterioles from both groups were isolated and pressurized to 60 cmH_2O for *in-vitro* pharmacological studies. Those include the assessment of the K_V channel contribution to the arteriolar response to the vasodilator 2-chloroadenosine. Pharmacological blockade of K_V channels by 4-aminopyridine reduced the arteriolar sensitivity to 2-chloroadenosine in both control and early stage metabolic syndrome groups. This result suggests that Kv channel regulation of the arteriolar diameter was still preserved at the early stage of the modeled metabolic syndrome. In contrast, blockade of Kir6 (K_{ATP}) channels (see below) with glibenclamide reduced the arteriolar sensitivity to 2-chloroadenosine in the control group only. Therefore, the involvement of K_V channels in the arteriolar responses to 2-chloroadenosine is resistant to the described diet.

A more complex scenario was observed in work by Heaps *et al* on a Yucatan miniature swine model that was placed on high-fat/high-cholesterol diet for 20 weeks [22-23]. Already after 4 weeks, blood cholesterol and LDL levels were increased on the average by 6 times when compared to the pre-diet and to the group on control diet levels. At the end of a 20 week-long

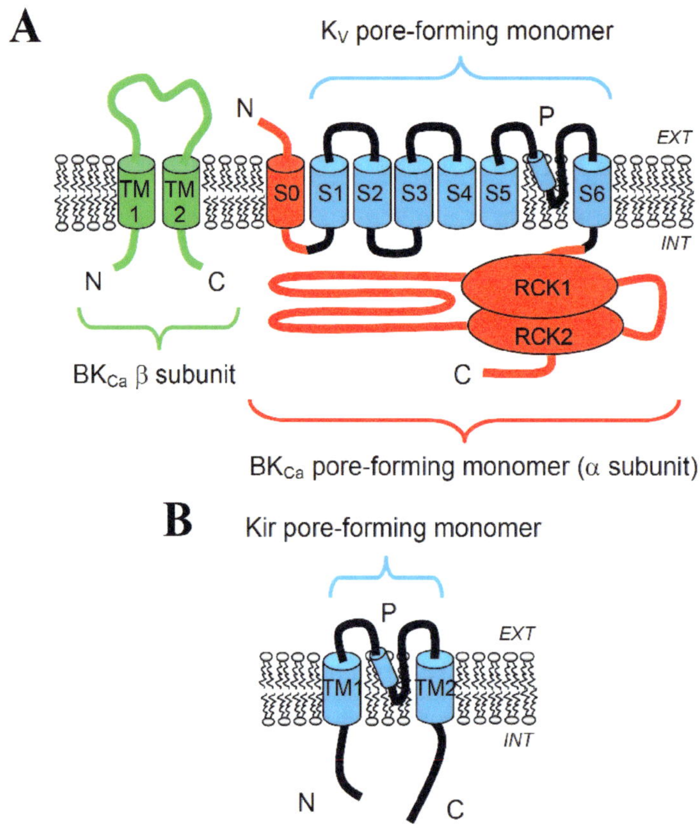

Figure 2. Schematic structures of K_v, K_{Ca}, and Kir channels. (A) Schematic structure of voltage-gated and voltage-/calcium gated potassium channel subunits. TM: transmembrane domain of b subunit; S: transmembrane domain of a subunit; RCK: regulator of conductance of potassium; EXT: extracellular media; INT: intracellular media. (B) Schematic structure of inwardly rectifying potassium channel subunit. TM1 is the outer transmembrane helix and TM2 is the inner transmembrane helix.

diet, *coronary vascular reactivity* was assessed. Coronary microvessels were removed, cannulated, pressurized at 40 mmHg and the luminal diameter was monitored. In this experimental setting, 4-aminopyridine attenuated adenosine-induced dilation of coronary arterioles in the control group, but did not affect adenosine-induced arteriole dilation in the group subjected to high-fat/high-cholesterol diet. Therefore, adenosine activation of K_V channels is attenuated during hypercholesterolemia. In contrast, Bender *et al* did not detect diet-induced changes in K_V channel contribution to the 2-chloroadenosine-induced dilation of swine coronary arterioles [26]. This controversy may be attributed to several differences between the two studies. For instance, in the study by Bender et al., animals were subjected to a high-fructose diet in addition to high-fat/high-cholesterol food. Second, Bender *et al* were studying the consequences of brief (only 9 weeks) dieting as opposed to Heaps *et al* who placed the animals on a 20 weeks diet. It is therefore likely that a longer duration of diet is needed for K_V channels to lose their sensitivity to adenosine application. Loss of K_V channel contribution to adenosine-mediated vasodilation was studied further at the level of coronary arteriole smooth muscle K_V currents. Outward K^+ currents were recorded in whole-cell configuration from freshly isolated arteriole myocytes. Noteworthy, the intracellular calcium was chelated to eliminate the calcium-dependent component from the whole-cell K^+ currents. K_V currents from myocytes in the high-cholesterol diet group were significantly smaller compared to the control [22-23]. Therefore, reduction in K^+ currents may underlie the attenuation of the K_V component in adenosine-induced arteriole dilations. Treatment of membrane patches with different concentrations of the non-selective potassium channel blocker tetraethylammonium (TEA) revealed that high-cholesterol diet primarily altered K_V channel isoforms with high sensitivity to TEA. RT-PCR experiments determined that $K_V3.1$ and $K_V3.3$ channel isoforms were expressed in coronary arterioles. However, expression levels of $K_V3.1$ and $K_V3.3$ were not changed by the diet. In contrast, it was shown that arteriole dilation caused by the receptor-independent activator of adenylyl cyclaseforscolin was abolished in the high-fat/high-cholesterol diet group. Furthermore, the K_V channel blocker 4-aminopyridine and the non-selective blocker of potassium channels TEA significantly attenuated forscolin-mediated vasodilation in control, but not in the high-fat/high-cholesterol diet group. Taken together, these data suggest that hypercholesterolemia-mediated ablation of adenosine-induced vasodilation of coronary arterioles could be attributed to the impairment of the adenylyl cyclase pathway coupled to highly TEA-sensitive K_V channel isoforms.

These data showing a reduced K_V component in the whole-cell outward potassium current are consistent with another report that focused on potassium currents in swine coronary artery smooth muscle cells [25]. The animals were placed on a high-fat diet for 20 weeks. The diet significantly increased the total blood serum cholesterol level and triglycerides. Remarkably, the increase in both blood lipid components was higher in female swines. 4-aminopyridin-sensitive component of the whole-cell outward potassium current recorded from the isolated coronary artery smooth muscle cells was significantly diminished in the high-cholesterol diet group of male swines. In females, however, no significant reduction in K_V 4-aminopyridine-sensitive (K_V component) was detected [25]. This report suggests that the effect of high-cholesterol diet on the function of K_V channels may be gender-specific.

Loss of K_V channel current and its contribution to vasodilatory responses has not only been documented in coronary arteries, but also in the *middle cerebral artery*. In the latter work, New Zealand rabbits were placed on chow supplemented with 1% cholesterol for 8 weeks [20]. The total blood serum cholesterol increased close to 30 times at the end of the diet. In the vasodilatory response study, the middle cerebral arteries were dissected, mounted and pre-contracted with a high-K^+ (50 mM) physiologic saline solution. In the pre-contracted arteries isolated from control animals, acetylcholine produced artery relaxation. In the arteries from the high-cholesterol diet group, similar concentrations of acetylcholine induced less relaxation. In the control group, neither TBA, an inhibitor of K_{Ca} channels, nor glibenclamide, an inhibitor of K_{ATP} channels, significantly affected the concentration-response to acetylcholine, whereas 4-aminopyridine, a blocker of K_V channels, strongly inhibited this relaxation. In the high-cholesterol diet group, TBA, glibenclamide or 4-aminopyridine did not significantly affect the response to acetylcholine [20]. Loss of 4-aminopyridine effect on acetylcholine-induced cerebral artery dilation suggests that either the function of K_V channels or their sensitivity to acetylcholine-activated pathway is diminished.

Apart from the vascular system, the effect of a high-cholesterol diet on K_V channels was studied in the *heart* itself [24]. Rabbits were subjected to a high-cholesterol diet (1.5% cholesterol) for 8 weeks. The diet resulted in an approximately 14 times increase in blood serum cholesterol level. RT-PCR studies were used to determine the impact of the high-cholesterol diet on the left ventricular mRNA expression level of several potassium channels that play a key role in the contractility of the heart. High-cholesterol diet significantly decreased the expression of $K_V4.2$, but did not alter the level of $K_V4.3$. Notably, a significant decrease and a significant increase in mRNA levels were detected for $K_V11.1$ (ERG1) and $K_V7.1$ (K_{VLQT1}) channels, respectively [24]. These data document that that a high-cholesterol diet differentially affects the expression of voltage-gated potassium channels, with decrease, increase and "no-effect" being detected for this group of channels. The authors suggested that the arrhythmogenic nature of the hypercholesterolemia may be mediated by changed expression levels of the examined channels.

Calcium-activated potassium (K_{Ca}) channels. The effect of a high-cholesterol diet on calcium-sensitive potassium channels (K_{Ca}) is well described for calcium- and voltage-gated potassium channels of large conductance (BK). Fully functional BK channels result from the tetrameric association of 125-140 kDa polypeptides termed α, slo or slo1 subunits. Slo1 subunits share significant homology with K_V channels of the six transmembrane domain (TM6) family, with the S1-S4 regions contributing to voltage-sensing and the S5-S6 helices forming the activation gate-pore region (Figure 2A) [12, 56-57]. Unlike purely voltage-gated K_V channels, in addition to the S1-S6 core, BK slo1 subunits contain an additional transmembrane helix S0 leading to an extracellular N-terminus [58] and a large cytosolic tail domain (CTD) [59-61]. The CTD includes two domains that Regulate the Conductance of K^+ (RCK). RCKs contain sites for sensing intracellular Ca^{2+} levels and allow BK channels to increase channel activity in response to an increase in intracellular Ca^{2+} physiological levels [59-60]. In most tissues, BK channels usually result from the association of slo1 proteins with auxiliary β subunits. Four types of BK β subunits, β1-4, have been identified. BK β subunits share an overall topology of two TM segments joined by a large extracellular loop, plus two short intracellular N and C termini [62]. Expression of β subunits is tissue-specific, with the β1 subunit being prevalent in smooth muscle, including vasculature [62-63]. The functional role of BK channels is similar to K_V channels: upon membrane depolarization BK channels generate outward potassium currents to oppose depolarization and favor the return of the transmembrane voltage to its resting level.

Several animal models have been used to document that plasmalemma BK channels are sensitive to dietary-induced hypercholesterolemia [64]. Considering the ample evidence linking hypercholesterolemia to cardiovascular disease, and the key role of BK channels in regulating vascular tone [65], most of the studies describe the effect of a high-cholesterol diet on BK channel function in the vascular system. One of the early studies addressed changes in endothelium-dependent and independent components *in-vitro* relaxation of carotid artery rings obtained from rabbits following administration of a 12 week-long high-cholesterol diet (0.5% cholesterol). Evaluation of isometric tension in carotid artery rings was performed in the presence of nitric oxide (NO), sodium nitroprusside and 8-bromoguanosine 3′, 5′-cyclic monophosphate (8-Brc-GMP). The responses to all three chemicals remained unaltered by dietary-induced hypercholesterolemia [45]. After application of a BK channel blocker, NO-mediated artery relaxation was significantly reduced in the hypercholesterolemic group. These findings could imply that BK channel contribution to the regulation of arterial tension during hypercholesterolemia is enhanced. It has been repeatedly suggested that dietary-induced hypercholesterolemia may lead to a compensatory increase in BK channel activity [45, 66]. Considering that smooth muscle BK channels are critical regulators of the arterial diameter, the compensatory increase in BK channel function during the course of high-cholesterol diet could take place in the arterial smooth muscle [45, 66]. Alternatively, BK channel activity could be reduced by hypercholesterolemia, in which case BK channels would be more available for activation [64], and would contribute more to an NO-induced decrease in vascular tension. However, the latter scenario is unlikely as an increase in vascular smooth muscle BK channel activity has been reported in cell-attached recordings from the area affected by the athero-sclerotic plaque formation [67]. This difference is lost when BK channel function is evaluated in cell-free patches excised from the cells [67]. Thus, increased smooth muscle BK channel activity associated with atherosclerotic plaque likely requires the involvement of the intracel-lular organelles and/or freely diffusible cytosolic signals.

Hypercholesterolemia-driven increase in arterial K_{Ca} channel function compared to control chow was also reported in diabetic pigs receiving high-fat/high-cholesterol (2%) diet [21]. Patch-clamp recording of whole-cell outward potassium currents revealed increased density of the K_{Ca}-component in the high-cholesterol diet group. Western blot failed to detect a significant increase in the amount of the K_{Ca} pore-forming protein. In addition, intracellular calcium concentration did not differ in control versus high-cholesterol diet groups. The data indicated that diabetic hypercholesterolemia leads to an increased functional coupling between K_{Ca} and intracellular calcium release.

In contrast to the above *in-vitro* studies, *in-vivo* work conducted on hypercholesterolemic rabbits showed a reduction in NO-induced vasodilation as determined by monitoring the hindlimb vascular conductance in response to acetylcholine and bradykinin [27]. In this set of experiments, rabbits were fed high-cholesterol (0.5% cholesterol) diet for 16 weeks. The NO-independent vasodilation in response to acetylcholine and bradykinin, however, was larger in animals on high-cholesterol diet. Development of this NO-independent component of vasodilation was blocked by either TEA or by a mixture of the K_{Ca} channel blocker charybdo-toxin and the small conductance K_{Ca} channels blocker apamin. Thus, the authors concluded that hypercholesterolemia impaired K_{Ca} channel-mediated vasodilation [27].

Another study using hypercholesterolemic rabbits to test acetylcholine-induced vasorelaxa-tion focused on renal artery. Rabbits were subjected to a high-cholesterol diet (0.5% cholesterol) for 5 weeks. This diet resulted in an over 50 fold increase in the total blood cholesterol and an almost 40-fold increase in LDL-cholesterol [28]. Contrary to the findings in the hindlimb circulation, acetylcholine-induced dilation of phenylephrine pre-constricted renal arteries was not changed by the high-cholesterol diet. However, the NO-independent (N(G)-nitro-l-arginine-resistant) component of this relaxation was significantly enhanced in arteries from hypercholesterolemic animals. This component totally vanished after endothelial removal in both control and hypercholesterolemic groups, yet was only reduced significantly in the hypercholesterolemic group when an artery with endothelium was incubated in BK and the intermediate conductance K_{Ca} channel blocker charybdotoxin [28].

Studies on rat cerebral arteries yielded results that are in agreement with the conclusions obtained in the hindlimb of rabbits. Specifically, rat middle cerebral arteries obtained from a Sprague-Dawley strain on control versus high-cholesterol (2% cholesterol supplement for either 10 or 18-23 weeks) were dissected, de-endothelialized, cannulated and pressurized at 60 mm Hg. A blood lipid profile revealed a significant increase in the total serum cholesterol, LDL, and triglyceride levels only at 18-23 weeks of diet (Figure 1). The arterial responses to a depolarizing solution containing 60 mM KCl were similar in control and in all hypercholesterolemic arteries. However, treatment of arteries from either one of the high-cholesterol diet groups with the selective BK channel blocker paxilline resulted in vasoconstriction that was significantly smaller compare to the control group (Figure 3A). BK channel function seemed to be altered rather selectively: arterial diameter responses to the K_V channel blocker 4-aminopyridine were similar in control versus hypercholesterolemic animals (Figure 3A). First, these results demonstrated that the general contractile capability of the artery (as tested by a high KCl-containing solution) was largely preserved during the high-cholesterol diet. Second, endothelium-independent vasodilation that is mediated by the activity of smooth muscle BK channels was diminished during hypercholesterolemia [30, 31]. Moreover, the fact that reduced sensitivity to paxilline was observed after 10 weeks on a high-cholesterol diet, well before the changes in the blood lipid profile took effect (Figure 1) suggested that BK channels were highly sensitive to dietary cholesterol levels, independent of the increase in blood cholesterol.

Further experimentation took place in an effort to unveil molecular mechanisms that enable the sensitivity of BK channels to dietary cholesterol. First, it was shown that cholesterol accumulation in the wall of de-endothelialized cerebral arteries of hypercholesterolemic rats followed the pattern of increase in blood cholesterol level. In particular, the cholesterol level in cerebral artery tissue was only increased significantly during weeks 18-23 on diet, but not earlier (Figure 3B) [31]. Therefore, the direct accumulation of cholesterol in the vicinity of the BK channel might not be the sole reason for depressed BK channel sensitivity to paxilline during a high-cholesterol intake. The reduction in paxilline-induced cerebral artery constriction by hypercholesterolemia might result from a decreased number of BK channels in arterial smooth muscle. In particular, hypercholesterolemia may down-regulate accessory, smooth muscle-type β subunit (β1) (Figure 2A). Indeed, cerebral arteries of β1 (*KCNMB1)* knock-out mice were reported to be insensitive to selective BK channel block by the peptide blocker iberiotoxin [68]. Moreover, hypercholesterolemia-induced changes in BK β1 subunit level have been studied in circular smooth muscle strips from the sphincter of Oddi in rabbits fed by high-cholesterol food (1 g cholesterol per day) for 4 weeks [29]. Immunohistochemical and Western blot protein analysis using a BK β1 subunit-specific polyclonal antibody showed a decreased level of the BK β1 protein in the cholesterol-fed group. Thus, in the sphincter of Oddi high-cholesterol diet down-regulated BK β1 subunits [29]. However, in rat cerebral artery myocytes high-cholesterol diet did not down-regulate, but actually significantly increased the fluorescent signal associated with selective labeling of BK β1 subunits (Figure 3C, left panel). Since β1 subunits themselves do not form functional channels, diminished responses of the artery to paxilline may be indicative of the reduction in the amount of the BK pore-forming (α) subunit protein. However, no significant differences between the BK α subunit-associated fluorescence signal in cerebral artery myocytes from rats on control versus high-cholesterol diet were detected (Figure 3C, right panel). Therefore, ablated paxilline-induced cerebral artery constriction observed in pressurized cerebral arteries from hypercholesterolemic rats could not be attributed to down-regulation of BK protein surface presence on myocyte membranes. Alternatively, ablated paxilline-induced cerebral artery constriction may arise from diminished functional properties of the BK channel itself. These may include but are not limited to the coupling (both, physical association and functional communication) between the BK pore-forming α subunit and the accessory β1 subunits, changes in the gating pattern of the channel making the protein less responsive to paxilline binding. Alternatively, reduction in paxilline-induced cerebral artery constriction may not be a reflection of decreased BK channel function but rather be explained by changes in the affinity of the channel to paxilline. The latter possibility needs to be further studied as several BK channel blockers other than paxilline block BK channel with different efficacy depending on the presence of the accessory β1 and β4 subunits [69]. Theoretically, an increased amount of the BK β1 protein by high-cholesterol diet may preclude paxilline from reaching its site in the BK α subunit and therefore, may result in a decreased paxilline effect. The most unequivocal evidence of the effect of a high-cholesterol diet on BK channel function must come from direct electrophysiological evaluation of BK voltage- and calcium-dependent gating following a high-cholesterol diet. The intrinsic mechanism(s) that underlie(s) alteration in BK channel function during a high-cholesterol diet is currently under investigation.

Remarkably, dietary cholesterol does not only alter the paxilline-sensitivity of the channel but also protects against ethanol-induced BK channel-mediated constriction of cerebral arteries. It was shown that BK channels represent a major target for ethanol in the cerebral vessels. Upon ethanol application, BK channel function is diminished, and cerebral artery constriction is observed [70]. The protective role of a high-cholesterol diet against alcohol-induced constriction of cerebral arteries was demonstrated *in-vivo* using a closed cranial window on anesthetized rats receiving conventional chow versus high-cholesterol (2% cholesterol) diet for 18-23 weeks [31]. Control or ethanol-containing solutions were infused into the cerebral circulation via a catheter in the carotid artery of the rat, and the diameter of the pial arterioles was determined. Infusion of 50 mM ethanol (e.g. the amount of ethanol detected in the blood during moderate-to-heavy alcohol intake in humans) into the cerebral circulation of control rats rendered a significant, 20% decrease in the pial arteriole diameter (Figure 4A). In contrast to the control group, infusion of 50 mM ethanol into the cerebral circulation of rats on a high-cholesterol diet resulted in no more that a 10% decrease in the pial arteriole diameter. To rule out the contribution of circulating factors in the observed protective effect of a high-cholesterol diet, the experiment was repeated using isolated cerebral arteries that were pressurized *in-vitro* at 60 mmHg. As observed with pial arterioles *in-vivo*, application of 50 mM ethanol to pressurized middle cerebral arteries from control rats resulted in up to 12% decrease in the

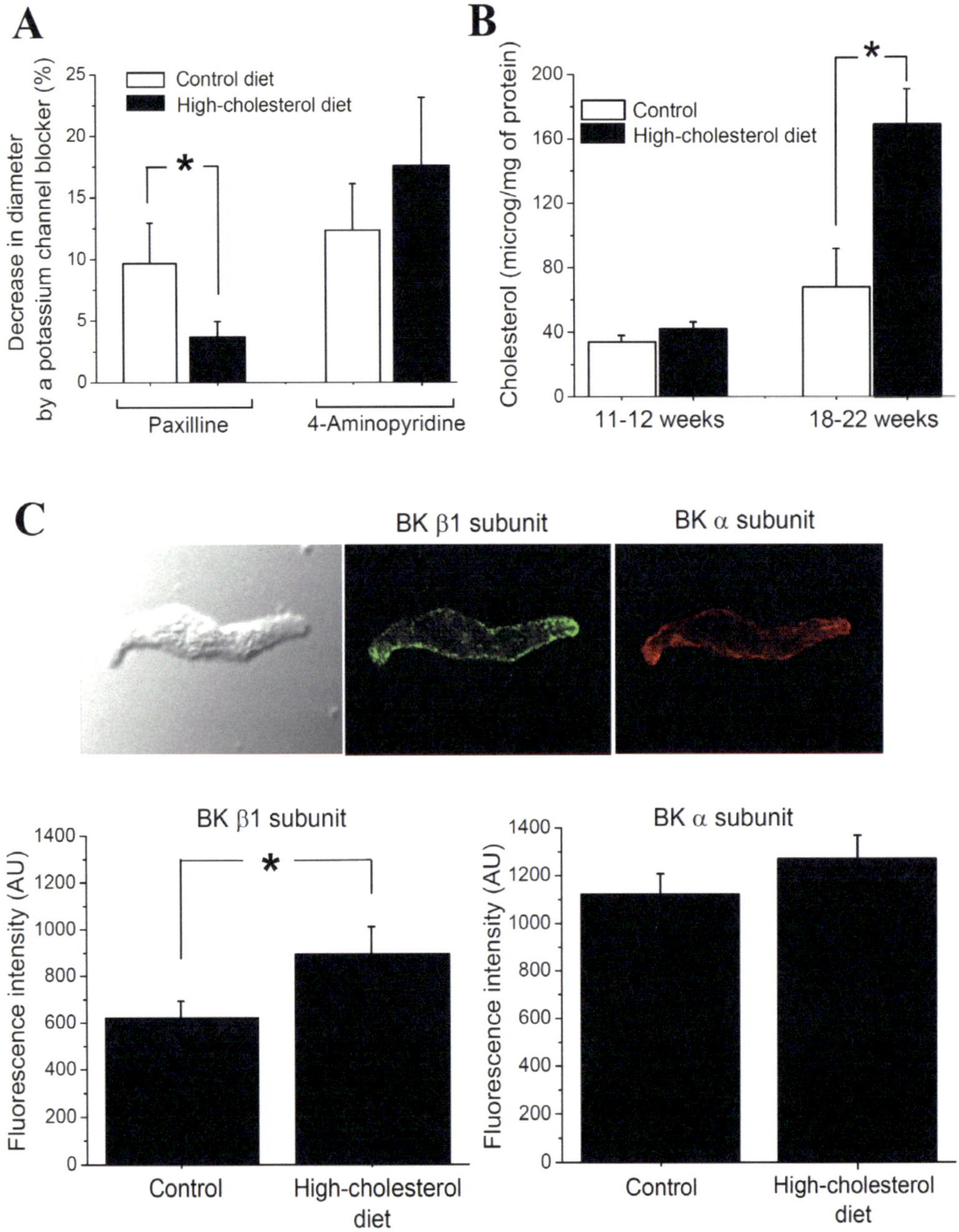

Figure 3. Effect of high-cholesterol diet on rat cerebral artery BK channel function. (A) Average data showing a decrease in arterial diameter by the selective BK channel blocker paxilline. (B) Cholesterol level in de-endothelialized cerebral arteries from rats fed control versus high-cholesterol diet. (C) Representative confocal microscope images showing an isolated cerebral artery myocyte and its fluorescence labeling of BK β1 and α subunits. (D) Averaged fluorescence intensity associated with BK β1 subunit. (E) Averaged fluorescence intensity associated with BK α subunit. (With modifications from [94]).

arterial diameter. In contrast, application of 50 mM ethanol to pressurized middle cerebral arteries from rats on a high-cholesterol diet resulted in only a 6-7% decrease in the arterial diameter (Figure 4B). Remarkably, the protective effect of a high-cholesterol diet against ethanol-induced constriction of cerebral arteries was similar in arteries with intact endothelium and in de-endothelialized vessels. Accordingly, dietary cholesterol-driven protection did not require the presence of functional endothelium and/or endothelium-derived vasoactive factors. Moreover, accumulation of cholesterol within the arterial wall was shown to play a major role in the observed protection by high-cholesterol diet against ethanol-induced constriction of cerebral arteries. In particular, after removal of the cholesterol that was accumulated in the cerebral artery tissue in the course of a high-cholesterol diet, ethanol-induced constriction was restored and reached the control value (Figure 4C) [31]. The molecular mechanisms by which membrane cholesterol affects the function of a major ethanol target in the artery, namely the BK channel, are still under investigation and are discussed in great detail elsewhere [71].

Inwardly rectifying potassium (Kir) channels. The effect of high-cholesterol diet on Kir channel function has been demonstrated for several members of the Kir family. Kir channels regulate important functions including membrane excitability, heart rate, vascular tone, insulin release and salt flow across epithelia (see, for example, reviews [10, 11, 13]). Structurally, they are comprised of four homo- or heteromeric subunits, each with two membrane spanning helices and intracellular N- and C- termini (Figure 2B). Fifteen Kir channels have been identified and classified in seven subfamilies (Kir1–7) [72]. Among these, it has been shown that a high-cholesterol diet affects the function of Kir2 channels, Kir3.1/Kir3.4 (K_{ACh}) channels and Kir6 (K_{ATP}) channels.

The effect of a high-cholesterol diet on Kir2 channels has been determined in different animal models and cell types. In earlier studies of Kir2 channels expressed in endothelial cells, hypercholesterolemia was induced by administering an atherogenic diet (0.5% cholesterol, 10% lard, and 1.5% sodium cholate) to castrated male Yorkshire pigs [18]. The properties of endothelial Kir2 channels and the values of the membrane potentials were compared in porcine aortic endothelial cells freshly isolated from the pig aortas. Cells isolated from hypercholesterolemic animals had significantly lower Kir currents than those isolated from control cells. Moreover, the membrane potential in hypercholesterolemic pigs was significantly more depolarized compared with that in control animals. More recently, the effect of a high-cholesterol diet on Kir2 channels expressed in cardiac myocytes was determined using a rat model [19]. In these experiments a group of 25-day-old male Sprague-Dawley rats was placed on a high-cholesterol diet (2% cholesterol in standard rodent food). Another group of the same age was fed an isocaloric, cholesterol-free diet from the same supplier. The rats were sacrificed as atrial tissue donors after 20-24 weeks on control or high-cholesterol diet. Notably, as a result of the high-cholesterol diet, in addition to an approximately 2.5-fold increase in serum LDL levels (see Figure 1), there was also an approximately1.8-fold increase in cholesterol levels in the atrial tissue itself (see Figure 5A). This increase in cholesterol levels in the atrial myocytes following the high cholesterol diet resulted in an approximately 60% decrease in Kir2 currents in atrial cardiomyocytes [19].

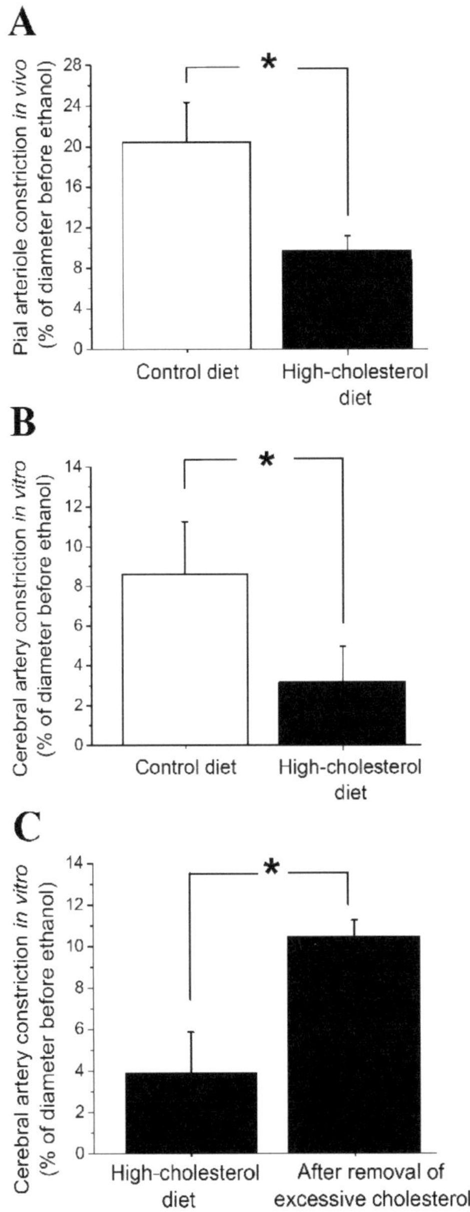

Figure 4. Cholesterol control of ethanol-induced constriction of cerebral artery. (A) Averaged data showing constriction of pial arterioles *in-vivo* in rats fed control versus high-cholesterol diet. (B) Ethanol-induced cerebral artery constriction in pressurized cerebral arteries *in-vitro* obtained from rats on control versus high-cholesterol diet. (C) Averaged data showing ethanol-induced cerebral artery constriction *in-vitro* in arteries from rats on a high-cholesterol diet before and after removal of excessive cholesterol using the cholesterol carrier methyl-β–cyclodextrin.(From [94]).

In addition to Kir2 channels, atrial myocytes also express Kir3 channels. In particular, atrial K_{ACh} channels are heterotetrameric proteins that consist of Kir3.1 and Kir3.4 [73]. Recent studies

http://dx.doi.org/10.5772/59761

[19] demonstrated that unexpectedly rats that were on a high-cholesterol diet for 18-22 weeks exhibited up to 2-3 fold increase in K_{ACh} currents that were sensitive to the selective $I_{K, ACh}$-blocker tertiapin (Figure 5B-5E). The summary data in Figure 5D-E show that the high-cholesterol diet affected both inward and outward currents in a similar manner. Thus, while the effect was more visible for the larger inward currents, the physiologically relevant smaller outward currents were also significantly affected by cholesterol. This result was surprising because an increase in channel function following an increase in cholesterol levels (as shown in Figure 5A) is rare. These data suggest that an increase in cholesterol levels in atrial myocytes may underlie the increase in K_{ACh} currents in hypercholesterolemic rats.

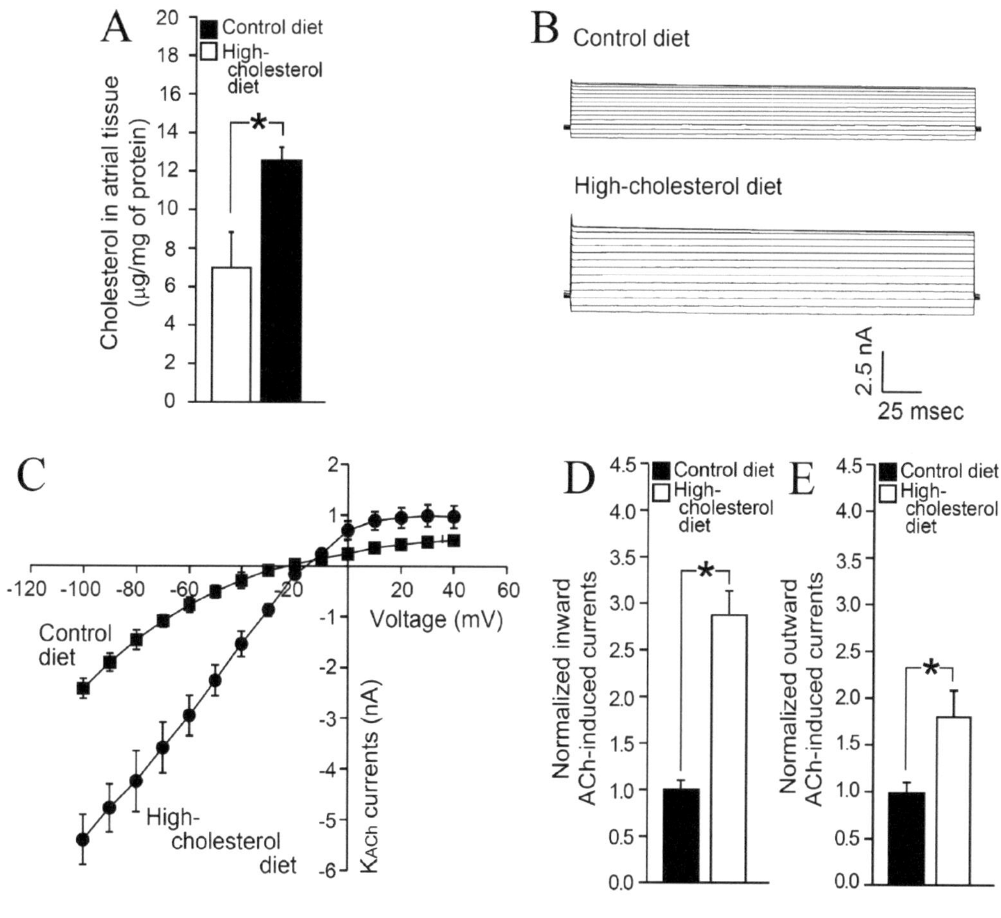

Figure 5. ACh-induced K_{ACh}currents in atrial cardiomyocytes are enhanced in hypercholesterolemic rats. (A) Cholesterol levels in atrial tissue of Sprague-Dawley rats fed a high-cholesterol diet compared to control. Tertiapin-sensitive currents (B) and I-V relationships (C) of ACh-induced current densities for atrial myocytes from control and hypercholesterolemic rats. Summary data: (D) inward ACh-induced current densities at -80 mV; (E) outward ACh-induced current densities at +40 mV. ((B)-(E) From [19]).

Several studies were also carried out to determine the effect of high-cholesterol diet on Kir6 channels. ATP-sensitive K^+ (K_{ATP}) channels are expressed in the sarcolemma of cardiomyocytes [74] and in the mitochondrial inner membrane [75]. Structurally, K_{ATP} channels are comprised of a pore forming Kir channel (Kir6.1 or Kir6.2) and an ATP-binding regulatory subunit, the sulfonylurea receptor (SUR1, SUR2A, or SUR2B).

Activation of K_{ATP} channels mediates coronary vasodilation during decreases in perfusion pressure within the autoregulatory range [76] and dilation of collateral and noncollateral vessels during ischemia [77]. However, dilation in response to the K_{ATP} channel activator aprikalim was not altered in monkeys following an atherogenic diet and reduction in dietary cholesterol [78].

In contrast, acidosis-induced coronary arteriolar dilation was impaired in hypercholesterolemic rabbits. When myocardial ischemia takes place [79], the interstitial pH of the heart rapidly decreases followed by an immediate decrease in coronary resistance by microvascular dilation [80]. It was shown that acidosis-induced coronary arteriolar dilation is mediated via the activation of pertussis toxin-sensitive G protein and consequent opening of the K_{ATP} channel [81-82]. Since hypercholesterolemia produces structural and functional abnormalities in blood vessels [83], its impact on coronary microvascular response to acidosis was investigated [84]. Coronary arterioles isolated from rabbit hearts were cannulated to micropipettes in a vessel chamber and microvascular responses were observed. The effect of the K_{ATP} channel blocker glibenclamide on the acidosis-induced microvascular responses was examined. Coronary arterioles significantly dilated as the pH was reduced and the dilation was significantly inhibited by glibenclamide. In another set of experiments, rabbits were randomly assigned to normal chow or high-cholesterol diet. After 8 weeks, the responses of isolated coronary arterioles to acidosis were examined in the two groups. Acidosis-induced dilation in the high-cholesterol group was significantly attenuated compared to the control group. These data suggest that K_{ATP} channels play an important role in the acidosis-induced dilation of rabbit coronary arterioles and that dilation of coronary arterioles is impaired in hypercholesterolemia. Notably, the impairment occurs upstream of K_{ATP} channel opening.

K_{ATP} channels play a key role in endogenous cardioprotective mechanisms [85-88]. Specifically, during cardiac ischemia, the levels of intracellular ATP may decrease. This would result in the opening of K_{ATP} channels that operate as molecular biosensors for coupling cellular energy metabolism and excitability [89]. The opening of K_{ATP} channels leads to increased influx of K^+, which then leads to shortening of the action potential duration and to reduction of the Ca^{2+} overload that occurs during ischemia-reperfusion induced injury [90-92]. Since hyperlipidemia has been shown to interfere with cardioprotective mechanisms, studies were carried out to investigate the interaction of hyperlipidemia with cardioprotection induced by pharmacological activators of K_{ATP} channels [93]. Hearts isolated from rats fed a 2% cholesterol-enriched or normal diet for 8 weeks were subjected to 30 min of global ischemia and 120 min of reperfusion in the presence or absence of K_{ATP} modulators. In normal diet-fed rats, activation of K_{ATP} channels either by the nonselective K_{ATP} activator cromakalim or the selective mitochondrial K_{ATP} channel opener diazoxide significantly decreased infarct size compared with vehicle-treated control rats.

Moreover, the cardioprotective effect was abolished by blocking the channels using the nonselective K_{ATP} blocker glibenclamide or the selective mitochondrial K_{ATP} channel blocker 5-hydroxydecanoate. In contrast, in cholesterol-fed rats, the cardioprotective effect was not observed following administration of K_{ATP} channel activators, demonstrating that cardioprotection by K_{ATP} channel activators is impaired in cholesterol-enriched diet-induced hyperlipidemia. Notably, whereas protein levels of Kir6.1 and Kir6.2 remained unchanged, cardiac expression of Kir6.1 was significantly downregulated in cholesterol-fed rats.

Together, these data demonstrate a wide range of effects of a high-cholesterol diet on the function of inwardly rectifying potassium channels and on their physiological implications. Whereas the function of Kir2 and Kir6 channels was suppressed in several cases following a high-cholesterol diet, atrial Kir3 channels were enhanced. Moreover, in the case of Kir6 channels, whereas K_{ATP}-mediated coronary vasodilation was not altered in atherosclerotic monkeys, a high-cholesterol diet resulted in impaired cardioprotection by K_{ATP} channel activators in rats and impaired K_{ATP}-mediated acidosis-induced coronary arteriolar dilation in rabbits.

4. Conclusive remarks

Different types of potassium channels have been shown to be affected by high-cholesterol diet in a variety of species. The modulation of potassium channel activity by high-cholesterol diet results in alterations of organ function *in-vitro* and *in-vivo*. Notably, the effect of high-cholesterol diet on potassium channels varies and may result in decreased or increased channel function. In a few cases, potassium channels were found to be insensitive to dietary cholesterol manipulation. Among the potassium channels that were affected by a high-cholesterol diet are included several voltage-gated potassium channels (K_V), calcium-activated potassium (K_{Ca}) channels, and inwardly rectifying potassium (Kir) channels. Among the channels studied, only the currents of the heterotetrameric Kir3.1/Kir3.4 (K_{Ach}) channels were consistently enhanced by high-cholesterol dietary intake. The structural and molecular bases for the diverse effect of high-cholesterol diet on potassium channels remain largely unknown. Thus, considering the critical role of potassium channels in physiology and pathology, an important aspect of future studies will be to elucidate the intrinsic mechanisms leading to dietary cholesterol modulation of channel function.

Acknowledgements

This work was supported by a Scientist Development Grant 11SDG5190025 from the American Heart Association (to A.R.-D.), the Alcoholic Beverage Medical Research Foundation grant for New Investigator (A.B.), and NIH Support Opportunity for Addiction Research for New Investigators R03 AA020184 (A.B.)

Author details

Anna N. Bukiya[3] and Avia Rosenhouse-Dantsker[1,2*]

*Address all correspondence to: dantsker@uic.edu

1 Department of Chemistry, University of Illinois at Chicago, Chicago, IL, USA

2 Departments of Medicine and Pharmacology, University of Illinois at Chicago, Chicago, IL, USA

3 Department of Pharmacology, The University of Tennessee Health Science Center, Memphis, TN, USA

References

[1] Yeagle PL. Cholesterol and the cell membrane. BiochimBiophysActa 1985;822 267-287.

[2] Yeagle PL. Modulation of membrane function by cholesterol. Biochimie 1991;73 1303-10.

[3] Kellner-Weibel G, Geng YJ, Rothblat GH. Cytotoxic cholesterol is generated by the hydrolysis of cytoplasmic cholesteryl ester and transported to the plasma membrane. Atherosclerosis 1999;146(2) 309-319.

[4] Ross R. Atherosclerosis--an inflammatory disease. N Engl J Med. 1999;340(2) 115-126.

[5] Kruth HS. Lipoprotein cholesterol and atherosclerosis. Current Molecular Medicine 2001;1(6) 633-653.

[6] Steinberg D. Atherogenesis in perspective: hypercholesterolemia and inflammation as partners in crime. Nat Med. 2002;8(11) 1211-1217.

[7] Maguy A, Hebert TE, Nattel S. Involvement of lipid rafts and caveolae in cardiac ion channel function. Cardiovasc Res. 2006; 69 798-807.

[8] Levitan I. Cholesterol and Kir channels. IUBMB Life 2009;61 781-90.

[9] Rosenhouse-Dantsker A, Mehta D, Levitan I. Regulation of ion channels by membrane lipids. ComprPhysiol. 2012;2 31-68.

[10] Nichols C, Lopatin A. Inward rectifier potassium channels. Annu Rev Physiol. 1997;59 268-277.

[11] Bichet D, Haass FA, Jan LY. Merging functional studies with structures of inward-rectifier K(+) channels. Nat Rev Neurosci. 2003;4 957-967.

[12] Salkoff L, Butler A, Ferreira G, Santi C, Wei A. High-conductance potassium channels of the SLO family. Nat Rev Neurosci 2006;7(12) 921-931.

[13] Hibino H, Inanobe A, Furutani K, Murakami S, Findlay I, Kurachi Y.Inwardly rectifying potassium channels: their structure, function, and physiological roles. Physiol Rev. 2010;90 291-366.

[14] Castle NA. Pharmacological modulation of voltage-gated potassium channels as a therapeutic strategy. Expert OpinTher Pat. 2010;20(11) 1471-503.

[15] González C1, Baez-Nieto D, Valencia I, Oyarzún I, Rojas P, Naranjo D, Latorre R. K^+ channels: function-structural overview. Compr Physiol. 2012;2(3) 2087-149.

[16] Jan LY, Jan YN. Voltage-gated potassium channels and the diversity of electrical signalling. J Physiol. 2012;590 2591-9.

[17] Ge L, Hoa NT, Wilson Z, Arismendi-Morillo G, Kong XT, Tajhya RB, Beeton C, Jadus MR. Big Potassium (BK) ion channels in biology, disease and possible targets for cancer immunotherapy.IntImmunopharmacol. 2014;22 427-443.

[18] Fang Y, Mohler ER 3rd, Hsieh E, Osman H, Hashemi SM, Davies PF, Rothblat GH, Wilensky RL, Levitan I. Hypercholesterolemia suppresses inwardly rectifying K^+ channels in aortic endothelium in vitro and in vivo. Circ Res. 2006;98 1064–1071.

[19] Deng W, Bukiya AN, Rodríguez-Menchaca AA, Zhang Z, Baumgarten CM, Logothetis DE, Levitan I, Rosenhouse-Dantsker A. Hypercholesterolemia induces up-regulation of KACh cardiac currents via a mechanism independent of phosphatidylinositol 4, 5-bisphosphate and Gβγ. J Biol Chem. 2012;287(7) 4925-35.

[20] Ghanam K, Javellaud J, Ea-Kim L, Oudart N. Effects of treatment with 17beta-estradiol on the hypercholesterolemic rabbit middle cerebral artery. Maturitas. 2000;34(3) 249-60.

[21] Mokelke EA, Hu Q, Song M, Toro L, Reddy HK, Sturek M. Altered functional coupling of coronary K^+ channels in diabetic dyslipidemic pigs is prevented by exercise. J Appl Physiol. 2003;95(3) 1179-93.

[22] Heaps CL, Tharp DL, Bowles DK. Hypercholesterolemia abolishes voltage-dependent K^+ channel contribution to adenosine-mediated relaxation in porcine coronary arterioles. Am J Physiol Heart Circ Physiol. 2005;288(2) H568-76.

[23] Heaps CL, Jeffery EC, Laine GA, Price EM, Bowles DK. Effects of exercise training and hypercholesterolemia on adenosine activation of voltage-dependent K^+ channels in coronary arterioles. J Appl Physiol. 2008;105(6) 1761-71

[24] Varga A, Bagossi P, Tözsér J, Peitl B, Szilvássy Z. Effect of experimental hypercholesterolaemia on K^+ channel alpha-subunit mRNA levels in rabbit hearts. Eur J Pharmacol. 2007;562(1-2) 130-1.

[25] Yang Y, Jones AW, Thomas TR, Rubin LJ. Influence of sex, high-fat diet, and exercise training on potassium currents of swine coronary smooth muscle. Am J Physiol Heart Circ Physiol. 2007;293(3) H1553-1563.

[26] Bender SB, Tune JD, Borbouse L, Long X, Sturek M, Laughlin MH. Altered mechanism of adenosine-induced coronary arteriolar dilation in early-stage metabolic syndrome. ExpBiol Med (Maywood). 2009;234(6) 683-92.

[27] Jeremy RW, McCarron H. Effect of hypercholesterolemia on Ca(2+)-dependent K(+) channel-mediated vasodilatation in vivo. Am J Physiol Heart CircPhysiol 2000;279(4) H1600-H1608.

[28] Taniguchi J, Honda H, Shibusawa Y, Iwata T, Notoya Y. Alteration in endothelial function and modulation by treatment with pioglitazone in rabbit renal artery from short-term hypercholesterolemia. VasculPharmacol. 2005;43(1) 47-55.

[29] Du P, Cui GB, Wang YR, Zhang XY, Ma KJ, Wei JG. Down regulated expression of the beta1 subunit of the big-conductance Ca^{2+} sensitive K^{+} channel in sphincter of Oddi cells from rabbits fed with a high cholesterol diet. ActaBiochimBiophys Sin (Shanghai). 2006;38(12) 893-9.

[30] Bukiya A, Dopico A. Endothelium-independent, smooth muscle BK channel-mediated dilation of resistance-size cerebral arteries is significantly impaired in rats on a high-cholesterol diet. ArteriosclerThrombVasc Biol. 2008;28 e107.

[31] Bukiya AN, Vaithianathan T, Kuntamallappanavar G, Asuncion-Chin M, Dopico AM. Smooth muscle cholesterol enables BK β1 subunit-mediated channel inhibition and subsequent vasoconstriction evoked by alcohol. ArteriosclerThrombVasc Biol. 2011;31(11) 2410-23.

[32] Howell WH, McNamara DJ, Tosca MA, Smith BT, Gaines JA Plasma lipid and lipoprotein responses to dietary fat and cholesterol: a meta-analysis. Am J ClinNutr. 1997;65 1747–1764.

[33] Asemi Z, Tabassi Z, Samimi M, Fahiminejad T, Esmaillzadeh A. Favourable effects of the Dietary Approaches to Stop Hypertension diet on glucose tolerance and lipid profiles in gestational diabetes: a randomised clinical trial. Br J Nutr 2013;109 2024–2030.

[34] Hadjiev DI, Mineva PP, Vukov MI. Multiple modifiable risk factors for first ischemic stroke: a population-based epidemiological study. Eur J Neurol. 2003;10(5) 577-82.

[35] Ivan A, Azoicăi D, Stefanache F, Manole A, Hodorog D, Trifan M, Cuciureanu DI, Matei M. [Prospective epidemiologic and clinical observations on the prevalence of risk factors for stroke, performed on 374 inpatients, during the period of June 2001-June 2004]. Rev Med ChirSoc Med Nat Iasi. 2004;108(3) 561-5.

[36] Weikert C, Berger K, Heidemann C, Bergmann MM, Hoffmann K, Klipstein-Grobusch K, Boeing H. Joint effects of risk factors for stroke and transient ischemic attack in a German population: the EPIC Potsdam Study. J Neurol. 2007;254(3) 315-21.

[37] Castilla Guerra L, del Carmen Fernández Moreno M, López Chozas JM, Jiménez Hernández MD. Statins in stroke prevention: what an internist should know. Eur J Intern Med. 2008;19(1) 8-14.

[38] Cui R, Iso H, Toyoshima H, Date C, Yamamoto A, Kikuchi S, Kondo T, Watanabe Y, Koizumi A, Inaba Y, Tamakoshi A; JACC Study Group. Serum total cholesterol levels and risk of mortality from stroke and coronary heart disease in Japanese: the JACC study. Atherosclerosis 2007;194(2) 415-20.

[39] Uchiyama S, Shibata Y, Hirabayashi T, Mihara B, Hamashige N, Kitagawa K, Goto S, Origasa H, Shimada K, Kobayashi H, Isozaki M, Ikeda Y; J-TRACE Investigators. Risk factor profiles of stroke, myocardial infarction, and atrial fibrillation: a Japanese Multicenter Cooperative Registry. J Stroke Cerebrovasc Dis. 2010;19(3) 190-7.

[40] Stella F, Banzato CE, GasparettoSé EV, Scudeler JL, Pacheco JL, Kajita RT. Risk factors for vascular dementia in elderly psychiatric outpatients with preserved cognitive functions. J Neurol Sci. 2007;257(1-2) 247-9.

[41] Babiak J, Rudel LL. Lipoproteins and atherosclerosis. BaillieresClinEndocrinolMetab. 1987;1(3) 515-50.

[42] Ayajiki K, Fujioka H, Torii R, Toda N, Okamura T. Endothelial and neuronal functions in cerebral and temporal arteries from monkeys fed a high-cholesterol diet. J CardiovascPharmacol. 2002;40(3) 456-66.

[43] Chan YC1, Leung FP, Tian XY, Yung LM, Lau CW, Chen ZY, Yao X, Laher I, Huang Y. Raloxifene improves vascular reactivity in pressurized septal coronary arteries of ovariectomized hamsters fed cholesterol diet. Pharmacol Res. 2012;65(2) 182-8.

[44] Amran AA, Zaiton Z, Faizah O, Morat P. Effects of Garciniaatroviridis on serum profiles and atherosclerotic lesions in the aorta of guinea pigs fed a high cholesterol diet. Singapore Med J. 2009;50(3) 295-9.

[45] Najibi S, Cohen RA. Enhanced role of K^+ channels in relaxations of hypercholesterolemic rabbit carotid artery to NO. Am J Physiol. 1995;269(3 Pt 2) H805-811.

[46] Irie H, Koshiba H, Koyama M, Asakura E, Shibata H, Kimura K, Naito K, Yamauchi T, Yada K, Hanamura T, Hanada S, Abe Si, Nakamura N. Effects of recombinant human macrophage colony-stimulating factor on atherosclerotic lesions established in the aorta of high cholesterol-fed rabbits. J Biochem. 2001;129(5) 717-24.

[47] Liu RY, Gu R, Qi XL, Zhang T, Zhao Y, He Y, Pei JJ, Guan ZZ. Decreased nicotinic receptors and cognitive deficit in rats intracerebroventricularly injected with beta-amyloid peptide(1-42) and fed a high-cholesterol diet. J Neurosci Res. 2008;86(1) 183-93.

[48] Balkanci ZD, Pehlivanoğlu B, Bayrak S, Karabulut I, Karaismailoğlu S, Erdem A. The effect of hypercholesterolemia on carbachol-induced contractions of the detrusor smooth muscle in rats: increased role of L-type Ca2+ channels. NaunynSchmiedebergs Arch Pharmacol. 2012;385(11) 1141-8.

[49] El-Sayyad HI, Khalifa SA, Fouda YA, Yonis AS Effects of diabetes and/or hypercholesterolemia on skin development of rat fetuses. Nutrition 2012;28 698–706.

[50] Yeap SK, Beh BK, Kong J, Ho WY, MohdYusof H, Mohamad NE, Hussin AB, Jaganath IB, Alitheen NB, Jamaluddin A, Long K. In Vivo Hypocholesterolemic Effect of MARDI Fermented Red Yeast Rice Water Extract in High Cholesterol Diet Fed Mice. Evid Based Complement Alternat Med. 2014;2014 707829.

[51] Kushwaha RS, McGill HC Jr. Diet, plasma lipoproteins and experimental atherosclerosis in baboons (Papio sp.). Hum Reprod Update. 1998;4(4) 420-9.

[52] Beynen AC, Katan MB, Van Zutphen LF. Hypo- and hyperresponders: individual differences in the response of serum cholesterol concentration to changes in diet. Adv Lipid Res. 1987;22 115-71.

[53] Rosenbaum MA, Chaudhuri P, Graham LM. Hypercholesterolemia inhibits re-endothelialization of arterial injuries by TRPC channel activation. J Vasc Surg. 2014;pii S0741-5214(14)00834-9.

[54] Awayda MS, Awayda KL, Pochynyuk O, Bugaj V, Stockand JD, Ortiz RM. Acute cholesterol-induced anti-natriuretic effects: role of epithelial Na^+ channel activity, protein levels, and processing. J Biol Chem. 2011;286 1683-95.

[55] Hille B. Ion channels of excitable membranes. 3rd Edition. Sinauer Associates, Inc; 2001.

[56] Latorre R, Brauchi S. Large conductance Ca^{2+}-activated K^+ (BK) channel: activation by Ca^{2+} and voltage. Biol Res. 2006;39(3) 385-401.

[57] Lee US, Cui J. BK channel activation: structural and functional insights. Trends Neurosci. 2010;33(9) 415-423.

[58] Wallner M, Meera P, Toro L. Determinant for beta-subunit regulation in high-conductance voltage-activated and Ca^{2+}-sensitive K^+ channels: an additional transmembrane region at the N terminus. ProcNatlAcadSci U S A. 1996;93(25) 14922-14927.

[59] Wei A, Solaro C, Lingle C, Salkoff L. Calcium sensitivity of BK-type K_{Ca} channels determined by a separable domain. Neuron 1994;13(3) 671-681.

[60] Cox DH. The BKCa channel's Ca^{2+}-binding sites, multiple sites, multiple ions. J Gen Physiol 2005;125(3) 253-255.

[61] Yuan P, Leonetti MD, Pico AR, Hsiung Y, MacKinnon R. Structure of the human BK channel Ca^{2+}-activation apparatus at 3.0 A resolution. Science 2010;329(5988) 182-186.

[62] Orio P, Rojas P, Ferreira G, Latorre R. New disguises for an old channel: MaxiK channel beta-subunits. News Physiol Sci. 2002;17 156-161.

[63] Brenner R, Jegla TJ, Wickenden A, Liu Y, Aldrich RW. Cloning and functional characterization of novel large conductance calcium-activated potassium channel beta subunits, hKCNMB3 and hKCNMB4. J Biol Chem. 2000;275(9) 6453-6461.

[64] Sobey CG. Potassium channel function in vascular disease. ArteriosclerThrombVasc Biol. 2001;21(1) 28-38.

[65] Brayden JE, Nelson MT. Regulation of arterial tone by activation of calcium-dependent potassium channels. Science 1992;256(5056) 532-535.

[66] Najibi S, Cowan CL, Palacino JJ, Cohen RA. Enhanced role of potassium channels in relaxations to acetylcholine in hypercholesterolemic rabbit carotid artery. Am J Physiol. 1994;266(5 Pt 2) H2061-H2067.

[67] Wiecha J, Schläger B, Voisard R, Hannekum A, Mattfeldt T, Hombach V. Ca^{2+}-activated K^+ channels in human smooth muscle cells of coronary atherosclerotic plaques and coronary media segments. Basic Res Cardiol. 1997;92(4) 233-239.

[68] Brenner R, Peréz GJ, Bonev AD, Eckman DM, Kosek JC, Wiler SW, Patterson AJ, Nelson MT, Aldrich RW. Vasoregulationby the beta1 subunit of the calcium-activated potassium channel. Nature. 2000;407(6806) 870-6.

[69] Meera P, Wallner M, Toro L. A neuronal beta subunit (KCNMB4) makes the large conductance, voltage- and Ca^{2+}-activated K^+ channel resistant to charybdotoxin and iberiotoxin. ProcNatlAcadSci U S A. 2000;97(10) 5562-7.

[70] Liu P, Xi Q, Ahmed A, Jaggar JH, Dopico AM. Essential role for smooth muscle BK channels in alcohol-induced cerebrovascular constriction. ProcNatlAcadSci U S A. 2004;101(52) 18217-22.

[71] Dopico AM, Bukiya AN, Singh AK. Large conductance, calcium- and voltage-gated potassium (BK) channels: regulation by cholesterol. PharmacolTher. 2012;135(2) 133-50.

[72] Reimann F, Ashcroft FM. Inwardly rectifying potassium channels.CurrOpin Cell Biol. 1999;11 503-8.

[73] Krapivinsky G, Gordon EA, Wickman K, Velimirović B, Krapivinsky L, Clapham DE. The G protein-gated atrial K^+ channel IKACh is a heteromultimer of two inwardly rectifying K^+ channel proteins. Nature 1995;374 135–141.

[74] Noma A. ATP-regulated K^+ channels in cardiac muscle. Nature 1983;305 147–148.

[75] Inoue I, Nagase H, Kishi K, Higuti T. ATP-sensitive K^+ channel in the mitochondrial inner membrane. Nature 1991;352 244-247.

[76] Komaru T, Lamping KG, Eastham CL, Dellsperger KC. Role of ATP-sensitive potassium channels in coronary microvascularautoregulatory responses. Circ Res. 1991;69 1146-1151.

[77] Lamping KG, Bloom EN, Harrison DG. Regulation of native collateral vessel dilation following coronary occlusion in the dog. Am J Physiol. 1994;266 H769-H778.

[78] Lamping KG, Piegors DJ, Benzuly KH, Armstrong ML, Heistad DD. Enhanced coronary vasoconstrictive response to serotonin subsides after removal of dietary cholesterol in atherosclerotic monkeys. ArterioscIerThromb. 1994;14(6) 951-7.

[79] Momomura S, Ingwall JS, Paker JA, Sahagian P, Ferguson JJ, Grossman W. The relationships of high energy phosphates, tissue pH, and regional blood flow to diastolic distensibility in the ischemic dog myocardium. Circ Res. 1985;57 822–835.

[80] Lee JC, Halloran KH, Taylor JF, Downing SE Coronary flow and myocardial metabolism in newborn lambs: effects of hypoxia and acidemia. Am J Physiol. 1973;224 1381–1387.

[81] Ishizaka H, Kuo L. Acidosis induced coronary arteriolar dilation is mediated by ATP-sensitive potassium channels in vascular smooth muscle. Circ Res. 1996; 78 50–57

[82] Ishizaka H, Gudi SR, Frangos JA, Kuo L. Coronary arteriolar dilation to acidosis. Role of ATP-sensitive potassium channels and pertussis toxin-sensitive G proteins. Circulation 1999;99 558–563.

[83] Vanhoutte PM. Endothelial dysfunction and atherosclerosis. Eur Heart J. 1997;18(suppl) E19–E29.

[84] Shioiri H, Komaru T, Sato K, Takahashi K, Takeda S, Kanatsuka H, Watanabe J, Shirato K. Impact of hypercholesterolemia on acidosis-induced coronary microvascular dilation. Basic Res Cardiol. 2003;98 76-83.

[85] Kevelaitis E, Oubenaissa A, Peynet J, Mouas C, Menasche P. Preconditioning by mitochondrial ATP-sensitive potassium channel openers: an effective approach for improving the preservation of heart transplants. Circulation 1999;100(19 Suppl) II345–II350.

[86] Ferdinandy P, Schulz R, Baxter GF. Interaction of cardiovascular risk factors with myocardial ischemia/reperfusion injury, preconditioning, and postconditioning. Pharmacol Rev. 2007;59 418–458.

[87] Wang L, Cherednichenko G, Hernandez L, Halow J, Camacho SA, Figueredo V, Schaefer S. Preconditioning limits mitochondrial Ca^{2+} during ischemia in rat hearts: role of KATP channels. Am J Physiol HeartCirc Physiol. 2001;280 H2321–H2328.

[88] Wang Y, Kudo M, Xu M, Ayub A, Ashraf M. Mitochondrial KATP channel as an end effector of cardioprotection during late preconditioning:triggering role of nitric oxide. J Mol Cell Cardiol. 2001;33 2037–2046.

[89] Zingman LV, Alekseev AE, Hodgson-Zingman DM, Terzic A. ATPsensitive potassium channels: metabolic sensing and cardioprotection. JAppl Physiol. 2007;103 1888–1893.

[90] Loussouarn G, Pike LJ, Ashcroft FM, Makhina EN, Nichols CG. Dynamic sensitivity of ATP-sensitive K^+ channels to ATP. J Biol Chem. 2001;276 29098–29103.

[91] Puskas LG, Nagy ZB, Giricz Z, Onody A, Csonka C, Kitajka K, Hackler L Jr, Zvara A, Ferdinandy P. Cholesterol diet-induced hyperlipidemiainfluences gene expression pattern of rat hearts: a DNA microarraystudy. FEBS Lett. 2004;562 99-104.

[92] Olson TM, Terzic A. Human KATP channelopathies: diseases of metabolic homeostasis. Pflügers Arch. 2010;460 295–306.

[93] Csonka C1, Kupai K, Bencsik P, Görbe A, Pálóczi J, Zvara A, Puskás LG, Csont T, Ferdinandy P. Cholesterol-enriched diet inhibits cardioprotection by ATP-sensitive K^+ channel activators cromakalim and diazoxide. Am J Physiol Heart Circ Physiol. 2014;306(3) H405-13.

[94] Bukiya A, Dopico AM, Leffler CW, Fedinec A. Dietary cholesterol protects against alcohol-induced cerebral artery constriction. Alcohol ClinExp Res. 2014 ;38(5) 1216-26.

Chapter 6

Hypercholesterolemia as a Risk Factor for Catheterization-Related Cerebral Infarction — A Literature Review and a Summary of Cases

Yusuke Morita, Takao Kato and Moriaki Inoko

Additional information is available at the end of the chapter

http://dx.doi.org/10.5772/59282

1. Introduction

Hypercholesterolemia is one of the major risk factors of atherosclerotic disease. Treatment with statins reduces serum levels of low-density lipoprotein cholesterol, and attenuates atherosclerotic plaque formation in the carotid artery, coronary artery, and thoracic aorta.

During diagnostic angiography or interventions for coronary artery diseases, catheterization can lead to devastating complications, including stroke. Previous studies reported stroke rates of 0.1–0.4% [1-9]. Catheterization-related acute stroke is associated with high in-hospital mortality and prevalence of overall major complications [5,10,11].

Because only new neurological complications are classified as stroke, clinically unapparent cerebral embolisms are not taken into account. Asymptomatic cerebral infarction is thought to be related to the incidence of symptomatic cerebral infarction, cognitive decline, and dementia [12], and may thus represent a significant complication of catheterization procedures.

Here, we summarize our review of published literature, present two case studies in our cardiovascular center, and summarize our data on hypercholesterolemia and catheterization-related stroke.

2. A review of published literature on hypercholesterolemia and catheterization-related stroke

Previously published data on catheterization-related acute stroke is summarized in Figure 1. Previous studies have reported stroke rates of 0.1– 0.4% [1-9], and rates of stroke and transient ischemia attack (TIA) after catheterization do not appear to have decreased over time (Figure 1). Much of the published data is limited to stroke. Stroke is defined as cerebral infarction or hemorrhage with a neurological deficit lasting >24 h; TIA is a neurological deficit lasting <24 h.

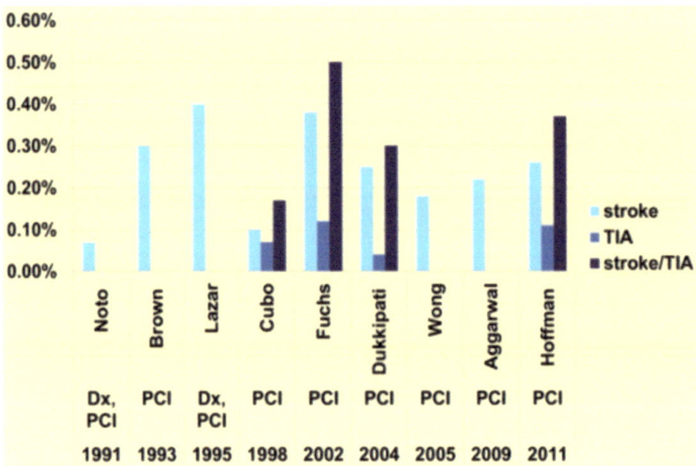

Figure 1. Rates of stroke and transient ischemic attack (TIA) after catheterization have not reduced overtime [1-9].

Magnetic resonance imaging (MRI) can be used to detect asymptomatic cerebral infarction related to catheterization. Diffusion-weighted MRI (DW-MRI), in particular, represents a highly sensitive tool for detecting acute cerebral ischemic lesions [13,14]. New lesions appear as focal high-intensity cerebral lesions on diffusion-weighted imaging (DWI) and have a low signal on apparent diffusion coefficient (ADC) maps [15].

Several prospective studies of silent cerebral infarction have been performed in a small number of patients. Bendszus et al. used DW-MRI before and after angiography of cerebral vessels to assess embolic events in 100 consecutive angiographies (66 diagnostic and 34 interventional) in 91 patients [16]. In their report, published in *The Lancet* in 1999, they showed that 23% of procedures caused silent embolic cerebral infarction: 42 bright lesions were observed in 23 patients after 23 procedures (17 diagnostic, six interventional), in a pattern consistent with embolic events, and in the absence of any new neurological deficit. More contrast medium, a longer fluoroscopy time, more frequent additional catheters, and having more vessels that were difficult to approach were the risks of silent embolic cerebral infarction. Patients' mean age did not differ between patients with lesions and those without lesions, but their mean age was relatively young (around 50 years old) compared to patients who are receiving cardiac catheterization.

Lund et al. monitored cerebral microemboli during catheterization in 42 unselected patients using multifrequency transcranial Doppler alongside cerebral DW-MRI and neuropsychological assessments. Measurements were taken on the days before and after catheterization [17]. Their report, published in the *European Heart Journal* in 2005, showed that new cerebral lesions were present in 15.2% of transradial catheterization patients, but in none of the transfemoral catheterization patients. These lesions were significantly associated with a higher number of solid microemboli and a longer fluoroscopy time. Approximately 80% of patients were male and had hyperlipidemia or were statin users; approximately 40% of patients had a previous history of myocardial infarction.

In 2005, Karen et al., using MRI before and after catheterization procedures, reported focal cerebral infarction without any symptoms in 15% of 48 patients [18]. In this prospective study, definitive conclusions could not be drawn owing to the small sample size, but procedure duration appeared to predict cerebral infarction following catheterization. Patients with cerebral infarction were also found to have a history of smoking, hyperlipidemia, hypertension, and obesity.

It is often difficult to acquire MR images before and after procedures in prospective studies. In 2011, Kojuri et al. reported in *BMC Cardiovascular Disorders* the prevalence of retinal emboli after diagnostic and therapeutic catheterization during retinal examination: 6.3% of 300 patients and only 1 patient developed vision disorder [19].

Patients who undergo aortic stenosis (AS) procedures that involve crossing of the aortic valve carry a high risk of cerebral infarction. In 2003, Omran et al. reported in the *Lancet* that 22% of 101 AS patients undergoing retrograde catheterization of the left ventricle had new lesions on MRI, and 3 patients had symptomatic cerebral infarction [20]. A total of 152 patients with AS undergoing cardiac catheterization were randomized to receive catheterization with or without retrograde passage of the aortic valve in a ratio of 2:1. An additional 32 patients without AS were also assessed as healthy controls. In patients without retrograde passage of the aortic valve, and in healthy controls, there was no MRI or clinical evidence of cerebral embolism.

Although these studies used relatively small sample sizes, the incidence of asymptomatic cerebral infarction following catheterization, as assessed by MRI or other methods, appears to remain relatively high. Following improvements in catheter design (rendering them more slender) and in techniques, catheterization-related cerebral infarctions were expected to decrease, though this may be counterbalanced by the increased risk profile of patients who undergo catheterization.

3. Two cases of asymptomatic and symptomatic cerebral infarction related to catheterization

Here we present two cases of cerebral infarction with and without symptoms which was related to cardiac catheterization.

Case 1: A 73-year-old man with hyperlipidemia, hypertension and diabetes underwent percutaneous coronary intervention (PCI) via the right radial artery. An initial diagnostic procedure was performed using 4F catheter; a 6F catheter was subsequently used to perform PCI for the left anterior descending artery (LAD). Due to the tortuosity of the LAD, the procedure time was 58 min and 275 ml contrast medium was used. MRI was performed 5 days later for MR angiography to detect carotid and intra-cranial lesions. MRI was not performed prior to the procedure; however, new lesions appeared as focal high-intensity cerebral lesions on DWI (Figure 2A) and gave a low signal on ADC maps (Figure 2B). ADC maps represent a useful tool for detecting acute ischemic infarct lesions [16].

Case 2: A 69-year-old woman with hyperlipidemia and diabetes underwent diagnostic catheterization for left ventricular systolic dysfunction of unknown etiology, with 45% ejection fraction. On the day after catheterization, the patient complained of dizziness. DW-MRI revealed a spotty high-intensity signal (Figure 2C).

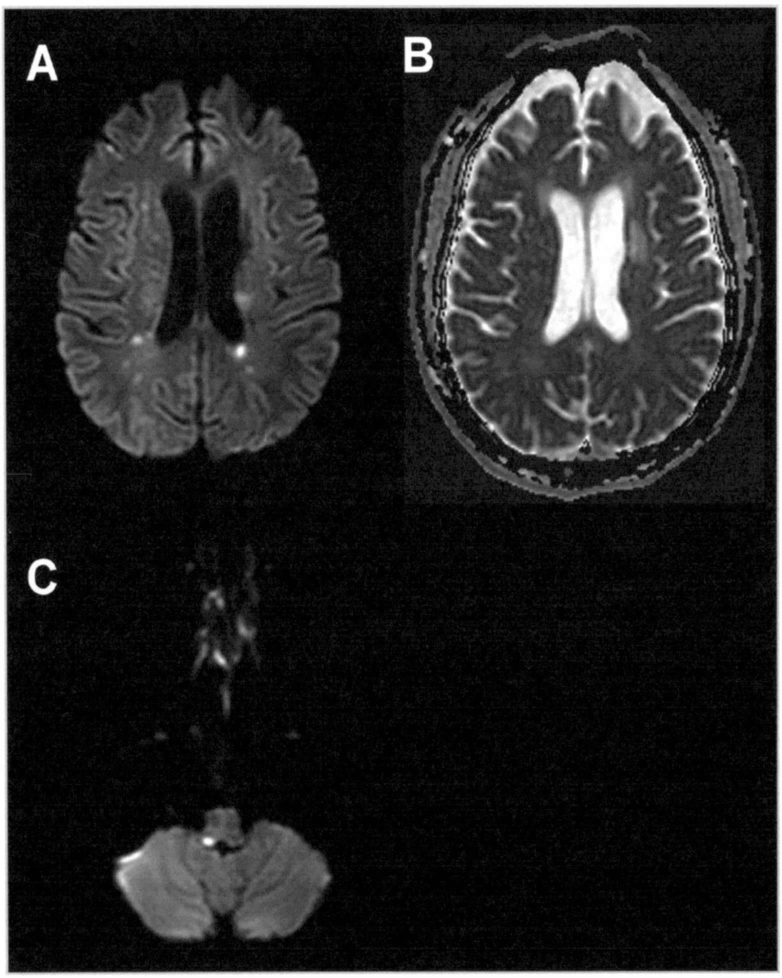

Figure 2. Magnetic resonance imaging (MRI) in two cases of asymptomatic and symptomatic cerebral infarction related to catheterization. (A) Diffusion-weighted MR image of Case 1. (B) Apparent diffusion coefficient (AMC) map of Case 1. (C) DW-MR image of Case 2.

4. A single center retrospective analysis of catheterization-related cerebral infarction

We next present the summarized results of a single center analysis of catheterization-related cerebral infarction in our cardiovascular center. A total of 84 patients who had undergone 1237 consecutive catheterizations with follow-up MRI within 14 days, between 2010 and 2011, were retrospectively analyzed. Of these, 10 symptomatic patients underwent MRI to check for cerebral infarction. The remaining 74 patients were asymptomatic, and underwent MRI for preliminary assessment before coronary artery bypass graft (35%), valvular surgery (18%), or aortic repair (6.8%). MRI revealed cerebral infarction in 5 out of 10 symptomatic patients (50%), and in 22 out of 74 asymptomatic patients (29.7%). Patient background characteristics are presented in Tables 1 and 2. In univariate analysis, the prevalence of dyslipidemia, the number of atherosclerotic risk factors, the number of catheters used, the procedure time, urgent settings, and reasons for intervention differed significantly between patients with and without cerebral infarction (Tables 1 and 2). Dyslipidemia and the number of catheters used were identified as predictive of catheterization-related cerebral infarction by multivariate analysis (odds ratio [OR], 4.66; 95% CI, 1.32–20.2; P=0.02 and OR, 2.04; 95% CI 1.02–4.35; P=0.04, respectively). Overall, the rate of asymptomatic catheterization-related cerebral infarction detected by DW-MRI was high (29.7%). This may be partially due to selection bias because MRI was performed in candidates for cardiac surgery for atherosclerotic disease. The rate of catheterization-related symptomatic ischemic stroke recorded in this study (0.24%) is roughly equivalent to those reported in previous studies [1-9].

	Infarction group	**No infarction group**	**P value**
	(n=27)	(n=57)	
Age, yr	74.1±6.6	70.4±9.4	0.08
Male, %	66.7	59.6	0.54
Risk factors			
Hypertension, %	77.8	71.9	0.57
Dyslipidemia, %	81.5	52.6	0.01
Diabetes, %	55.6	36.8	0.11
Smoking, %	63	57.9	0.66
Family history, %	29.6	15.8	0.14
No. of risk factors	3.03±1.26	2.32±1.19	0.014

Table 1. Baseline characteristics

	Infarction group	No infarction group	P value
	(n=27)	(n=57)	
No. of catheters used	2.85±1.1	2.12±0.9	0.003
Catheter size, F	4.44±0.8	4.25±0.6	0.3
Contrast volume, ml	128±55	120±55	0.48
Fluoroscopy time, min	22.7±14	17.1±12	0.04
LV angiogram, %	48.2	43.9	0.71
Aortic angiogram, %	11.1	14	0.71
Urgent, %	22.2	7	0.04
IABP, %	3.7	0	0.14
Purpose of procedure			
Diagnostic, %	74.1	91.2	0.04
Interventional, %	25.9	8.8	0.04
Approach site			
Radial or brachial, %	81.5	80.7	0.93
Femoral, %	18.5	19.3	0.93

Table 2. Procedural characteristics

5. Conclusions

Despite improvements in procedural techniques and catheter design, patients undergoing catheterization remain at greater risk of atherosclerosis. While ischemic or hemorrhagic stroke is the most debilitating complication of such procedures, conferring significant comorbidity and mortality, asymptomatic cerebral infarction, which has been associated with cognitive decline, is also a significant complication. Intervention against atherosclerotic risk factors is needed along with careful procedural planning, in order to reduce rates of catheterization-related cerebral infarction. Hypercholesterolemia is one of risks of catheterization-related cerebral infarction.

Acknowledgements

This work is supported from the AstraZeneca Research Grant and Grant from the Tazuke Kofukai Reseach Institute.

http://dx.doi.org/10.5772/59282

Author details

Yusuke Morita, Takao Kato* and Moriaki Inoko

*Address all correspondence to: takao-kato@kitano-hp.or.jp

Cardiovascular Center, the Tazuke Kofukai Medical Research Institute, Kitano Hospital, Ogimachi, Kita-ku, Osaka, Japan

References

[1] Noto TJ Jr, Johnson LW, Krone R, Weaver WF, Clark DA, Kramer JR Jr, Vetrovec GW. Cardiac catheterization 1990: a report of the Registry of the Society. Cathet Cardiovasc Diagn. 1991 Oct;24(2):75-83.

[2] Brown DL, Topol EJ. Stroke complicating percutaneous coronary revascularization. Am J Cardiol. 1993 Nov 15;72(15):1207-9.

[3] Lazar JM, Uretsky BF, Denys BG, Reddy PS, Counihan PJ, Ragosta M. Predisposing risk factors and natural history of acute neurologic complications of left-sided cardiac catheterization. Am J Cardiol. 1995 May 15;75(15):1056-60.

[4] Cubo E, Estefania CM, Monaco M, Monaco E, Gonzalez M, Egido JA, Gonzalez JL, Macaya C. Risk factors of stroke after percutaneous transluminal coronary angioplasty. Eur J Neurol. 1998 Sep;5(5):459-462.

[5] Fuchs S, Stabile E, Kinnaird TD, Mintz GS, Gruberg L, Canos DA, Pinnow EE, Kornowski R, Suddath WO, Satler LF, Pichard AD, Kent KM, Weissman NJ. Stroke complicating percutaneous coronary interventions: incidence, predictors, and prognostic implications. Circulation. 2002 Jul 2;106(1):86-91.

[6] Dukkipati S, O'Neill WW, Harjai KJ, Sanders WP, Deo D, Boura JA, Bartholomew BA, Yerkey MW, Sadeghi HM, Kahn JK. Characteristics of cerebrovascular accidents after percutaneous coronary interventions. J Am Coll Cardiol. 2004 Apr 7;43(7): 1161-7.

[7] Wong SC, Minutello R, Hong MK. Neurological complications following percutaneous coronary interventions (a report from the 2000-2001 New York State Angioplasty Registry). Am J Cardiol. 2005 Nov 1;96(9):1248-50.

[8] Aggarwal A, Dai D, Rumsfeld JS, Klein LW, Roe MT; American College of Cardiology National Cardiovascular Data Registry. Incidence and predictors of stroke associated with percutaneous coronary intervention. Am J Cardiol. 2009 Aug 1;104(3): 349-53.

[9] Hoffman SJ, Routledge HC, Lennon RJ, Mustafa MZ, Rihal CS, Gersh BJ, Holmes DR Jr, Gulati R. Procedural factors associated with percutaneous coronary intervention-related ischemic stroke. JACC Cardiovasc Interv. 2012 Feb;5(2):200-6.

[10] Hoffman SJ, Holmes DR Jr, Rabinstein AA, Rihal CS, Gersh BJ, Lennon RJ, Bashir R, Gulati R. Trends, predictors, and outcomes of cerebrovascular events related to percutaneous coronary intervention: a 16-year single-center experience. JACC Cardiovasc Interv. 2011 Apr;4(4):415-22.

[11] Singh M, Rihal CS, Gersh BJ, Roger VL, Bell MR, Lennon RJ, Lerman A, Holmes DR Jr. Mortality differences between men and women after percutaneous coronary interventions. A 25-year, single-center experience. J Am Coll Cardiol. 2008 Jun 17;51(24): 2313-20.

[12] Vermeer SE, Prins ND, den Heijer T, Hofman A, Koudstaal PJ, Breteler MM. Silent brain infarcts and the risk of dementia and cognitive decline. N Engl J Med. 2003 Mar 27;348(13):1215-22.

[13] Fiebach JB, Schellinger PD, Jansen O, Meyer M, Wilde P, Bender J, Schramm P, Jüttler E, Oehler J, Hartmann M, Hähnel S, Knauth M, Hacke W, Sartor K. CT and diffusion-weighted MR imaging in randomized order: diffusion-weighted imaging results in higher accuracy and lower interrater variability in the diagnosis of hyperacute ischemic stroke. Stroke. 2002 Sep;33(9):2206-10.

[14] Gass A, Ay H, Szabo K, Koroshetz WJ. Diffusion-weighted MRI for the "small stuff": the details of acute cerebral ischaemia. Lancet Neurol. 2004 Jan;3(1):39-45.

[15] Fiehler J, Knudsen K, Kucinski T, Kidwell CS, Alger JR, Thomalla G, Eckert B, Wittkugel O, Weiller C, Zeumer H, Rother J. Predictors of apparent diffusion coefficient normalization in stroke patients. Stroke. 2004 Feb;35(2):514-9.

[16] Bendszus M, Koltzenburg M, Burger R, Warmuth-Metz M, Hofmann E, Solymosi L. Silent embolism in diagnostic cerebral angiography and neurointerventional procedures: a prospective study. Lancet. 1999 Nov 6;354(9190):1594-7.

[17] Lund C, Nes RB, Ugelstad TP, Due-Tønnessen P, Andersen R, Hol PK, Brucher R, Russell D. Cerebral emboli during left heart catheterization may cause acute brain injury. Eur Heart J. 2005 Jul;26(13):1269-75.

[18] Büsing KA, Schulte-Sasse C, Flüchter S, Süselbeck T, Haase KK, Neff W, Hirsch JG, Borggrefe M, Düber C. Cerebral infarction: incidence and risk factors after diagnostic and interventional cardiac catheterization--prospective evaluation at diffusion-weighted MR imaging. Radiology. 2005 Apr;235(1):177-83.

[19] Kojuri J, Mehdizadeh M, Rostami H, Shahidian D. Clinical significance of retinal emboli during diagnostic and therapeutic cardiac catheterization in patients with coronary artery disease. BMC Cardiovasc Disord. 2011 Jan 21;11:5.

[20] Omran H, Schmidt H, Hackenbroch M, Illien S, Bernhardt P, von der Recke G, Fimmers R, Flacke S, Layer G, Pohl C, Lüderitz B, Schild H, Sommer T. Silent and apparent cerebral embolism after retrograde catheterization of the aortic valve in valvular stenosis: a prospective, randomized study. Lancet. 2003 Apr 12;361(9365):1241-6.

Section 2

Role of Phytochemicals and Statin on Hypercholesterolemia

Chapter 7

Medicinal Values of Selected Mushrooms with Special Reference to Anti-Hypercholesterolemia

Choong Yew Keong

Additional information is available at the end of the chapter

http://dx.doi.org/10.5772/59424

1. Introduction

1.1. Hypercholesterolemia

Hypercholesterolemia is a known major risk factor in the development of athereosclerosis [29, 32, 51]. This circumstance is caused by internal homeostasis due to foods consumed. The hypercholesterolemia may be related to high cholesterol diet or regular saturated fatty acids intake [42]. The incidence of Chronic Heart Disease (CHD) remains high despite blood pressure being controlled in hypertensive patients. Thus, in hypercholesterolemia patient's LDL (Low Density Lipoprotein) concentration increases, and the lipoprotein is more aged and more susceptible to oxidative modifications than LDL from healthy subjects [50]. These patients have been diagnosed with disability of LDL excreation and very low LDL receptor activity. The most potent inhibitors of cellular cholesterol synthesis are inhibitors of 3-hydroxy-3-methyglutaryl coenzyme A (HMG-CoA) reductase and consequently elevated the cellular LDL receptors synthesis, resulting in significant reduction of plasma LDL levels. [66].

1.1.1. Relation of hypercholesterolemia with atherosclerosis

Atherosclerosis is the disease caused by accumulation of foam cells originated from the monocytes which are transformed into macrophages that engulf excessive oxidized lipoprotein cholesterol. There was an increased foam cell formation which leads to intimal thickening after migration of smooth muscle cells to the intima and lamellar calcification under the endothelium. Finally a typical plaque characterized (Voet and Voet, 1990). The lumen of the arteries was narrowed and high blood pressure induced. The formation of plaque occurrs internally and raises the risk of cardiovascular diseases (CVDs) and strokes while remaining asymptomatic.

Cholesterol is an important component and needed in development of metabolism cell, but the excess of cholesterol content in serum could be problematic. Preclinical and clinical studies have shown that high cholesterol diet is regarded as a main factor in the development of hypercholesterolemia, atherosclerosis and ischemic heart disease [14]. The cholesterol content in hypercholesterolemia cases produced extremely high risk agents such as oxygen free radicals in serum as well as erythrocytes, platelets and endothelial cells. The elevation of total serum cholesterol and LDL cholesterol along with generation of reactive oxygen species (ROS) play a key role in the development of coronary artery disease and atherosclerosis.

In term of mechanism, these vascular problems of atherosclerosis, hypercholesterolemia and hypertension are all correlated to each other. The formation of plaque is associated with a period of time and relies on homeostasis of each individual in dealing with good cholesterol (HDL: high-density lipoprotein) and bad cholesterol (LDL).

Today, strategies and remedies are available to combat CVDs. Even though changing life style with appropriate dietary intake remains the first line of defence advocated by the healthcare workers, drug treatment is still widely used because of the rapid effect especially in treating severe cases [7]. Hence, most research today focuses on screening and identifying compounds exhibiting anti-hypercholesterolemic properties.

To date, several cholesterol lowering medications were discovered and used singly or in combination to lower the LDL cholesterol and triglycerides, a type of fats in the blood that also increases the risk of atherosclerosis. Concomitantly increase of HDL cholesterol often offers protection from CVDs [21]. These types of drug include, bile acid binding resins, cholesterol absorption inhibitor, combination cholesterol absorption inhibitor and statins such as ezetimibe-simvastatin, fibrates, niacin and omega-3 fatty acids. However, almost all the anti-hypercholesteromia drugs have been reported as having various adverse effects [46]. Several side effects such as constipation, nausea, diarrhea, stomach pain, cramps, muscle soreness, pain and weakness are reported; while more severe side-effects such as facial and neck flushing, nausea, vomiting, diarrhea, gout, high blood sugar etc. are also known. The side effects of statin and niacin are similar to each other. In addition, adverse drug reactions are always encountered in multiple diseases treated with a number of drugs. If hypercholesterolemia is accompanied by other diseases, these diseases may have an impact on the response of the body to anti-hypercholesterolemia drugs and the metabolic processes of the body may be affected negatively. Later on, increased dosages may be required, which in turn would only worsen the cholesterol medication drugs. The search for cholesterol lowering medication has now turned to complementary traditional medicine. However, the traditional use of herbs in lowering cholesterol is often not verified scientifically. On the other hand, even if proven effective, such herbs should be investigated on their mechanisms of action.

1.1.2. Mushrooms as medicinal-functional food against hypercholesterolemia

Medicinal mushrooms have been scientifically proven to be safe, efficacious, and novel anti-hypercholesterolemia therapeutic agents of natural source. An abundance of scientific research

http://dx.doi.org/10.5772/59424

and studies on medicinal mushrooms or edible mushrooms shed light on them as functional food due to their broad spectrum of therapeutic efficacy beside culinary demand [80].

The original term "functional food" has been defined by Martirosyan (1992) as "a natural or processed food that contains known biologically-active compounds which when in defined quantitative and qualitative amounts provides a clinically proven and documented health benefit, and thus, an important source in the prevention, management and treatment of chronic diseases of the modern age".

Medicinal Mushrooms (macrofungi), mostly members of the class Basidiomycetes fulfil the requirement of functional foods. Recently, they have become increasingly attractive as functional foods for their potential beneficial effects on human health. Hence, the food industry is especially interested in cultivating these mushrooms. The wild edible mushrooms have gained their reputation as health food due to their geographical origin in natural unpolluted environment. Nonetheless the cultivation of medicinal mushrooms using modern technology and the quality of the extracted product are crucial factors determining them as functional-medicinal food.

A plethora of potent therapeutic components in medicinal mushrooms such as fibers, phytosterols, saponins, polyphenols, flavanoids, terpenes and polysaccharides confer antihypercholesterolemic, antioxidant and anti-atherosclerotic properties [80].

The intensive study of [33] reported the hypocholesterolemic effect of the mushroom fruiting bodies and several types of these extracts exhibited different mechanisms of action, such as impairing dietary cholesterol absorption or inhibiting the endogenous cholesterol metabolism. Other reports showed that medicinal mushrooms are rich in chitin (dietary fibre) and specific β-glucans which may inhibit cholesterol absorption by increasing the faecal excretion of bile acids and reducing the amount of serum LDL-cholesterol [19, 28].

Among the most studied mushroom species are *Tricholoma giganteum* (giant mushroom), *Marasmius androsaceus* (horsehair parachute mushroom), *Grifola frondosa* (maitake mushroom), *Pleurotus* species (oyster mushroom), *Lentinula edodes* (shiitake mushroom), *Ganoderma lucidum* (reishi or lingzhi mushroom), *Sparassis crispa* (cauliflower mushroom), *Pholiota adiposa* (black tiger's paw mushroom), *Sarcodon aspratus* (yellow cap mushroom), *Hypsizygus marmoreus* (shimeji/buna shimeji mushroom), *Flammulina velutipes* (enoki mushroom), *Hericium erinaceus* (lion's mane mushroom), and *Agaricus bisporus* (button mushroom) [65].

The objectives of this article are to review the possible anti-hypercholesterolemic mechanisms of some putative bioactive compounds extracted from well known medical mushrooms particularly *G. lucidum*.

2. Selective mushrooms as anti-hypercholesterolemia agent

Ganoderma species are Basidiomycetes belonging to Polyporaceae (or Ganodermataceae) of Aphyllophorales. They differ from the ordinary mushrooms and are categorized in the order

Agaricales in that they have pores rather than gills on the surface of the fruiting bodies. *G. lucidum* has been reported to have multi-beneficial values and concerted medicinal effects in the treatment of various diseases. The recent application of modern analytical techniques has, in a number of cases, provided a scientific basic for these earlier empirical observation. Thus, many putatively effective compounds are isolated and identified from *G. lucidum*. The pharmacological activities of *G. lucidum* have been attributed mainly to its polysaccharides and triterpenes [24].

2.1. *Ganoderma* polysaccharides

As fungal wall constituents, bioactive polyglycans (polysaccharides), such as β-glucans in *G. lucidum*, are found in all parts of the mushroom, including the mycelium (Bartnicki-Garcia, 1968). Fungal polyglycans can also be secreted into the growth medium and become extracellular (Buck *et al.*, 1968). Bioactive polyglycans in *G. lucidum* comprise neutral polysaccharides (β-1,3, β-1,6 homo D-glucan), acidic glucan and polyglycan [60], protein-bond heteroglucan [58], arabinoxyoglucan, a highly branched heteroglucan [61], with a heteroglycan with β-(1,4) core [62], and peptidoglycan: ganoderan A, B, C [35] in the fruiting body [84], β-D glucan [72] and lucidan, a protein-bond heteroglycan [44], as well as other polyglycans in the mycelia which have not been characterized.

In fact, *Ganoderma* glucans, β-(1,3), β-(1,6)-D-glucan is blocked by basic unit of β-(1,3)-D-glucopyronan which consists of 1-15 units of β-(1,6) monoglucosyl side chains (Mizuno, 1991). Numerous reports show that β-(1,3), β-(1,6)-D-glucans with molecular weight of 10^4-10^6 Daltons exhibit antitumor activity (Mizuno, 1991). It seems that the higher the molecular weight, the more effective anti-hypercholesterolemia activity. Anti-hypercholesterolemia activity is also linked to the frequency of polysaccharide branching which varies during different stages of mycelial growth. Different extraction and purification processes yield a variety of bioactive glycans. Identification of these large and highly complex bioactive *Ganoderma* polysaccharides, whose precise structures have not been elucidated, involved expensive process.

2.2. *Ganoderma* Triterpenes

Triterpenes are relatively simple molecules which are easy to isolate and quantify. They can be used as a measure of the quality of different *Ganoderma* samples [24] (Stavinoha, 1995). Twenty or so bioactive triterpenes have been isolated from *G. lucidum* although over one hundred with known chemical compositions and molecular configurations have been reported to occur in *G. lucidum*.

Triterpenes are produced in the fruiting body. They can also be induced in the mycelial mat on solid medium (Nishitoba *et al.*, 1987) or in the still liquid culture of late stationary phase [86]. Limited amount of triterpene is formed in the mycelial pellets of liquid shaking culture [76]. It is said that strains producing basidiocarps with a light yellow underside may contain a high amount of triterpenes in their caps. Such observation has been used to grade commercial *Ganodema* fruiting bodies in Asia [37]. [75] found that the highest concentration of *Ganoderma* triterpenes was in the spore scrapings obtained from the underside of the mushroom in the

1-2 mm tube region (the hymenial layer). Only 18-58 mg of bioactive triterpenes were obtained from 1000 g of *Ganoderma tsugae* basidiocarps, while 4.5% (w/v) of crude ethanol extract was obtained from the sample [77]; thus, Stavinoha *et al.* (1993) used spore scrapings from the mushroom underside instead of the whole mushroom for extracting bioactive triterpenes.

The bitter taste of *G. lucidum* as a traditional Chinese medicine or tonic is attributed to its highly oxygenated polar triterpenes [54]. Triterpenes as secondary metabolites are more strain specific in *G. lucidum* [64]. High temperature and prolonged oxidation should be avoided during extraction to retain intact structures of these volatile compounds [37].

3. Mechanism on different biomedical application of *Ganoderma lucidum*

There are many studies on *G. lucidum* worldwide due to its superior therapeutic value in tackling many types of diseases. However the mechanisms involved have yet to be clarified and fully understood. This review is undertaking to specify the anti-hypercholesterolemia mechanisms of different *G. lucidum* medicinal compounds.

Excretion of second metabolism products of the mushroom are used for self protection in extremely severe environment condition. The second metabolism products of *G. lucidum*, which included β-glucans and triterpenes have been known to possess a broad spectrum of health benefits from disease prevention and maintenance of health to the regulation or treatment of chronic as well as acute life threatening illness [16]. The anti-hypercholesterolemia therapeutics of *G. lucidum* extracts involved several types of mechanisms.

3.1. Mechanism of inhibitory effect of ganoderic acid on HMG-CoA reductase

Previous research by [85] focused on the oxygenated lanostanoid triterpenes isolated from *G. lucidum*. The pure isolated triterpenes taste bitter and some are cytotoxic. Their unique chemical structures have been studied in detail. The derivatives of these terpenes type compounds (Figure 1) were obtained through chemical conversion during inhibition of cholesterol biosynthesis.

These mushroom triterpenes inhibited histamine release from rat mast cells. Compound VI with 7-oxo and 15 α-hydroxy groups at 40 μM showed highly potential inhibition of cholesterol synthesis from [24,25-3H]-24,25-dihydrolanosterol (18 μM). This encouraging result was obtained by testing 24, 25-dihydrolanosterol on rat hepatic subcellular 10,000 xg supernatant fraction. The triterpene involved is ganoderic acid C methyl ester. Its derivative is synthesized by a complicated reaction included the yield of tri β-methoxyethoxymethyl ether (MEM) derivative under Wolff-Kishner condition to allow the 7-oxo-11-deoxo derivative further decarboxylation and deprotection of the hydroxyl group. The whole structure of compound VI has no functional group in the side chain and has both 7-oxo and 15 α-hydroxy groups on the same skeleton and showed potent inhibitory effect compared with other derivatives with carboxyl groups at the side chain.

Compound I and II showed the other derivatives with oxo group at C-23 and decarboxyl compounds at the side chain had moderate inhibitory effects. Derivatives of compond IV and

V has carboxyl group at C-25 in the side chain showed almost no inhibitory effect. These results provided an excellent clue and fundamental of specific side of triterpenes on the discovery of other *G. lucidum* bioactive triterpenes in anti-hypercholesterolemic study.

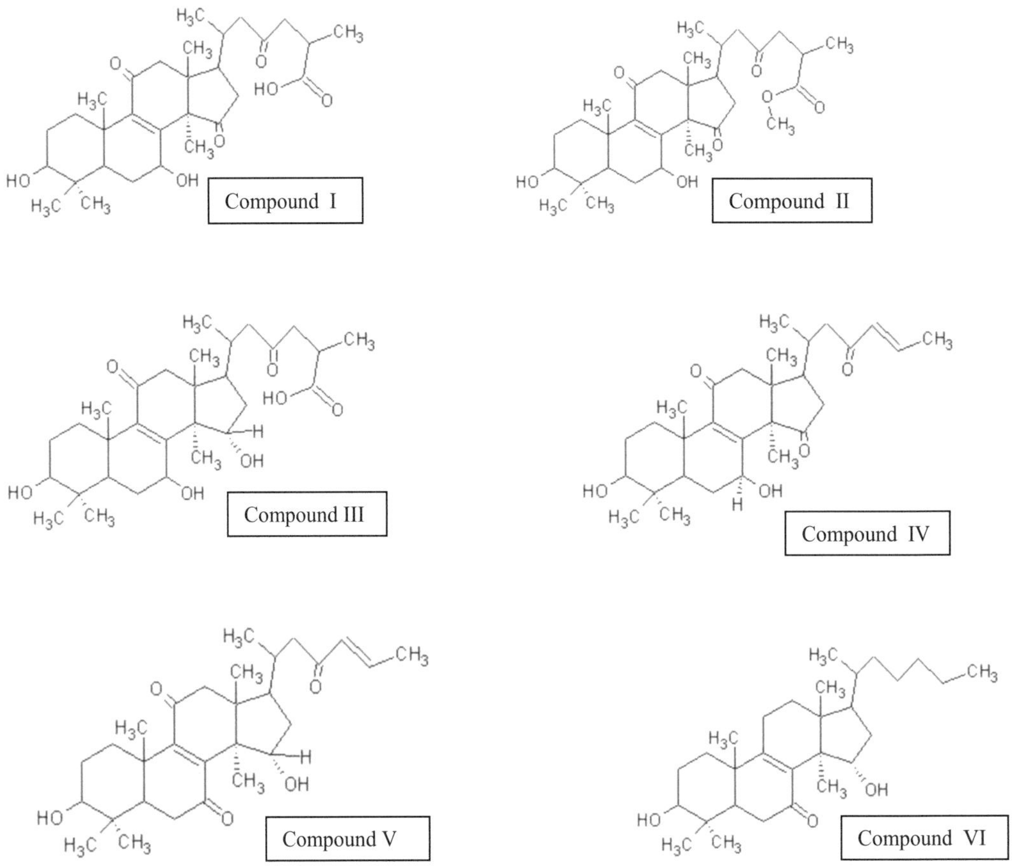

(Source: [84]

Figure 1. Ganoderic acid B methyl ester (compound II) was obtained by treating compound I with ethereal diazomethane. Decarboxylated compounds IV and V were synthesized by the reaction of compound I and III with lead tetraacetate in the presence of cupric acetate containing a drop of pyridine in refluxing benzene. In the case of V derived from III, the 7β-hydroxyl group was further oxidized to the carbonyl group.

3.1.1. Mechanism

Figure 2 showed the statins as HMG-CoA reductase inhibitor drug playing its key role in the pathway of blocking the biosynthesis mevalonate from the HMG-CoA. The mechanism involved the statin by interrupting the structure of HMG-CoA reductase binding to NADPH in HMG-CoA to produce mevalonate. Therefore the metabolic pathway that produces cholesterol and other isoprenoids has terminated.

http://dx.doi.org/10.5772/59424

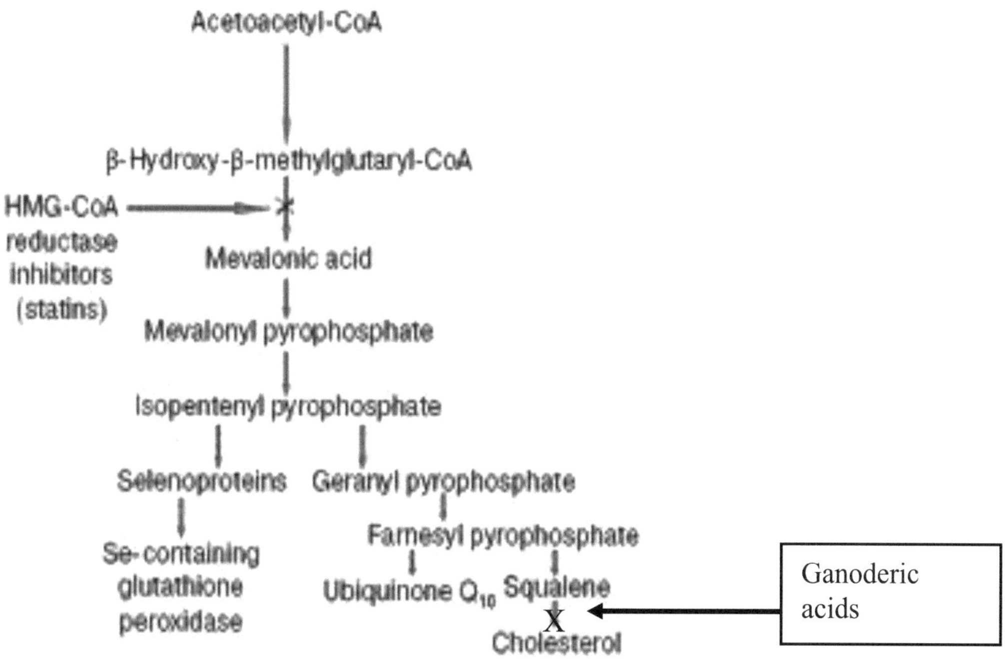

(Source: [84]; (Akira Endo, 1971)

Figure 2. Figure 2 showed the statins as HMG-CoA reductase inhibitor drug play its key role in the pathway of blocking the biosynthesis mevalonate from the HMG-CoA. Whereby ganoderic acid inhibit the cholesterol formation by competed with squalene oxido-cyclase at the last stage of cholesterol synthesis.

Akira Endo and his group discovered statins in 1976, and these HMG-CoA reductase inhibitors showed competitive effect on inhibiting HMG reductase due to their very close molecular structure to HMG-CoA. The use of statins is able to reduce the blood cholesterol levels significantly as HMG reductase is the first committed enzyme in the sequence of cholesterol synthesis cumulative process. However, since mevalonic acid (MVA) is a common precursor for many isoprenoids, blocking of MVA formation may induce undesired side effects besides inhibiting sterol synthesis. More specific inhibition of cholesterol synthesis may be attained by inhibition at some later stage of cholesterol synthesis. In this case, lanosterol was chosen in the ganoderic acid test as it originally converts from squalene by squalene oxido-cyclase at the end of cholesterol synthesis (Figure 2).

3.1.2. Comparison of structure of statins and ganoderic acid derivatives

These renowned drugs have been studied for their functional anti-hypercholesterolemic mechanism as a model for preliminary comparison of undefined natural products based on the results of the laboratory and the spectroscopy elucidation of their structure. Therefore the highest percentage of similarity of both compound structures implied similar highest effectiveness. This theory has been validated when the structure of HMG-CoA and the binding site of competitor lovastatin drug in HMG-CoA reductase inhibition was compared (figure 3).

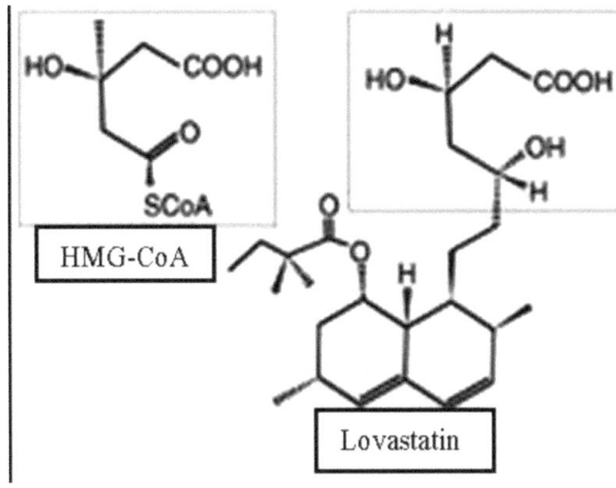

Figure 3. Comparison structure of HMG-CoA and the binding site of competitor lovstatin drug in HMG-CoA reductase inhibition.

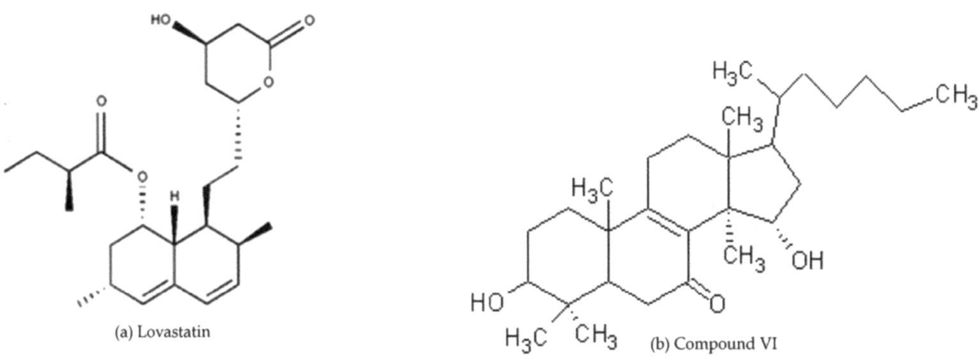

Figure 4. Comparative molecular structure of lavastatin as pharmaceutical drug and compound VI as triterpene derivative of ganoderic acid.

The active side of lovastatin is circled in box, while the structure site of the ganoderic acid derivatives automatically refers to the site chain for comparison. The important difference is statin inhibited the earlier stage of cholesterol formation whereby ganoderic acid inhibited at the late stages of cholesterol formation. Figure (4a) showed that lavostatin has 5 carbons in aromatic ring when the reaction of carboxyl group and the hydroxyl group occurred. The active sites mostly rely on the double bond of oxide group and the beta hydroxyl group. The position of both active sites is separated and impossible to react intra-molecularly. Conversely the site chain of ganoderic acid derivatives (figure 4b) is aliphatic whereby the position of carboxyl group and double bond could possibly interact. Compound IV and V (in figure 1) has close double bond at C-23 and 24 and this contribute to instability. Structure of figure (VI) shows that it is a potent inhibitor but is surprisingly without any carboxyl and double bond at the site chain. Its competitor effect could be due to the interaction of C-7 and C-15 with the binding site of 24, 25-dihydrolanosterol. The binding site of ganoderic acids with 24, 25-dihydrolanosterol is essentially similar to ganoderic acid and hence no side effect to the patient will result.

3.2. Mechanism as angiotensin converting enzyme inhibitor in rennin angiotension-aldosterone system

The other mechanism that could apparently be involved is the inhibition of angiotensin converting enzyme (ACE) in renin-angiotensin system. This system is indirectly related to hypercholesterolemia. Atherosclerosis is the main contributory factor in this case but it may result in high blood pressure due to the narrowing of lumen of blood arteries. Therefore the regulatory mechanism of blood pressure by vasoconstriction and vasodilation may attenuate the hypercholesterolemia impact.

[62] identified five novel lanostane triterpenes, namely ganoderal A; ganoderols A and B; ganoderic acids K and S in the methanolic extract. These compounds were tested for their ACE inhibitory effect by a modification of the method described by Friedland and Silverstein (1976) and expressed in terms of IC_{50} (the amount of samples needed to inhibit 50% of ACE activity). All the newly discovered lanostane triterpenes showed IC_{50} of the order of 10^{-5} M which is considered potent. However, the earlier reported ganoderic acid F (figure 5) achieved the highest inhibitory effect with IC_{50} of 4.7×10^{-6} M.

In 2012, Abdullah *et al.* reported that the hot water extract of *G. lucidum* exhibited the best ACE inhibitory effect compared to other culinary-medicinal mushrooms. Normally the hot water extract consists of polar compounds. It has been proposed that the multitudes of phenolic substances present in *G. lucidum* contributed to this inhibitory action [62]. In addition the anti-ACE activity of the hot water extract of *G. lucidum* was enhanced when the mushroom was grown on the germinated brown rice [35].

3.2.1. Mechanism of Renin-Angiotensin System (RAS) of G. lucidum extract

The RAS is important for the aldosterone hormone system in kidneys and lung. Consequently, the blood pressure and water (fluid) balance is regulated.

Briefly, when the blood volume is low in the circulation, this scenario would be sensed by the juxtaglomerular cells at the afferent arterioles of the renal glomeruli [11] in kidneys and concurrently activate the prorenin which converts to renin directly into circulation. Plasma rennin hydrolyzes its substrate, angiotensinogen released by the liver to produce a decapeptide known as angiotensin I, which is then rapidly converted to an octapeptide, angiotensin II, by a circulating angiotensin-converting enzyme found in the lungs. Angiotensin II is a potent vasoconstrictor peptide that stimulates the cells of the zona glomerulosa of adrenal cortex to produce aldosterone [10] and [41] which causes blood vessels to constrict, resulting in increased blood pressure. When the re-intake of sodium and water in the kidneys tubules is caused by Aldosterone, the body fluid eventually increases resulting in increase of blood pressure. [4].

3.2.2. ACE inhibitor

Interrupting the RAS effectively control the constriction of blood vessels. When the arteries are confronted with the problem of narrowing lumen caused by the formation of plaque in hypercholesterolemia, the treatment of using ACE inhibitor or compound that blocks the activity of ACE could reduce some risk drastically via vasodilation. Most of the synthetic pharmaceutical drug for the treatment of hypertension has no curative effect, and in fact needs prolonged administration for congestive heart failure protection. These types of drugs are usually used in combination with other medication and are usually well-tolerated by most individuals. Nevertheless, side effects such as cough, headache, drowsiness, weakness, abnormal taste (metallic or salty taste), rash are very common. By testing the active ingredient(s) in *G. lucidum*, it is possible to identify ACE inhibitor(s) which may be devoid of side effect.

3.2.3. Comparative structure of ACE inhibitor captopril and ganoderic acid F

Captopril (figure 5) is a ACE inhibitor used for the treatment of hypertension and some types of congestive heart failure. Captopril plays its role in blocking the conversion of angiotensin I to angiotensin II. Both captopril and ganoderic acid F are highly active ACE inhibitor. In term of structure, captopril contains a side chain with 3 carbons with different functional groups and an aromatic ring formed with 4 carbons and a nitrogen atom as the main attachment to the side chain. The molecule is small with a molecular weight of 217 Daltons. In contrast, ganoderic acid F is a natural product. Its structure is huge with 7 carbons at the side chain attached to the main skeleton which contains 4 aromatic rings. Its molecular weight is 2.6 times more than captopril. Both compounds have the carboxyl, ketone and methyl functional groups except captopril which, in addition has a sulphate group at the tail. There is no sulphate and nitrogen atom in ganoderic acid F.

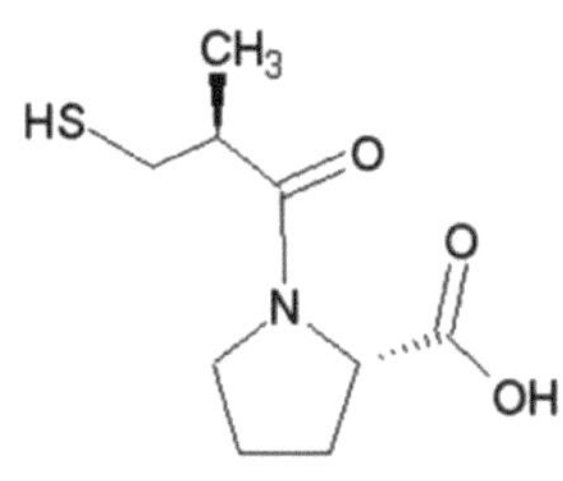

Captopril

Figure 5. Comparative molecular structure of captopril as a commercial pharmaceutical drug and ganoderic acid F extracted from *G. lucidum*.

Comparison of the molecular structure cannot really ascertain the effectiveness of both compounds in term of anti-hypertension or indirectly on anti-hypercholesterol activity. In addition, there are many other differences in term of their configurations and binding site of both compounds. Moreover, there could be many other factors influencing the mechanism of RAS system. As the comparison is based on the isolated and characterized *G. lucidum* lanostane triterpenes which have shown ACE-inhibitory activity, this wound provide some hints on the working structure. The effect of captopril on hypertension is rapid but comes with side effect. While ganoderic acid F is a natural product, experimental studies and clinical trials are still needed. The findings from this present review contrasted the conclusion by [8] that the compounds responsible for anti-hypertensive activity have molecular weights of more than 1,000,000 Daltons, based on their in vivo data in Spontaneously Hyoertensive rats.

3.3. Mechanism of inhibition of oxidative damage

Extracts prepared from either mycelial or fruiting body of *G. lucidum* have been accorded a prominent role as a source of natural antioxidants [57]. The antioxidant activity of these extracts was found mainly correlated with their polysaccharide content as well as with their phenolic content [21]. Several scientific reports [26, 38, 45] have proven that the mechanism involved is direct inhibition of the process of oxidation at the cell membrane of the host. The reactive compounds react directly with the free radicals and neutralize the oxidation effect in reducing oxi LDL which forms the key precursor in cardiovascular diseases included hypercholesterolemia. The physiological effects of these extracts was shown to depend on the strain and the nature of cultivation [65].

$(1 \rightarrow 6)$ or $(1 \rightarrow 3)$-β-D-glucans from *G. lucidum* are reportedly potential drugs against oxidation. These substances seem to enhance the activity of the immune system, but there is no accepted mechanism of action nor agreement on the parameters which influence the activity (Werner *et al.*, 1997). Therefore, glucans with different structures and/ or varying molar mass were characterized by spectroscopy, spectrometry coupled with size-exclusion chromatography in order to obtain the molar mass distribution and to gain an idea of the structure in solution. The activity of polysaccharides is determined by their conformation, composition and size [13]. Additionaly, polysaccharides may contribute to the oxidation properties, depending on their molecular structure, the sugar unit and conformation in whole. [78]

Many synthetic chemicals such as phenolic compounds are found to be strong radical scanvengers but they usually have side effects [33]. Most of the 2,2-diphenyl-1-picrylhydrazyl (DPPH) scavenging activities of *G. lucidum* crude extract were compared with those of the well-known antioxidants such as vitamin C. At all concentrations tested, the *G. lucidum* polysaccharides exhibited a dose-dependent DPPH radical-scavenging activity. [19]

3.3.1. *The mechanism of scavenging DPPH radicals*

Crude hot water extract of *G. lucidum* showed its maximum scavenging activity (94.8%) at 2.5 mg/mL. However a declining tendency was also noted with higher concentrations (till 10 mg/mL). This could be caused by limitation of solubility, and increased hydrogen bonding once the concentration of polysaccharide is increased. [43] reported that the concentration of available hydroxyl groups is responsible for the scavenging ability of polysaccharides. [56] supported the direct relationship between monosaccharide composition and conformation of side chains with scavenging ability of polysaccharides. In this case, the scavenging of DPPH radicals is conducted by the arabinose linked by 1, 4 linkages of the side-chain and glucose linked to the 1,6 glycosidic linkage respectively [57].

3.3.2. *Inhibition of Lipid Peroxidation (LPO)*

LPO is regarded as one of the basic mechanisms of cellular damage caused by free radicals [68]. The relationship between LPO and hypercholesterolemia is well recognized. A cholesterol rich diet results in increased LPO by the induction of free radical production [3]. Hypercholesterolemia and lipid peroxidation are believed to be critically involved in development of atherosclerosis [9].

G. lucidum extract expressed the same pattern in prevention of linoleic acid peroxidation. In such experiment, the antioxidant activity of *G. ludicum* extract increased from 0.1 to 10.0 mg/mL and reached a plateau of 77.2–77.3% at 10.0–20.0 mg/mL. [56] measured the inhibition of lipid peroxidation by conjugated diene method. They concluded that strong relationship existed between monosaccharide ratio and antioxidant activity. Antioxidant activity increased with increasing concentrations of mannose and rhamnose,whereas the activity decreased with corresponding increases in concentration of arabinose and glucose.

3.3.3. Reducing power

G. lucidum polysaccharide extract exerted a high potential in hydrogen-donating ability in the ferric–reducing antioxidant power assay [57]. This extract showed promising reducing power gradually when the concentration was increased from 0.1 to 0.5 mg/mL and achieved a relative stable level of 3.2–3.4 at 5.0–20.0 mg/mL. The effectiveness of *G. lucidum* extract in reducing power test was obvious when compared to ascorbic acid tested as positive control which had a reducing power of 3.5 at 20.0 mg/mL.

[70] reported xanthan and methylcellulose showed hardly any hydrogen donating activity compared with the very huge activity of ascorbic acid. [56] also reported that weak relationship was found between monosaccharide composition and reducing ability. In fact the non-polysaccharide components of the *Ganoderma* extract play the main role in reducing power. These components could react with free radicals and eventually stabilize and block chain reactions.

3.3.4. Chelating ability on ferrous ions

The molecular masses of the polysaccharide fractions are important for the chelating ability [43]. The ferrous ions chelating ability of polysaccharides extract of *G. lucidum* is 11.0–64.6% at 0.1–20 mg/mL and achieved a maximum of 68.9 % at 10 mg/mL. A mole number of poly-saccharide is required to chelate a mole number of ferrous (Fe^{2+}) ions. The absolute chelating power is inversely related with the mean molecular mass, showing that higher molecular weight of polysaccharide exhibits higher chelating ability. However, this rule excludes amylopectine and starch which have no chelating effect despite their higher molecular weight. Therefore glycoside linkage of β-D-glucan exhibited higher ranking in chelating ability compared to α-D-glucan.

3.4. Mechanism of inflammation — Hepatoprotective effect

Total triterpenes extract from *G. lucidum* have been tested on two different experimental liver injury mice models induced by carbon tetrachloride and D-galactosamine [69]. In this test model, the extract showed inhibition of liver triglyceride and serum alanine aminotransferase levels significantly. Such result is encouraging when compared to a known reference sub-stance, malotilate for this form of protective effects. Both superoxide dismutases (SOD) activity and the glutathione content have been antagonized and decreased by *G. lucidum* extract. This corresponds to the reduction of malondialdehyde content in the carbon tetrachloride and D-galactosamine liver-injured mice. (Andréia *et al.*, 2013).

These data indicated that peptides and ganoderic acids which have been isolated from *G. lucidum* have a powerful protective effect against liver damage induced by carbon tetrachloride and D-galactosamine. The increased activity of free radical scavenging enzymes could be related to the hepatoprotective effects and, thus, enhancing the effectiveness of anti-oxidation.

However the other experiments revealed administration of *G. lucidum* polysaccharides dose-dependently significantly enhanced antioxidant enzymes activities in the serum of rats fed with polysaccharides compared to model group [73]. Another report reported that rats fed with ergosterol-rich and nicotinic acid-rich extract had significantly higher serum glutathione peroxidase and SOD activities (Andréia, 2013).

The liver is the main organ of detoxification and is the site of metabolic conversion of endogenous and exogenous compounds. Another major function of the liver is to synthesize bile acids from cholesterol and to secrete these compounds from the hepatocytes into the intestine, thereby generating bile flow and facilitating dietary fat emulsification and absorption [82]. The studies on hepatoprotective effect of *G. lucidum* relied on many types of substrates. Since the liver is the main organ of metabolism, many biochemical pathway are related, thus more than one substrates are involved in the respective mechanism.

3.4.1. Mechanism of hepatoprotective effect of Ganoderma extract

Whatever substrates are involved, the basic of this mechanism is promoting the release of SODs into the blood stream. Kurt and Stefan (2014) reported that plasma clearance of human extracellular-superoxide dismutase C (EC-SOD C) in rabbits was initiated in the liver which contained the most 125I-EC-SOD C, followed by kidney, spleen, heart, and lung. This scenario shows that almost all 125I-EC-SOD C in the organs was deposited on endothelial cell surfaces and was not associated with any other tissue cell surfaces, or present within the cells. [47].

Pathology studies on the hepatocytes that the SODs are a family of metalloenzymes which need mineral copper as integral component. About 50–80% copper absorption is maximal in the duodenum and may be absorbed from the stomach. Within the intestinal mucosal cells, copper can react with metallothionein, a sulfhydryl group-rich protein that binds copper through the formation of mercaptide bonds. Factors affecting copper absorption include gender, the chemical form and certain dietary constituents.

The rich and multi nutrient ingredient of ganoderma extract has provided sufficient natural supplement in enhancing the liver metabolism. Besides beta-glucan, coumarin, mannitol, and alkaloids, triterpenes isolated from *G. lucidum* included ganodenic acid which have a molecular structure similar to steroid hormones and ganoderol, ganoderenic acid, ganoderiol, ganodermanontriol, lucidadiol, and ganodermadiol which is believed to stimulate the metabolism of liver to achieve the detoxifying effect. Combination of different substrates and components also provoke the synergic in term of efficacy. It is interesting that phytochemistry profile of *G. lucidum* includes 18 types of amino acids and more than 10 minerals which could be the vital ingredient of 50–80 % cupper and other minerals absorbed from duodenum and stomach in men.

There are three types of SODs in eukaryotic cells catalysing the same reaction. They are copper and zinc-containing SOD (CuZnSOD) exists in cytosol, an manganese-containing SOD (MnSOD) which is encoded in the nucleus, synthesized in the cytosol and imported post-translationally into the mitochondrial matrix, and an extracellular CuZnSOD.

Basically 90% of the cell's oxygen is consumed by MnSOD at the mitochondria matrix. Thus mitochondria are sensitive to oxidative damage, especially inducible by environment oxidative stress. Most probability due to mitochondria are lack of histones and an efficient DNA repair [12].

The SODs are playing their role in the initial stage of cellular anti-oxidant defense by the dismutation of the superoxide radical into hydrogen peroxide and molecular oxygen. Superoxide is the one-electron reduction product of molecular oxygen.

There are two possible equations of SOD-catalysed dismutation of superoxide where the oxidation state of the metal cation oscillates between n and n+1. The half-reactions could be written as :

$$M^{(n+1)+}\text{-SOD} + O_2^- \rightarrow Mn^+\text{-SOD} + O_2$$

$$M^{n+}\text{-SOD} + O_2^- + 2H^+ \rightarrow M^{(n+1)+}\text{-SOD} + H_2O_2$$

The H_2O_2 will be disproportionating to H_2O and O_2 by catalase which is excreted from hepatocytes to complete the oxygen radical detoxification process [12]

The mechanisms of the hepatoprotective effects of *G. lucidum* have been largely undefined. However accumulating evidences suggest most of the identified substrates of *G. lucidum* extract are able to enhance the release of SOD or other anti-oxidant enzymes from the cytosolic and extracellular which have potential hepatoprotective effect. They play their role in modulation of hepatic phase I and II enzymes, modulation of nitric oxide production, and maintenance of hepatocellular calcium homeostasis [81].

3.5. Mechanism on immunostimulation with *Ganoderma* polysaccharides

Many bioactive components in *G. lucidum* are biological response modifiers which stimulate the host's own defense system [54] by evoking favorable immune responses. The cell surface is the *Ganoderma* bioactivity target site in terms of receptors and membrane alternation. In contrast to starch and a number of other naturally occurring polysaccharides, bioactive *Ganoderma* glycans are not degraded into their component sugars in animals or humans. Thus, such fungal polysaccharides are able to produce therapeutic effects. Starch, on the other hand, is decomposed enzymatically into its component sugar, glucose, and can be used as an energy source [37].

Of great interest is the discovery of β-D-glucan receptors on the surface of a number of white blood cells (leukocytes, monocytes, macrophages, natural killer (NK) cells, and other lymphocytes) in animals and humans [17, 22]. The broad stimulatory effects of *Ganoderma* β-glucans, via transduced cell surface receptors in the immune system, lead to the release of cytokines and lymphokines (cell mediators), such as IL-1, IL-2, IL-4 (interleukins), interferon and TNF (tumor necrosis factor). Many immune parameters are improved, e.g., increase of T-cell functions and antibody production. Potential benefits and low toxicity make *Ganoderma* polysaccharides desirable for boosting the immune system of patients undergoing chemotherapy, radiation therapy or during recovery from major surgery [17]. Immunomodulatory effects of *Ganoderma* polysaccharides may also be useful in atherosclerosis, hypercholesterolemia and heart failure prevention.

[64] reported activation of T-cell by administering *Ganoderma* polysaccharides orally. Stimulation of cytokines [15] and activation of cytotoxic NK cells [83] by *Ganoderma* polysaccharides were subsequently reported. The major polysaccharide fraction, β-1,3 glucan has been shown to exhibit a wide-based adjuvant stimulatory activity on macrophages and T-cells, leading to IL-1 [39], IL-2 [15, 87], and TNF production [88] which play a role in antitumor immune surveillance [49]. *Ganoderma* has been reported to have some effects on immunofunctions which can stimulate the activity of acid phosphatase and β-glucuronidase of peritoneal macrophages in mice (Liu, 1993). It is also observed that there is a significant increase in plague forming cell and agglutination titer of anti-sheep erythrocytes (SRBC) antibody as well as the activity of γ interferon of mice [52]. The activity of crude *Ganoderma* extract on NK cells was of specific interest. Firstly, the effectiveness of a water soluble *Ganoderma* polysaccharide fraction derived from mycelium was shown to enhance splenic NK activity in normal mice when administered via intraperitoned, intravenous or oral route. The fraction also restored depressed NK cytotoxicity in tumor-bearing mice [83]. Secondly, the capacity of *Ganoderma* polysaccharide in activating macrophages [89] and lastly the polysaccharides markedly enhanced the cytotoxicity of T-lymphocytes [52]. The last two activities are established tumoricidal affector pathways of the host immune system.

3.6. Mechanism — *Ganoderma lanostane*-type triterpenes as potent Farnesoid-X-Receptor (FXR) agonists

[79] reported the application of *in silico* tools for the identification of natural products, namely *Ganoderma lanostane*-type triterpenes as potent FXR agonists. Intriguingly, three lanostanes secondary metabolites from *G. lucidum*, that is, ergosterol peroxide, ganodermanontriol, and ganoderiol F, dose-dependently induced FXR in the low micromolar range in a reporter gene assay.

The relevance of FXR as bile acid (BA) activated receptor was illustrated with regard to the treatment of atherosclerosis and its counter-regulatory role in immunity and inflammation. FXR exhibits a regulating function in many endogenous pathways. Its active site contains specific features which are well-characterized. These important characteristics have contributed to the attractiveness of this nuclear receptor as an atypical drugable target for the development of novel therapaeutic agents which may be effective in the prevention and treatment of, including, the metabolic syndrome, dyslipidemia and atherosclerosis. Chenodeoxycholic acid (CDCA) and other BA are natural ligands for FXR.

A dose-dependent FXR-inducing activity showed the EC_{50} of the most active lanostanes identified from *G. lucidum* activated FXR at even lower concentrations than control, the ranking from the most active is ergosterol peroxide (0.85l M), ganodermanontriol (2.5l M), ganoderiol F (5.0l M) and the control CDCA (16.8 lM). The tested *Ganoderma* compounds significantly decreased the levels of cholesterol 7α- hydroxylase (CYP7A1) mRNA. The degree of inhibition was similar to that induced by the positive control CDCA.

3.6.1. Comparative molecular structure of active lanostanes and CDCA

Four of the compounds have the basic molecular structure with 3 benzene rings and a penta ring, and the side chain is completely different (Figure 6). In term of number of carbon, ergosterol peroxide has the higher number of carbons at the side chain which is 4 carbons more than CDCA. The other two compounds contain same number of carbon. Ergosterol peroxide has 4 methyl groups at the side chain excluding hydroxyl group. The rest contain at least a hydroxyl group at the side chain with the possibility of intermolecular bond forming. Only ergosterol peroxide and ganoderiol F formed double bond at their side chain but at different position. This is important as double bond is favoured in binding and activating the compound. The position of double bond of ergosterol peroxide is ideal compared with ganoderiol F, because there is no other functional group beside the double bond. There is a carbonyl group at the side chain of CDCA compared with others. This interpretation is comparable with the possible mechanism of inhibition of HMG-CoA reductase by ganoderic acid derivatives, as the compound with carboxyl group at the side chain has lower inhibitory potential. In the component of aromatic ring, the position of carbon 7 determines the activity of the compound. In this case, ergosterol peroxide showed double bond within carbon 6 and 7. Ganodermanontriol and ganoderiol F formed double bond at carbon 7 but within carbon 8 and both compounds have another double bond of which the configuration is not as stable as ergosterol peroxide and CDCA. The interesting point is, only ergosterol peroxide showed the binding of oxygen between carbon 5 and 8 which stablises the compound and equivalent the active side of double bond between carbon 6 and 7 in the ring.

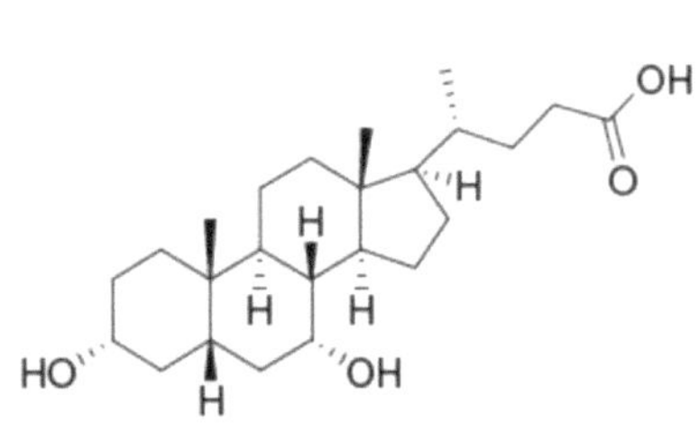

chenodeoxycholic acid (CDCA)

Figure 6. Comparative molecular structure of chenodeoxycholic acid and three types of bioactive lanostanes extracted from *G. lucidum*.

3.6.2. Mechanism

Farnesoid X receptor (FXR; NR1H4) plays a role in the pathogenesis of cardiovascular disease [28]. It is a ligand-induced transcriptional activator and is expressed at high level in liver, intestine, kidney, adrenal glands, and also in the vasculature. It targets the enterohepatic recycling and detoxification of BA. When activated, FXR translocates to the cell nucleus, forms a heterodimer with retinoid-X-receptor and binds to hormone response elements on DNA, which produces either repression or an up regulation of gene transcription. The resulting mechanisms are affected by antagonist or agonist character of the respective ligand [79].

On the other hand, both (*CYP7A1*) and sterol response element binding protein 1c (*SREBP1c*) have shown their expression by elevation of oxysterol-induced liver X receptor-α (LXR-α) activation. This may result in increased triglyceride and BA biosynthesis, whereby the FXR-α-mediated induction of small heterodimer partner (SHP), will interrupt the activity of (LXR-α) to induce *CYP7A1* and *SREBP1c*, and hence inhibits BA and lipogenesis synthesis. Supernumerary, FXR-α-mediated induction of intestinal mouse fibroblast growth factor 15 is a surrogate SHP-independent signal from the gut to the liver to inhibit BA biosynthesis [18].

4. Conclusion

These mechanisms are possibly valid due to the promising results by comparing the treated and the control group. The activity of isolated compounds mentioned herein is very convincing and the working mechanisms mentioned above are involved. However, it is likely more than one mechanism may interplay. The method of extracting the bioactive compounds or the fraction used is closely related to the anti-hypercholesterolemia effect. There are several factors that may influence the possible mechanisms. The effective dosage of *G. lucidum* extract have yet to be standardized in animal and human clinical trial. Although many reports showed the favourable effects of *G. lucidum* extract to patients in China, such reports are anecdotal. In the absence of case-control studies, these reports could not be validated. The duration of administration of *G. lucidum* for its anti-hypercholesterolemia activity is also arguable. The mechanism responsible for the inhibition of cholesterol synthesis is also unclear, as the test subjects were provided with high cholesterol diet during the course of trial which did not reflect the real situation. Hence, to date, the effectiveness of *G. lucidum* on the hypercholesterolemia patients is still undefined. There is a lack of evidence to prove that *G. lucidum* successful dislodge the cholesterol plaque from the affected blood vessels. Whether other mechanisms are also playing a part in cholesterol lowering activity is still unclear. Another compounding factor is the different absorption rate of each test subject. In addition, the effectiveness data of *G. lucidum* acquired from testing in rats could not be applied to human, as the dosage is based on body weight. Moreover, the strain of *Ganoderma* used is also an important factor in determining the rate and type of mechanism involved, since different strain produces different contents in the extract. This becomes more prominent when the mushroom is harvested from different geographical regions.

Synthetic anti-hypercholesterolemia drug works by affecting an array of intermediate precursors which could be important for health. Therefore the side effect of such drug would be more severe than someone taking a mixture of active components present in *G. lucidum* since *G. lucidum* extract most probably exerts its inhibitory effects at the late stage of the pathway.

Author details

Choong Yew Keong

Address all correspondence to: yewkeong11@yahoo.co.uk

Phytochemistry Unit, Herbal Medicine Research Centre, Institute for Medical Research, 50588 Jalan Pahang, Kuala Lumpur, Malaysia

References

[1] Abdullah, N., Ismail, S.M., Aminudin, N., Shuib, A.S., Lau, B.J. (2012) Evaluation of selected culinary-medicinal mushrooms for antioxidant and ACE inhibitory activities. *Evidence-Based Complementary and Alternative Medicine*. Doi : 10.1155/2012/464238.

[2] Adaramoye O.A., Nwaneri V.O., Anyanwa K.C. (2005) Possible anti atherogenic effect of kolaviron (a Garcinia kola seed extract) in hypercholesterolemic rats. *Clin. Exp. Pharmacol. Physiol*. 32: 40-46.

[3] Alan H. Yee, DO, Joseph D. Burns, Eelco F.M. Wijdicks. (2010) Cerebral Salt Wasting: Pathophysiology, Diagnosis, and Treatment. *Neurosurg Clin N Am*. 21 339–352.

[4] Akira Endo, Masao Kuroda and Kazuhiko Tanzawa. (1976). Competitive Inhibition of 3-hydroxy-3-methylglutaryl coenzyme a reductase by ML-236A and ML-238B fungal metabolites,having hypocholesterolemic activity. FEBS LETTERS. (Dec 1976) Volume 72, number 2. Review: A historical perspective on the discovery of statins. *Proc. Jpn. Acad., Ser.* B 86 (2010): 484-493.

[5] Andréia Assunção Soares , Anacharis Babeto de Sá-Nakanishi , Adelar Bracht , Sandra Maria Gomes da Costa , Eloá Angélica Koehnlein , Cristina Giatti Marques de Souza and Rosane Marina Peralta . (2013) Hepatoprotective effects of mushrooms. *Molecules*. 18: 7609-7630; doi:10.3390/molecules18077609.

[6] Appel L.J. (2003) Lifestyle modification as a means to prevent and treat high blood pressure. *Journal of the American Society of Nephrology*; 14 (Suppl 3): S99-S102.

[7] Arichi S, T. Tani, M. Kuba, H.Matsuda, N. Yoshimura and N. Kirigaya. (1979) *Kiso To Rinsho*. 13: 4239.

[8] Aviram, M and Fuhrman. B. (1998). Poluphenolic flavonoids inhibit macrophage-mediated oxidation of LDL and attenuate atherogenesis. *Atherosclerosis.* 137 (suppl). S45-S50.

[9] Baxter, J.O., Perloff, D., Hsuch, W., Biglieri, E.G. (1987) The endocrinology of hypertension. In: Endocrinology and Metabolism. 2nd ed. P. Felig. *et al.*, Eds. *New York, McGraw-Hill.* 693-772.

[10] Biglieri, E.G., Kater, C.E. (1992). Mineralocorticoids. In : Basic and Clinical Endocrinology, 3rd ed. F.S. Greenspan. P.H. Forsham, Eds. East Norwalk, C.T. *Appleton & Lange.* 310-325.

[11] Borgstahl G.E., Parge H.E., Hickey M.J., Beyer W.F. Jr, Hallewell R.A., Tainer J.A. (1992). The structure of human mitochondrial manganese superoxide dismutase reveals a novel tetrameric interface of two 4-helix bundles. *Cell.* 71 (1): 107–18.

[12] Bohn, J.A. and BeMiller, J.N. (1995) (1-3)-β-D-Glucan as biological response modifiers: a review of structure–functional activity relationships. *Carbohydrate Polymers.* 28: 3–14.

[13] Braunwald E. (1997) Shattuck lecture-cardiovascular medicine at the turn of the millennium : triumphs, concerns and opputunities. *New Eng. J. Med.* 337: 1360-1369.

[14] Chang, H., Y. Tung, T. Tung. (1988) Effect of *Ganoderma lucidum* extract on interleukin-2 production in mice. *J. Chinese Oncol. Soc.* 4: 13-22.

[15] Chang, S.T. (1995) *Ganoderma*- the leader in production and technology of mushroom nutriceuticals. Recent advances in *Ganoderma lucidum* research, Seoul, Korea: *The Pharmaceutical Soc. Of Korea.* 43-52.

[16] Chang, R. (1996). The Central Importance of the β-glucan receptor as the basis of immunologic bioactivity of *Ganoderma* polysaccharides, In Reishi, Mizuno T, Kim BK (eds), II *Yang Press, Seoul.* 177-179.

[17] Charles Thomas, Roberto Pellicciari, Mark Pruzanski, Johan Auwerx, Kristina Schoonjans .(2008) Targeting bile–acid signalling for metabolic diseases. *Nature Reviews Drug Discovery.* 7: 678-693.

[18] Chen, G., Luo, Y.C., Ji, B.P., Li, B. Guo,Y., Li.Y., Su W., Xiao Z.L. (2008) Effect of polysaccharide from *Auricularia auricula* on blood lipid metabolism and lipoprotein lipase activity of ICR mice fed a cholesterol- enriched diet. *Journal of Food Science.* 73(6), H 103-H108.doi: 10.1111/j.1750-3841.2008.00821.x

[19] Chen XiaoPing, Chen Yan , Li ShuiBing , Chen YouGuo , Lan JianYun , Liu LanPing. (2009) Free radical scavenging of *Ganoderma lucidum* polysaccharides and its effect on antioxidant enzymes and immunity activities in cervical carcinoma rats. *Carbohydrate Polymers.* 77: 389–393.

[20] Cheung, L.M., Cheung, P.C.K., Ooi, V.E.C. (2003) Antioxidant activity and total phenolics of edible mushroom extracts. *Food Chemistry.* 81, 249–255.

[21] Chobaniar, A.V.,Bakris, G.L., Black,H.R., Cushman, W.C, Green, L.A. & IzzoJr. Et al., (2003). The seventh report of the joint national committee on prevention, detection, evaluation, and treatment of high blood pressure: The JNCT report. The Journal of the American Medical Association. 289(19), 2560-2571.

[22] Crop, J.K. and J. Kay. (1991). Isolation and characterization of β-glucan receptors on human mononuclear phagocytes. J. Exp. Med. 173:1511-1520.

[23] Dharmananda, S. (1988) Medicinal mushrooms. *Bestways Magazine*, July, 54-58.

[24] Donald Voet and Judith G.Voet. (1990) Biochemistry. *John Wiley & Sons. Inc.* 308-310.

[25] Elmastas, M., Isildak, O., Turkekul, I., Temur, N. (2007) Determination of antioxidant activity and antioxidant compounds in wild edible mushrooms. *Journal of Food Composition and Analysis.* 20: 337-345.

[26] Fiorucci, S.; Rizzo, G.; Donini, A.; Distrutti, E.; Santucci, L. (2007) Targeting farnesoid X receptor for liver and metabolic disorders. *Trends Mol. Med.* 13: 298-309.

[27] Forman, B. M., Goode, E., Chen, J., Oro, A. E., Bradley, D. J., Perlmann, T., Noonan, D. J., Burka, L. T., McMorris, T., Lamph, W. W., Evans, R. M.,Weinberger, C. (1995) Identification of a nuclear receptor that is activated by farnesol metabolites. *Cell.* 81(5): 687-693.

[28] Fukashima M, Nakano M, Morti.Y, Ohashi T, Fujiwara Y, Sonoyama K. J. (2000) Hepatic LDL Receptor mRNA in Rats Is Increased by Dietary Mushroom (Agaricus bisporus) Fiber and Sugar Beet Fiber. *The American Society for Nutritional Sciences.* 130: 2151-2156.

[29] Gerd Assmarm MD and Helmut S. (1992) Relationship of high density lipoprotein cholesterol and triglycerides to incidence of atherosclerotic coronary artery disease. *American Journal of Cardiology.* 70: 733-37.

[30] Goldstein JL, Brown MS. (1987) Regulation of low-density lipoprotein receptors: implications for pathogenesis and therapy of hypercholesterolemic and atherosclerosis. *Circulation.* 76(3): 504-507.

[31] Gordon T, Castelli WP, Hiortland MC, Kannel WB and Dawber TR. (1977) High density lipoprotein as a protective factor against coronary heart disease. The Framingham study. *American Journal of Medicine.* 707-14.

[32] Grice, H.C. (1988) Safety evaluation of butylated hydroxyanisole from the perspective of effects on forestomach and oesophageal squamous epithelium. *Food and Chemical Toxicology.* 26: 717–723.

[33] Guillamor, A., Gracia- Latuente, Ana, Lozano, M., D'Arrigo., M, Rostango, M.A., Villares,A., Martinez, J.A. (2010). Edible mushrooms : Role in the prevention of cardiovascular disease. *Fitoterapia*. 81: 715-723.

[34] Hasnat, M. A., Pervin, M., & Lim, B.O. (2013) Acetylcholinesterase inhibition and in vitro and in vivo antioxidant activities of *Ganoderma lucidum* grown on germinated brown rice. *Molecules*. 18: 6663-6678.

[35] Hikino, H., C. Konno, Y. Mirin and T.Hayashi. (1985) Antidiabetes drugs: isolation and hypoglycemic activity of ganoderan A and ganoderan B, Glycans of *Ganoderma lucidium* fruit bodies. *Planta Medica*. 51:339-340.

[36] Hseu, R.Y. (1993) An overview on *Ganoderma* mushrooms. Taichung, Taiwan: *Wann Nian Publishing Co*. 141 (in Chinese).

[37] Huang, D., Ou, B., Prior, R.L. (2005) The chemistry behind antioxidant capacity assays. Journal of Agricultural of Food Chemistry. 53: 1841-1856.

[38] Jia, Y.F., Xu, W.M., Ren J., Yinm X., Zhang, L. (1993). Effects of Ling Zhi on the production of Interleukin-1 (IL-1)-immunopharmacological study. In: The research on *Ganoderma* (part 1). Zhu S. and M. Mori. (eds). Shanghai: *Shanghai Medical University Press*. 254-258.

[39] Kabir, Y., Kimura, S., Tamura, T. (1988) Dietary effect of *Ganoderma lucidum* mushroom on blood pressure and lipid levels in spontaneously hy pertensive rats (SHR). *J. Nutr. Sci. Vitaminol*. 34: 433-438.

[40] Kaplan, N.M. (1992) Endocrine hypertension: In: Williams Textbooks of Endocrinology .J.D.Wilson, D.W. Fester, *Eds.Philadelphia, W.B.Saundes*. 707-731.

[41] Kamsiah Jaarin and Nafeeza MI. (1999) Effect of Nicardipine on fasting plasma lipids and a polipoproteins in male New Zealand white rabbits. *Malaysian Journal of Medical Sciences*, Vol. 6, No. 2, July 1999 (5-11).

[42] Ker, Y.B., Chen, K. C., Chyau, C.C., Chen, C.C., Guo,J.H., Hsien C.L., Wang,H.E., Peng. C.C., Chang, C.H., Peng,R.P. (2005) Antioxidant caspability of polysaccharides fractionated from submerge-cultured Agaricus blazei Mycelia. *Journal of Agricultural and Food chemistry*. 53: 7052-7058.

[43] Kim, B.K., H.W.Kim and E.C.Choi. (1993) Anti-HIV activities of *Ganoderma lucidium*. 5th International Symposium on *Ganoderma lucidium*, Seol, Korea. 67-69.

[44] Klaus, A., Kozarski, M., Niksic, M., Jakovljevic, D., Todorovic, N., Van Griensven, I.J.I.D. 2011. Antioxidative activities and chemical characterization of polysaccharides extracted from the basidiomycetes schizophyllum commune. LWT. *Food Science and Technology*. 44: 2005-2011.

[45] Ko, D.T., Hebert, P. R., Coffey, C.S., Curltis, J.P, Joody, J.M., Sediakyan, A., Krumbolz, H.M.(2004) Adverse effects of β-blocker theraphy for patients with heart failure.

A quantitative overview of randomized trials. *Archives of International Medicane*, 164(13), 1389-1394.

[46] Kurt Karlsson and Stefan L.Marklund.(1988). Plasma Clearance of Human Extracellular –Superoxide Dismutase C in Rabbits. *The Journal of Clinical Investigation*. Doi: 10: 1172/JCI 113676. Volume 82, September 1988, 762-766.

[47] Lankin V. Z., A. K. Tikhaze, V. I. Kapel'ko, G. S. Shepel'kova, K. B. Shumaev, O. M. Panasenko, G. G. Konovalova, Yu. N. Belenkov. (2007) Mechanisms of Oxidative Modification of Low Density Lipoproteins under Conditions of Oxidative and Carbonyl Stress. © Pleiades Publishing, Ltd., ISSN 0006-2979, *Biochemistry (Moscow)*. 72(10): 1081-1090.

[48] Lattime E., and O. Stutman. (1991) Antitumor immune surveillance by tumor necrosis factor producing cells. *Immunology Research*. 10: 104-113.

[49] Lavy A, Brook JG, Dankner G, Ben Amotz A, Aviram M. (1991) Enhanced in vitro oxidation of plasma lipoproteins derived from hypercholesterolemic patients. *Metabolism*. 40: 794-799.

[50] Ledwozyw A, Michalak J, Stepien A, Kadziolka A. (1986) The relationship between plasma triacylglycerols, cholesterol, total lipids and lipid peroxidation products during human atherosclerosis. *Clinica Chimic. Acta*. 155: 275-84.

[51] Lei L.S., and Z.B. Lin. (1992). Effect of *Ganoderma* polysaccharides on T-cell subpopulations and production of interleukin 2 in mixed lymphocyte response. *Acta Pharm. Sinica* 27: 331-335.

[52] Lin, J.M., Lin, C.C. Chiu, H.F., Yanf, J.J. Lee, S.G. (1993). Evaluation of the anti-inflammatory and liver protective effects of anoectochilus formosanus *Ganoderma lucidum* and *Gynostemma pentaphyllum* in rats. *Am J Chi Med*. 21: 59-69.

[53] Lindequist, U. (1995). Structure and biological activity of triterpenes, polysaccharides and other constituents of *Ganoderma lucidum*, in Recent advances in *Ganoderma lucidum* research, Kim, B.K., I.H. Kim and Y.S. Kim (eds), Seoul, Korea: *Pharmaceutical Society of Korea*. 61-92.

[54] Liu Gen-Tao. (1993) Pharmacology and clinical uses of *Ganoderma* mushroom biology and mushroom products proceedings of the *First International Conference on MBMP*, 23-26 August, Hong Kong.

[55] Lo, T.C.T., Chang, C.A., Chiuc, K.H., Tsayd, P.K., Jena, J.F. (2011) Correlation evaluation of antioxidant properties on the monosaccharide components and glycosyl linkages of polysaccharide with different measuring methods. *Carbohydrate Polymers*. 86: 320-327.

[56] Maja Kozarski, Anita Klaus, Miomir Niksic, Miroslav M. Vrvic, Nina Todorovic (2012) Antioxidative activities and chemical characterization of polysaccharide extracts from the widely used mushrooms *Ganoderma applanatum*, *Ganoderma lucidum*,

Lentinus edodes and *Trametes versicolor*. *Journal of Food Composition and Analisis*. 26 : 144-153.

[57] Martirosyan , D.M. (2011) The 9th International Conference on " Functional Foods And Chronic Diseases : Science and Practice" University of Nevada, Las Vegas, USA.

[58] Mizuro, T. (1992) Comparative studies on the host-mediated antitumor polysaccharides isolated from the fruiting body and mycelium of three *Ganoderma* species fungi, *Ganoderma lucidum* , *Ganoderma tsugae* and *Ganoderma applanatum*. 4th *International Symposium on Ganoderma lucidum,* Seoul, Korea. 21-29.

[59] Mizuno, T., Kato, N., Totsuka, A., Takenaka, K., Shinkai, K. & Shimizu, M. (1984) Fractionation, structural features and antitumor activity of water-soluble polysaccharide from "Reishi", the fruit body of *Ganoderma lucidum*. *J. Agric. Chem. Soc. Jpn.* 58: 871-880.

[60] Miyazaki T. and Nishijima M. (1981) Studies on fungal polysaccharides, XXVII. Structural examination of a water-soluble, antitumor polysaccharide of *Ganoderma lucidum*. *Chem. Pharm. Bull.* 29: 3611-3616.

[61] Miyazaki T. and Nishijima M. (1982) Structural examination of an alkali-extracted, water-soluble heteroglycan of the fungus *Ganoderma lucidum*. *Carbohydrate Research.* 109: 290-294.

[62] Morigiwa A., Kitabatake K., Fujimoto Y., Ikekawa N.(1986) Angiotensin Converting Enzyme-Inhibitory Triterpenes from *Ganoderma lucidum*. *Chem. Pharm. Bull.* 34: 3025-3028.

[63] Nakashima, S., T. Uneda, and T. Kanada. (1979). Effects of polysaccharides from *Ganoderma applanatum* on immune responses. *Microbiol. Immunol.* 23: 501-513.

[64] Nishitob, T., Sato, H., Shirasu, S., Sakamura, S. (1986) Evidence on the strain-specific terpenoid pattern of *Ganoderma lucidum*. *Agricultural and Biological Chemistry.* 50: 2151-2154.

[65] Noor Fazila Mohamed Yahaya, Mohammad Azizur Rahman, Noorlidah Abdullah. (2014) Therapeutic potential of mushrooms in preventing and ameliorating hypertension. Trends in Food Science & Technology. 39(2): 104-116.

[66] Osamah Hussein, Sorina Schlezinger, Mira Rosenblat, Shlomo Keidar, Michael Aviram. (1997) Reduced susceptibility of low density lipoprotein (LDL) to lipid peroxidation after fluvastatin therapy is associated with the hypocholesterolemic effect of the drug and its binding to the LDL. Atherosclerosis 128: 11–18.

[67] Pracheta P., Sharma V, Singh L., Paliwal R, Sharma S, Yadav S, Sharma S. (2011) Chemopreventive effect of hydroethanolie ectract of Euphorbia neriifolia leaves against DENA-induced renal carcinogenesis in mice. *Asian Pacific J.Cancer Prev.* 12: 677-683.

[68] Shieh, Y.H., liu, C.F., Huang, Y.K., Yang, J.Y., Wu, I.L., Lin, C.H., Li, S.C. (2001). Evaluation of the hepatic and renal-protective effects of *Ganoderma lucidum* in mice. *Am. J. Chin. Med.* 29: 501-507.

[69] Shimada, K., Fujikawa, K., Yahara, K., Nakamura, T. (1992) Antioxidative properties of xanthan on the autoxidation of soybean oil in cyclodextrin emulsion. *Journal of Agricultural and Food Chemistry*. 40: 945-948.

[70] Smith, C.G., Vane, J.R. (2003) The discovery of captopril. *FASEB J.* 17(8): 788–9. doi: 10.1096/fj.03-0093life. PMID 12724335.

[71] Sone, Y. et al. (1985) Structures and antitumor activities of polysaccharides isolated from fruiting body and the growing culture of mycelium of *Ganoderma lucidum. Agric. Biol. Chem.* 49: 2641-2653.

[72] Sohn,D.H. (1995) Antifibrolic effect of polysaccharides from *Ganoderma lucidium* in experimental hepatic cirrhosis model. In: Recent advances in *Ganoderma lucidium* Research. Ed. By B.K. Kim, et al. Seol, Korea: *The pharmacol. Soc. Korea*. 29-41.

[73] Stanislaus CS. (1995). Lingzhi medicinal of kings. *New editions Health World*. 38-41.

[74] Stavinoha, W.B., B.J. Slama, S.T. Weintraub and P.L. Mobley. (1991). The anti-inflammatory activity of *Ganoderma lucidum*. 3rd International Symposium on *Ganoderma lucidum*, Seoul, Korea. 9-15.

[75] Su, C.H. (1991) Taxonomy and physiologically active compounds of *Ganoderma. J. Taipei Medical College*. 20: 1-16.

[76] Su, C.H., M.N. Lai and M.H. Chan. (1993) Hepato-p[rotective triterpenoids from *Ganoderma tsugae* Murell. In: Mushroom biology and mushroom producys, Eds. S.T. Chang et al., Hong Kong: *The Chinese University Press*. 275-283.

[77] Synytsya, A. Míčková, K. Synytsya, A. Jablonský, I. Speváček, J. Erban, V. Kováříková, E. Čopíková, J. (2009) Glucans from fruit bodies of cultivated mushrooms *Pleurotus ostreatus* and *Pleurotus eryngii*: structure and potential prebiotic activity. *Carbohydrate Polymers*. 76: 548–556.

[78] Ulrike Grienke, Judit Mihály-Bison, Daniela Schuster, Taras onyushkin, Markus Binder , Shu-hong Guan , Chun-ru Cheng , Gerhard Wolber , Hermann Stuppner , De-an Guo , Valery N. Bochkov , Judith M. Rollinger (2011). Pharmacophore-based discovery of FXR-agonists. Part II: Identification of bioactive triterpenes from *Ganoderma lucidum*. *Bioorganic & Medicinal Chemistry*. 19: 6779-6791.

[79] Wasser, S.P. (2011) Current findings, future trends and unsolved problems in studies of medicinal mushrooms. *Applied Microbiology and Biotechnology*. 89(5): 1323-1332.

[80] Wasser S.P. and Weis A.L. (1997a). In Medicinal mushrooms. Reishi mushroom *Ganoderma lucidum* (Curtis: Fr) P.Karst., *Nevo E., ed., Haifa, Peledfus Press*. 39.

[81] William F, Balistreri, M.D., Robert Rej. (1996) Liver function in Tietz Fundamentals of Clinical Chemistry. *W.B. Saunders Company*. 539.

[82] Won, S.J., Lee, S.S., Ke, Y.H., Lin, M.T. (1989) Enhancement of splenic N.K. cytotoxic activity by the extracts of *Ganoderma lucidum* mycelium in mice. *J. Biomed. Lab. Sci.* 2: 201-213.

[83] Yang, Q.Y., Fang, J.N., Yang, X.T. (1995) The isolation and identification of two polysaccarides of *Ganoderma lucidium* (GL-A, GL-B) In: *Ganoderma*: Systematics, phytopathology and pharmacology. P.K.Bachanan, R.S.Hseu and Monocalno(eds) Proceeding of Contributed Symposium 59, A,B,5th *International Mycological Congress, Vancouver*, 95-99.

[84] Yasuo Komoda, Masato Shimizu, Yoshiko Sonoda, Yoshihiro Sato. (1989) Ganoderic acid and its derivatives as cholesterol synthesis inhibitor. *Chem. Pharm. Bull.* 37 (2): 531-533.

[85] Yeh, S.F., K.C. Lee, M.S. Shiao. (1987) Sterols, triterpenes and fatty acid patterns in *Ganoderma lucidum. Proc. Natl. Sci. Counc, ROCCA*. 11:129-134.

[86] Zhang, L.X., H. Meng, Z.B. Zhon. (1993a) Effects of Lingzhi on the production of Interleukin-2 (IL-2)-immunolopharmaco-logical study (7). In: The research on *Ganoderma*(part I). Zhu S. and M. Mori (eds). Shanghai: *Shanghai Medical University Press*. 259-265.

[87] Zhang, L.X. and X.H. Xie. (1993b) Influence of Lingzhi on the production of tumor necrosis factor (TNF)- immunolo-pharmacological study (8). In: The research on *Ganoderma*(part I). Zhu S. and M. Mori. (eds). Shanghai: *Shanghai Medical University Press*. 266-272.

[88] Zhang L. and M. Yu. (1993c) Influence of Lingzhi on natural killer cells-immunopharmacological study (5). From The Research on *Ganoderma* (part I). Zhu S. and M. Mori. (eds). *Shanghai Medical University Press*. 246-253.

[89] Zhang, L.X., H.H. Miao, J. Shen. (1993d) Effects of Lingzhi on Macrophage phagocytosis and arbon clearance test-immunopharmacological study (4). In: The researsh on Ganoderma(part I). Zhu S. and M. Mori (eds). Shanghai: Shanghai Medical University Press. 241-245.

Chapter 8

Hypercholesterolemia — Statin Therapy — Indications, Side Effects, Common Mistakes in Handling, Last Evidence and Recommendations in Current Clinical Practice

Lucía Cid-Conde and José López-Castro

Additional information is available at the end of the chapter

http://dx.doi.org/10.5772/59622

1. Introduction

1.1. Pharmacology of statin

It is known as statins a group of drugs used to lower cholesterol in patients suffering from hypercholesterolemia and who have therefore increased risk of developing atherosclerosis and have episodes cardiovascular disease. From the pharmacological point of view, fall within the HMG-CoA reductase. Enzyme inhibition is precisely this which justifies the reduction of certain fractions of cholesterol in the body and explains its importance: their positive intervention on cardiovascular risk factors, leading to numerous cardiovascular diseases, which are the leading cause of death in the developed world [1,2]. Despite its short history (less than forty years) are many studies that have been done on statins and hundreds of thousands of patients who have taken these drugs. This has given rise to an extensive knowledge of the characteristics of these drugs has led to the synthesis of new substances that improve the properties of the above statins; in this line part of pharmaceutical research is still moving. However, it has also given rise to broadly meet the real toxicological profile for each substance. The phase IV studies have revealed the risks of using these substances for long periods or in certain basal conditions, which has led, among other things, the withdrawal of any member of the family due to their increased incidence of severe adverse reactions. Because of the variability in origin, the pharmacokinetics of statins differ greatly, however, its pharmacodynamic similarities allowed their joint study group them because, in terms of mechanism of action and effects of statins, and especially, regarding the clinical consequences of its use, there is an important congruence group, which has been widely studied (Table 1). All developed statins are used orally and absorbed by this route on a variable range from 30% of lovastatin to 35% of pravastatin, decreasing its absorption in the presence of food in the stomach. However, the changes in peak concentrations or the respective curves of assimilation have no impact on the final results in the modification of cholesterol levels, so it is generally advisable to take them at any time of day and in most cases with or without food. Also, there appears to be accumulation due to multiple doses, which is general consensus decision single dose. The recommendations do not drink grapefruit juice while being treated with statins is due to interference with the metabolism, not altered absorption. Generally, the bioavailability of the statins is low, ranging from 5% of lovastatin and 17% of pravastatin. Binding to plasma proteins is variable, but in general very high lines. Except 50% of pravastatin, all have a 95% binding to proteins. The tissue distribution is broad, crossing the blood-brain and placental barriers, even going to milk in lactating women. Liver specificity of these drugs is determined by its degree of lipophilicity and by the presence of some organic anion transporter proteins that allow more hydrophilic statins such as pravastatin and rosuvastatin, entering the hepatocyte [3]. Moreover, some statins may inhibit P-glycoprotein (multidrug resistance protein), a carrier protein of many drugs in the cell, which could predispose to drug interactions. [4]

PHARMACOLOGICAL CHARACTERISTICS OF STATIN							
	Sinvastatin	Pravastatin	Lovastatin	Fluvastatin	Atorvastatin	Rosuvastatin	Pitavastatin
Prodrugs	YES	NO	YES	NO	NO	NO	NO
Food and absorption	No influence	↓	↑	↓	↓	No influence	
Bioavailability	≤5%	17%	≤5%	24%	14%	20%	≥30%
Binding to plasma proteins	94%	50%	>95%	98%	98%	88%	-
Crosses blood-brain barrier	YES	NO	YES	NO	NO	NO	YES
Metabolism	CYP3A4	sulphation	CYP3A4	CYP2C9	CYP3A4	CYP2C9	CYP2C9 CYP2C8
Biliary excretion	60%	70%	83%	95%	-	90%	-
Urinary excretion	13%	20%	10%	5%	<2%	30%	3%
Elimination half-life	2-3h	0.8h	1-4h	2.5h	20h	20h	-

Table 1. Pharmacological characteristics of statin

The metabolism of statins is liver, undergoing first pass metabolism. In most, there are differences in the metabolism regarding sex and age, but not enough to change the doses in the absence of other pathologies. It seems clear that are substrates of CYP450: lovastatin, simvastatin and atorvastatin are metabolized exclusively by CYP3A4, and fluvastatin does exclusively by 2C9. For rosuvastatin, only 10% use the CYP2C9 and 2C19. Pitavastatin has a

http://dx.doi.org/10.5772/59622

low affinity for CYP2C9, so not a major metabolic pathway. Pravastatin is not metabolised by the cytochrome, but does so by enzymes present in the cytoplasm of hepatocytes. The metabolites may be hydroxylated derivatives, omega or beta-oxidized methylated glucuronide. The pharmacological activity of the same is very variable. Thus, the range is wide, from lovastatin, simvastatin, which are really a pharmacologically inactive lactones and performing their pharmacological activity through its metabolites, to fluvastatin, which has virtually inactive metabolites. For the most part, excretion in feces is due to its poor absorption. According to each type of statins, renal excretion ranges from 2% to 20%.

Statins are inhibitors of 3-hydroxy-3-methylglutaryl-coenzyme A (HMG-CoA) reductase. This enzyme catalyzes the conversion of HMG-CoA to mevalonate, which is a key metabolite in the biosynthesis of cholesterol. Blocking occurs due to the high structural resemblance with these drugs exhibit HMG-CoA. The affinity of the enzyme by statins is 1.000 to 10.000 times that of the natural substrate (Figure 1).

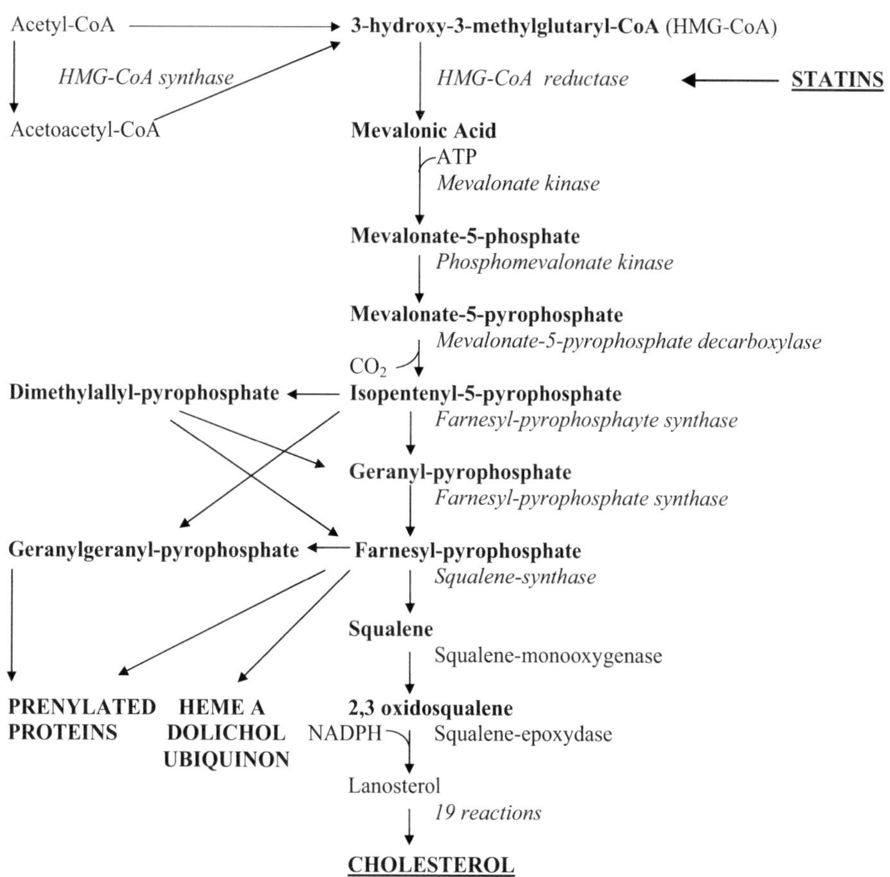

Figure 1. Biosynthesis of cholesterol

The blockade of hepatic cholesterol synthesis causes an activation of the regulatory proteins SREBP (sterol regulatory elements-binding proteins), which activate transcription of protein and thus result in higher expression of the LDL receptor gene and increased the number of functional receptors on hepatocytes [5]. Moreover, it has been shown that statins also produced inhibition associated antigen-1 with the function of lymphocytes (LFA-1: lymphocyte function-associated antigen-1) [6]. The LFA-1 is a glycoprotein integrin family expressed on the surface of leukocytes. When the LFA-1 is activated by certain receptors, binds to the intracellular molecule-1 adhesion (ICAM-1 or CD-54) and stimulates the extravasation of leukocytes and activation of T lymphocytes. This means that the LFA-1 is a proinflammatory agent and its inhibition is beneficial in conditions such as rheumatoid arthritis and rejection of homograft. It was shown that statins and particularly, lovastatin, bind to a site of LFA-1 domain, lovastatin currently designated site. This is the molecular mechanism by which lovastatin, simvastatin and other statin lesser extent inhibit the LFA-1 [7]. This would be one of the anti-inflammatory mechanisms and hence possessing antiatherogenic statins.

2. Effects of statins

The consequences of the inhibition of HMG-CoA may be grouped into two groups:

a. **Derivatives of interaction on cholesterol metabolism**: Lower levels of total cholesterol and LDL, substances closely related to atherosclerosis and increased cardiovascular risk. Density decreases LDL particles, increasing the size of these, leading to decreased atherogenesis [8]. Apolipoprotein B also falls substantially during treatment with statins. In addition, some statins modestly increase cHDL and reduces plasma triglycerides. As a result of these changes, the ratio of total cholesterol to HDL cholesterol and the ratio of LDL and HDL cholesterol are reduced. We have considered the combination of fibrate and enhancer preventing cardiac of statins, especially having no competitive metabolism pathways.

b. **Pleiotropic effects:** In addition to its effects on the lipid profile, statins have other beneficial cardiovascular effects, especially on the arterial wall, known as pleiotropic effects which explain the additional benefit not attributable to the reduction in cLDL observed in many studies intervention [9].

By inhibiting HMG-CoA reductase inhibitors, statins interfere with the formation of isoprenoids from mevalonate. [10] Isoprenoids are molecules such as farnesyl pyrophosphate (FPP) and geranylgeranylpyrophosphate (GGPP), derived from the metabolism of mevalonate, which serve as lipid-tags for the posttranslational modification of a variety of proteins, including the gamma subunit of G proteins and small GTP unidoras proteins. As a result, the prenylation of the G proteins (Rho, Rac, Ras and Rab Rac1) is reduced. Prenylation of these molecules is necessary for anchoring to the cell membrane and thus to exercise their mechanism of action related to migration, differentiation and cell proliferation. Generally, stimulate and inhibit proinflammatory pathways useful mechanisms for endothelial homeostasis. Through these potential effects on cellular proteins, statins may have a number of antiatherosclerotic and antithrombotic properties, such as inhibiting the growth of smooth muscle cells, cell adhesion, platelet activation and secretion of C-reactive protein among other. The mevalonic acid, may also act directly by inhibiting the synthesis of nitric oxide (NO) in a process dependent transferase inhibiting genilgeranil. NO is an essential molecule for proper function and vasodilatation of endothelium. To this should be added the effects resulting from inhibition of LFA-1, which in turn significantly impacting on endothelial function in blood vessels. These pleiotropic effects are constant source of research, since they can extend the usage profile of statins. Moreover, these drugs maintain and improve endothelial function to increase the bioavailability of NO, which is synthesized by the enzyme NO synthase (eNOS). NO is the principal regulator of the homeostasis of the arteries and endothelium-dependent vasodilation. The functions are, among others, inhibiting proinflammatory mechanisms and act as an antioxidant on lipoproteins [12].

Statins preserve and increase the bioavailability of NO in several ways:

1. Inhibition of Rho protein increases the expression of the enzyme nitric oxide synthase.
2. Increasing the half-life of the messenger RNA of the enzyme nitric oxide synthase.
3. Reduce excess caveolin molecule that acts as an inhibitor of nitric oxide synthase enzyme.
4. Inhibit the production of superoxide.
5. To protect the NO statins decrease platelet aggregation and reducing thromboxane A2 by platelets and thus limit the formation of unstable plaque.
6. Increasing the expression of tissue plasminogen activator and inhibit the expression of endothelin-1, a potent vasoconstrictor with mitogenic action [12].

The hypolipidemic action itself inherently reduces oxidative stress. However, of statins have their own antioxidant mechanisms that inhibit the production of superoxide anion radical. Superoxide is synthesized by NADPH oxidase, an enzyme which can be activated by the action of membrane receptor of angiotensin II, type I (R-1) receptors. Statins block the R-AT1 and also inhibit the phosphorylation of the NADPH oxidase, inactivating it [13].

Statins also block RhoA, one of the mediators of smooth muscle proliferation. The smooth muscle proliferation is a central phenomenon in the pathogenesis of vascular lesions, including post-angioplasty restenosis, transplant atherosclerosis and occlusion of the coronary vein grafts [14].

Atherosclerosis is a strong inflammatory component characterized by the presence of monocytes, macrophages and T cells in the plate. This process is induced by proinflammatory cytokines, free radicals and NO deficiency. Statins increase the bioavailability of NO and inhibit several proinflammatory cytokines [1].

A marker of inflammation and predictor of coronary heart disease risk is C-reactive protein (PCR). It is considered that PCR is also proinflammatory as joining the cLDL of the atheromatous, activates complement plate and induces the expression of inhibitor-1, plasminogen activator (PAI-1), reduces the expression of eNOS and increases the expression of adhesion molecules [15]. Therefore, it is valid to assume that the decrease in plasma CRP levels might be beneficial. Large studies with statins, as the AFCAPS/TexCAPS showed reduced blood PCR. For its anti-inflammatory action, statins increase the stability of the atheromatous plaque, and much of the reduction in coronary events attributable to the mechanism. Preclinical studies demonstrated that statins reduce the accumulation of macrophages in the atheromatous plaque and inhibit metalloproteinase production by activated macrophages. Metalloproteinases are capable of degrading proteins support and are therefore partly responsible for the accident plaque with thrombus formation [16].

Clinically the effects of statins lead to a reduction in cardiovascular risk, through the following mechanisms:

1. Directly decreasing cholesterol levels.
2. Improving endothelial function and inflammatory response.
3. Stabilizing atherosclerotic plaque.
4. Preventing thrombus formation.

Then offer recommendations for clinical practice for the treatment of hypercholesterolemia in adults and reduce the risk of atherosclerotic cardiovascular disease, which includes coronary heart disease, cerebrovascular disease, peripheral artery disease and other atherosclerotic probable origin.

3. Indications of statin in clinical practice

Statins are indicated as an adjunct to diet to reduce elevated total cholesterol, LDL cholesterol, apolipoprotein B and triglycerides; and to increase HDL cholesterol in patients with:

1. Primary hypercholesterolaemia.
2. Mixed dyslipidemia.
3. Homozygous familial hypercholesterolemia.

Also present clear indication in cardiovascular prevention [17]:

Primary prevention of coronary events: in hypercholesterolemic patients without clinical evidence of coronary heart disease.

1. Reduce the risk of myocardial infarction.
2. Reduce the risk of myocardial revascularization procedures.
3. Reduce the risk of cardiovascular mortality with no increase in death from non-cardiovascular causes.

Secondary prevention of cardiovascular events: in patients with clinical evidence of cardiovascular disease.

http://dx.doi.org/10.5772/59622

1. Reduce the risk of total mortality by reducing coronary death.
2. Reduce the risk of myocardial infarction.
3. Reduce the risk of myocardial revascularization procedures.
4. Reduce the risk of stroke and transient ischemic attacks (TIA).
5. Slow the progression of coronary atherosclerosis.

The latest evidence recommends an individualized approach (tailored treatment approach) identified four risk groups associated with therapeutic strategy (Figure 2). Groups that benefit from the use of statin therapy in moderate intensity: LDL reduction of 30-49% or high intensity, LDL reduction of >49% both demonstrate reduction cardiovascular risk (RCV) [17].

1. *Group 1*: Patients with clinical cardiovascular disease (secondary prevention): high intensity treatment with statins (<75 years) or moderate intensity (>75 years).
2. *Group 2:* Patients with LDL > 190 mg/dL: high intensity treatment.
3. *Group 3:* Diabetic patients between 40-75 years, LDL 70-189 mg/dL without cardiovascular disease: treatment of at least moderate intensity and high intensity probably if cardiovascular estimated 10-year risk ≥7.5%.
4. *Group 4:* Patients without diabetes and without clinical cardiovascular disease, with LDL between 70-189 mg / dl but with estimated 10-year risk> 7.5%: treatment of moderate to high intensity.

3.1. Types of statin therapy

The main therapeutic strategies are (Table 2),

High-intensity statin therapy	Moderate-intensity statin therapy	Low-intensity statin therapy
Daily doses lowers LDL on average >50%	Daily dose lowers LDL on average 30-50%	Daily dose lowers LDL on average 30%
Atorvastatin 40-80 mg *Rosuvastatin 20 -40 mg*	*Atorvastatin 10-20 mg* *Rosuvastatin 5-10 mg* *Simvastatin 20-40 mg* *Pravastatin 40-80 mg* *Lovastatin 40 mg* *Fluvastatin XL 80 mg* *Fluvastatin 40 mg BID* *Pitavastatin 2-4 mg*	*Simvastatin 10 mg* *Pravastatin 10-20 mg* *Lovastatin 20 mg* *Fluvastatin 20-40 mg* *Pitavastatin 1 mg*

Table 2. Low, moderate and high-intensity statin therapy categories in treating patients with varying risks.

Statin therapy of high, moderate and low intensity according to studies is classified:

1. *Statin therapy in high-intensity studies*: Atorvastatin 40-80 mg or rosuvastatin 20-40 mg.
2. *Statin therapy in moderate intensity*: Atorvastatin 10-20 mg, rosuvastatin 5-10 mg, simvastatin 20-40 mg (higher doses are not recommended by the incidence of adverse effects), pravastatin 40-80 mg, lovastatin 40mg, fluvastatin XL 80 mg, *Fluvastatin 40 mg bid and pitavastatin 2 to 4 mg.*
3. *Statin therapy in low-intensity*: Simvastatin 10 mg, * Pravastatin 10 mg-20 mg, lovastatin 20 mg, fluvastatin 20-40 mg and *Pitavastatin 1 mg.

* FDA approved but not tested in randomized controlled trials.

3.2. Specific risks

1. Primary prevention with LDL ≥ 160 mg/dL.
2. Genetic testing hyperlipidemias.
3. Family history of premature cardiovascular disease with onset <55years in a male first-degree relative or <65 years female.
4. C-reactive protein levels of high sensitivity (hs-CPR) >2 mg /L,
5. Coronary artery calcium (CAC) score ≥300 Agatston units or ≥ 75th percentile for age, sex and ethnicity.
6. Ankle-brachial index <0.9.

3.3. Treatment strategies

1. *Treat for goals*: It is the strategy most used in the past 15 years, but with 3 problems: Current randomized clinical trials do not specify what the best goal. The magnitude of the further reduction of the atherosclerotic cardiovascular disease than is obtained with a lower cholesterol goal another is unknown. Does not account the possible adverse effects of polypharmacy, which may be necessary to achieve a specific goal.
2. *"Lower is better":* This approach does not take into account the possible adverse effects of polypharmacy with an unknown magnitude reduction in atherosclerotic cardiovascular disease.
3. *Dealing with the level of atherosclerotic cardiovascular disease* (currently preferred): Consider both benefits in reducing cardiovascular risk and adverse effects of statin therapy. Hence the 4 groups that benefit, as previously mentioned, with the exception of use in individuals undergoing hemodialysis or heart failure with NYHA functional class III-IV out. This strategy is advocated today.
4. *Risk throughout life:* Are yet tracking data on >15 years, safety, reduction of atherosclerotic cardiovascular disease when statins are used for periods >10 years and treatment in individuals <40 years.

http://dx.doi.org/10.5772/59622

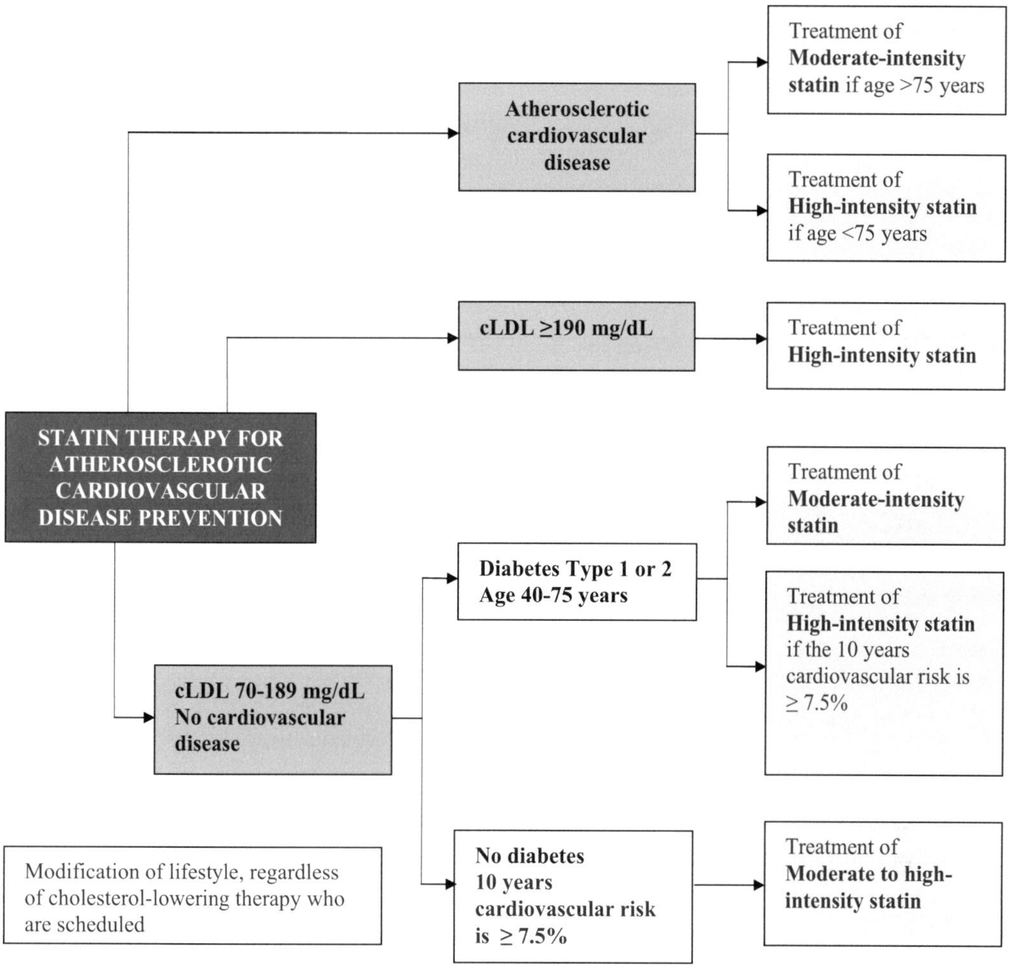

Figure 2. Statin therapy for atherosclerotic cardiovascular disease prevention

4. Side effects of statin and clinical management

4.1. Adverse effects of statins

In general, statins are well tolerated and the dropout rate in clinical trials as a result of any adverse effect is <10%, similar to that of patients taking placebo, and less than 1% are serious side effects (Table 3).

DIFFERENCES IN ADVERSE EFFECTS BETWEEN STATINS				
Adverse effects	**Incidence versus placebo**	**Dose-response relationship**	**Differences (favor/ against)**	**Statistically significant overall difference against**
Abandonment adverse impact	6%	yes	Simvastatin/atorvastatin Pravastatin/atorvastatin Pravastatin/rosuvastatin	-
Significantly relevant myalgia	2%	-	-	-
Relevant significantly increased transaminases	1%	yes	Simvastatin/atorvastatin Simvastatin/fluvastatin Pravastatin/atorvastatin Pravastatin/fluvastatin Rosuvastatin/atorvastatin Rosuvastatin/fluvastatin	Atorvastatin Fluvastatin
Relevant significantly increased CPK	0.6%	yes	Fluvastatin/others	Pitavastatin
Diabetes	9%	-	-	-

Table 3. Differences in adverse effects between statins

1. *Myotoxicity*: The most serious adverse effect associated with the muscular condition, which can range from myalgia (proximal muscle pain and/or weakness with a value of creatine kinase (CK) normal or slightly increased) to more severe forms, such as myopathy (pain and/or weakness over the presence of very high CK, usually >10 times normal) or rhabdomyolysis (serious muscle condition, with muscle weakness and pain, the presence of very high CK, myoglobinuria and renal failure) [18]. In general, the most common disorder is myalgia without elevated CK. Special mention should be cerivastatin withdrawal from the market, since it is the statin showed higher number of severe myopathy. The rate of fatal rhabdomyolysis associated with cerivastatin use at least 15 times higher than that produced by other statins, and was associated with the use of high doses of the drug (0.8 mg/day) or when coadministered with gemfibrozil [19].

   The drugs and clinical conditions that increase the risk of myopathy are,

   a. Chronic diseases (renal failure and diabetes).

   b. Multiple drugs.

   c. Surgical interventions.

   d. High doses of statins.

e. Statins in combination with:

- Fibrates.
- Nicotinic acid (not clearly stated)
- Cyclosporine.
- Antifungal azoles.
- Macrolide antibiotics
- Inhibitors of HIV protease.
- Verapamil.
- Amiodarone.
- Abuse of alcohol.
- Grapefruit juice (> 1/4 liter daily)

2. Hepatotoxicity: active hepatopathy or unexplained persistent elevations of serum transaminases (hypertransaminasemia). An elevation of three times the upper limit of normal transaminases in patients treated with statins occurs between 0.5% to 2% of cases and is directly related to the dose [20]. Hypertransaminasemia is reversible with drug discontinuation and progression to liver failure rarely occurs.

3. Hypersensitivity to any statin or any of the excipients of commercial presentations.

4. Dyspepsia.

5. Less common: sleep disturbances and memory, depression,....

4.2. Absolute contraindications to statins

1. Pregnancy and lactation.

2. Concomitant administration of potent inhibitors of CYP3A4 (itraconazole, ketoconazole, protease inhibitors, erythromycin, clarithromycin, telithromycin and nefazodone) or CYP2C9 (relative contraindication not dependent on CYP450 statins).

4.3. Relative contraindications to statins (but you can take a special medical supervision is required)

1. Elderly (age >70 years).

2. Renal failure.

3. Uncontrolled hypothyroidism.

4. Personal or family history of hereditary muscular disorders.

5. History of muscular toxicity with a statin or fibrate.

6. Alcoholism.

7. Concomitant weak inhibitors of CYP3A4 (Table 4)

OTHER DRUG THAT INTERACT WITH STATIN	
antacids	↓ absorption of statins
anticoagulants	↑ the anticoagulant effectiveness
Ion exchange resins	↓ absorption of statins
colchicine	↑ toxicity of colchicine
glibenclamide	↑ plasma levels of glibenclamide
oral contraceptives	↑ up to 30% in blood hormone levels

Table 4. Other drug that interact with statin

4.4. Recommendations to prevent adverse effects with statin use

Select the dose and type of statin, according to the type of patient cardiovascular risk and potential adverse effects.

Use moderate intensity therapy if the patient has renal or hepatic dysfunction including unexplained persistent transaminase elevations, history of muscular disorders or intolerance to statin use, ALT elevations >3 times the upper limit, concurrent use of medication known interactions with statin, age greater than 75 years, history of hemorrhagic stroke event, asian ancestry. This behavior can substantially reduce adverse events with statin use. The use of simvastatin is not recommended at doses of 80 mg/day because of the risk of toxicity. Liver function tests should be performed before starting statin therapy, with dose changes with the change of drug. During treatment should be monitored signs and symptoms of muscle toxicity.

Whenever a statin prescribing or replaced by another is important to analyze the other co-administered drugs due to the risk of clinically relevant interactions. In the absence of abnormal liver function and potential interactions with coadministered drugs, statins are all interchangeable. In the presence of inducing drugs or inhibitors of CYP3A4, fluvastatin, pravastatin and rosuvastatin are interchangeable. In the presence of inducers or inhibitors of CYP2C9 drugs, statins are all interchangeable, except fluvastatin. In the presence of drugs inducing activad or inhibitors of P-gp, fluvastatin and rosuvastatin are interchangeable. In the presence of inducers or inhibitors of OATP1B1 drugs, is not recommended therapeutic interchange of pravastatin and rosuvastatin. For all other statins, the exchange must be made with caution.

4.5. Analytical monitoring

Monitoring of CK at baseline in patients with or without a history of myopathy, have no solid evidence. It could only be recommended if the patient has muscle symptoms, weakness or fatigue. The only test that is fully justified, prior to initiating statin is the measurement of ALT. The liver function should be measured if the patient is suspected of hepatotoxicity statin use. With the same level of evidence is regular monitoring of blood glucose, the onset of diabetes mellitus associated with treatment [21].

4.6. Attitude pain, muscle stiffness, weakness or muscle fatigue statin taker

Clarify if the symptoms actually developed or intensified therapy. If there is a causal relationship apparent, and muscle symptoms are intolerable, discontinue medication. If rhabdomyolysis is suspected, measure CK-creatinine and urinalysis. If muscular symptoms are mild or moderate statin should be discontinued to reassess symptoms and assess whether the patient has conditions that increase risk of muscle symptoms (hypothyroidism, renal or hepatic dysfunction, polymyalgia rheumatica, steroid myopathy, vitamin D or primary) myopathies. If symptoms are resolved and there are no contraindications, restart the same statin at a lower dose. If symptoms relapse: start another statin at a lower dose and increase slowly. If after 2 months, the symptoms do not improve or CK levels do not decrease, consider alternative etiologies. If muscle symptoms persist after stopping statin or other clinical condition correspond to restart therapy [21].

In summary, the adverse events associated with statin therapy are uncommon. Statins are not associated with cancer risk, but on the contrary there is a greater chance of diabetes. Simvastatin and pravastatin appear to be safer and better tolerated than other statins [22]. It has not been able to show that there are real differences between the effects generic statin drug and reference mark to the modification of the lipid profile, nor in adverse reactions, assessed according to the elevation of transaminases and CPK [23,24].

5. Conclusions

Atherosclerotic cardiovascular disease is one of the most important public health problems of our time, both in Europe and in the rest of the world. Consistency of clinical care, incorporating new evidence and synthesis of recommendations from current practice is common task in various committees for clinical practice worldwide (Europe-ESC, American-AHA / ACC, British-NICE, Australian, Canadian...). This has generated discrepancies with the publication of the latest guidelines of the 2013 AHA/ACC compared to its European namesake 2011 ESC/ EAS. The innovation of greatest impact of the latest guidelines, has been the abandonment of the therapeutic strategy based on the target values LDL. The individualized strategy (tailored treatment approach) is recommended identifying four risk groups associated with therapeutic strategy. Are advised to use statins as well as healthy habits and lifestyle changes for all patients. The CK should not be measured routinely in patients on statins and there is no reason to monitor LDL levels.

Author details

Lucía Cid-Conde[1*] and José López-Castro[2]

*Address all correspondence to: lucidcon@hotmail.com

1 Department of Pharmacy, Hospital Comarcal Valdeorras. SERGAS. O Barco de Valdeorras-Ourense, Spain

2 Department of Internal Medicine, Hospital Comarcal Valdeorras. SERGAS. O Barco de Valdeorras-Ourense, Spain

Conflict of interest Not have any conflict of interest relating to the information in this article.

References

[1] Vaughan CJ, Gotto AM Jr., Basson CT. The evolving role of statins in the management of atherosclerosis. J Am Coll Cardiol 2000; 35(1):1–10.

[2] Torzewski J, Bowyer DE,Waltenberger J, Fitzsimmons C. Processes in atherogenesis: complement activation. Atherosclerosis 1997; 132(2):131–38.

[3] De Angelis G. The influence of statin characteristics on their safety and tolerability. Int J Clin Pract 2004; 58(10):945-55.

[4] Alonso Karlezi, RA, Mata Pariente N, Mata López P. Control de las hiperlipemias en la práctica clínica. Rev Esp Cardiol 2006; 6(G): 24 – 35.

[5] Nissen S, Tuzcu M, Schoenhagen P, Brown BG, Ganz P, Vogel RA, et al.. Effect of intensive compared with moderate lipid-lowering therapy on progression of coronary atherosclerosis: a randomized controlled trial. JAMA 2004; 291(9):1071-80.

[6] Frohlich ED. Target organ involvement in hypertension: a realistic primise of prevention and reversal. Me Clin North Am 2004; 88(1): 209-21.

[7] Kallen, J. et al. Structural basis for LFA-1 inhibition upon lovastatin binding to the CD11a I-domain. J Mol Biol 1999; 292(1): 1–9.

[8] Packard C, Caslake M, Shepherd J. The role of small, dense low density lipoprotein (LDL): a new look. Int J Cardiol 2000; 74(Suppl 1): S17-22.

[9] Davignon J.. The cardioprotective effects of statins. Curr Atheroscler Rep 2004; 6(1): 27-35.

[10] Liao JK.. Isoprenoids as mediators of the biological effects of statins. J Clin Invest. 2002; 110(3):285-8.

[11] Denicola A, Batthyany C, Lissi E, Freeman BA, Rubbo H, Radi R. Diffusion of nitric oxide into low density lipoprotein. J Biol Chem 2002; 277(2): 932-6.

[12] Hernandez-Perera O, Perez-Sala D, Navarro-Antolin J, Sánchez-Pascuala R, Hernández G, Díaz C et al. Effects of 3-hydroxy-3-methylglutaryl-CoA reductase inhibitors, atorvastatin and simvastatin, on the expression of endothelin-1 and endothelial nitric oxide synthase in vascular endothelial cells. J Clin Invest 1998; 101(12):2711–19.

[13] Wassmann S, Laufs U, Bäumer AT, Müller K, Ahlbory K, Linz W et al. HMG-CoA reductase inhibitors improve endothelial dysfunction in normocholesterolemic hypertension via reduced production of reactive oxygen species. Hypertension 2001; 37(6):1450–57.

[14] Laufs U, Marra D, Node K, Liao JK. 3-Hydroxy-3-methylglutaryl-CoA reductase inhibitors attenuate vascular smooth muscle proliferation by preventing rho GTPase-induced down-regulation of p27 (Kip1). J Biol Chem 1999; 274(31): 21926– 31.

[15] Danenberg HD, Szalai AJ, Swaminathan RV, Peng L, Chen Z, Seifert P et al. Increased thrombosis after arterial injury in human C-reactive protein-transgenic mice. Circulation 2003; 108(5): 512–15.

[16] Aikawa M, Rabkin E, Sugiyama S, Voglic SJ, Fukumoto Y, Furukawa Y et al. HMGCoA reductase inhibitor, cerivastatin, suppresses growth of macrophages expressing matrix metalloproteinases and tissue factor in vivo and in vitro. Circulation 2001; 103(2):276–83.

[17] Stone NJ, Robinson JG, Lichtenstein AH, Bairey Merz CN, Blum CB, Eckel RH et al. 2013 ACC/AHA Guideline on the Treatment of Blood Cholesterol to Reduce Atherosclerotic Cardiovascular Risk in Adults: A Report of the American College of Cardiology/American Heart Association Task Force on Practice Guidelines. J Am Coll Cardiol 2014; 63(25 Pt B): 2889-934.

[18] Davidson MH. Safety profiles for HMG-CoA reductase inhibitors. Drugs 2001; 61(2): 1917-206.

[19] Thompson P, Clarkson P, Karas RH. Statin-associated myopathy. JAMA 2003; 289(13): 1681-90.

[20] Pasternak C, Smith SC Jr, Bairey-Merz CN, Grundy SM, Cleeman JI, Lenfant C; American College of Cardiology; American Heart Association; National Heart, Lung and Blood Institute. ACC/AHA/NHLBI Clinical advisory on the use and safety of statins. Circulation 2002; 106(8):1024-1028.

[21] Expert Panel on Detection, Evaluation, and Treatment of High Blood Cholesterol in Adults. Executive Summary of the Third Report of the National Cholesterol Education Program (NCEP) Expert Panel on Detection, Evaluation, and Treatment of High Blood Cholesterol in Adults (Adult Treatment Panel III, or ATP III). JAMA 2001; 285:2486-2497.

[22] Bellosta S, Paoletti R, Corsini A. Safety of statins: focus on clinical pharmacokinetics and drug interactions. Circulation 2004; 109 (23 Suppl 1):III50-7.

[23] Agón Banzo PJ, Ejea Arquillué MV. Estudio comparativo entre estatinas genéricas y no genéricas, en relación a su uso terapéutico, efectos farmacológicos y reacciones adversas [Tesis Doctoral]. Universidad de Zaragoza 2013.

[24] Coscollar Santaliestra. Estatinización o el discreto encanto del colesterol LDL. AMF 2014; 10(1):59-60.

Chapter 9

Pleiotropic Effects of Statins

Sigrid Mennickent

Additional information is available at the end of the chapter

http://dx.doi.org/10.5772/59202

1. Introduction

Atherosclerosis is a multi-factorial condition involving dyslipidemia that can result in cardiovascular disease.

The 3-hydroxy-3-methylglutaryl coenzyme A reductase inhibitors or statins are potent inhibitors of cholesterol biosynthesis, and most of the benefits of statin therapy are owing to the lowering of serum cholesterol levels. Reduction of LDL-cholesterol leads to upregulation of the LDL receptor and increased LDL clearance. Statins are the principal drugs in the primary and secondary prevention of coronary heart disease. Recent evidence also shows that more intensive lowering of LDL-cholesterol by statins is associated with greater clinical benefits. The mechanisms attributed to lipid lowering with statin therapy include atheromatous plaque stabilization, modification of the atherosclerosis progression and improved endothelial functions.

Statins reduce cardiovascular events in not only hypercholesterolemic but also normocholesterolemic patients with coronary heart disease (CHD) or cardiovascular risks.

Moreover, clinical trials and clinical benefits have shown that statins' effects involved other pharmacological activities and not only changes in lipid levels. "Pleiotropic" effects of statins involve improving endothelial function, decreasing vascular inflammation and oxidative stress, and inhibiting the thrombogenic response. Moreover, some works shows statins' beneficial extrahepatic effects on the immune system, CNS, and bone. Many of these pleiotropic effects are mediated by inhibition of isoprenoids, which serve as lipid attachments for intracellular signaling molecules. In particular, inhibition of small GTP-binding proteins, Rho, Ras, and Rac, whose proper membrane localization and function are dependent on isoprenylation, may play an important role in mediating the pleiotropic effects of statins. By inhibiting the conversion of HMG-CoA to L-mevalonic acid, statins prevent the synthesis of the important isoprenoids mentioned above, and also farnesyl pyrophosphate (FPP) and geranylgeranyl pyrophosphate (GGPP), which are precursors of cholesterol biosynthesis. Isoprenylated proteins can modify diverse cellular functions, therefore, statins have additional effects cholesterol-independent. Indeed, recent studies suggest that statins might be involved in immunomodulation, neuroprotection, and cellular senescence.

Therefore, statins might exert cholesterol-independent or "pleiotropic" effects through direct inhibition of these small GTP-binding proteins.

2. HMG-CoA reductase inhibition

The 3-hydroxy-3-methylglutaryl coenzyme A reductase inhibitors or Statins (Figure 1) are potent inhibitors of cholesterol biosynthesis, and most of the benefits of statin therapy are owing to the lowering of serum cholesterol levels. Because 60-70% of serum cholesterol is derived from hepatic synthesis and HMG-CoA reductase is the crucial rate-limiting enzyme in the cholesterol biosynthetic pathway, inhibition of this enzyme by statins results in a dramatic reduction in circulating low-density lipoprotein (LDL)-cholesterol. Reduction of LDL-cholesterol leads to up-regulation of the LDL receptor and increased LDL clearance. Moreover, statins increases HDL levels and decreases triglyceride levels. Statins are the principal drugs in the primary and secondary prevention of coronary heart disease for more than 25 million people at risk of cardiovascular disease worldwide. The Scandinavian Simvastatin Survival Study (4S) was the first randomized controlled trial to show significant risk reduction in cardiovascular mortality in patients with coronary-artery disease. Many studies,, such as 4S, Cholesterol and Recurrent Events (CARE), Long-term Intervention with Pravastatin in Ischemia Disease (LIPID), West of Scotland Coronary Prevention Study (WOSCOPS), Air Force/Texas Coronary Atherosclerosis Prevention Study (AFCAPS/TexCAPS), and the Heart Protection Study (HPS), have demonstrated the beneficial effects of statins in the prevention of cardiovascular disease. These works have shown significant risk reduction in cardiovascular mortality in patients with coronary artery disease, due to reduction in cholesterol levels and, therefore, reduction in atherosclerotic lesion development. The mechanisms attributed to lipid lowering with statin therapy include atheromatous plaque stabilization, modification of the atherosclerosis progression, and improved endothelial functions. The lowering of serum cholesterol levels is therefore thought to be the primary mechanism underlying the therapeutic benefits of statin therapy in cardiovascular disease. As 60-70% of serum cholesterol is obtained from hepatic synthesis mediated by HMG-CoA reductase, inhibition of this enzyme by statins is a principal way of reducing circulating low-density lipoprotein (LDL) cholesterol [1, 5, 7, 11, 10, 13, 16, , 24, 27, 30, 36, 39].

Statins in use today are: lovastatine, simvastatine, pravastatine, fluvastatine, athorvastatine and rosuvastatine. Lovastatine, simvastatine, and pravastatine are natural compounds, obtained from the fungi *Aspergillus terreus*, and the other statins are synthetic compounds [1, 22, 30].

Another statin used in the past was cerivastatine, but it produced some fatal adverse effect of rhabdomyolysis. Therefore, this drug was discontinued in 2000 [4].

http://dx.doi.org/10.5772/59202

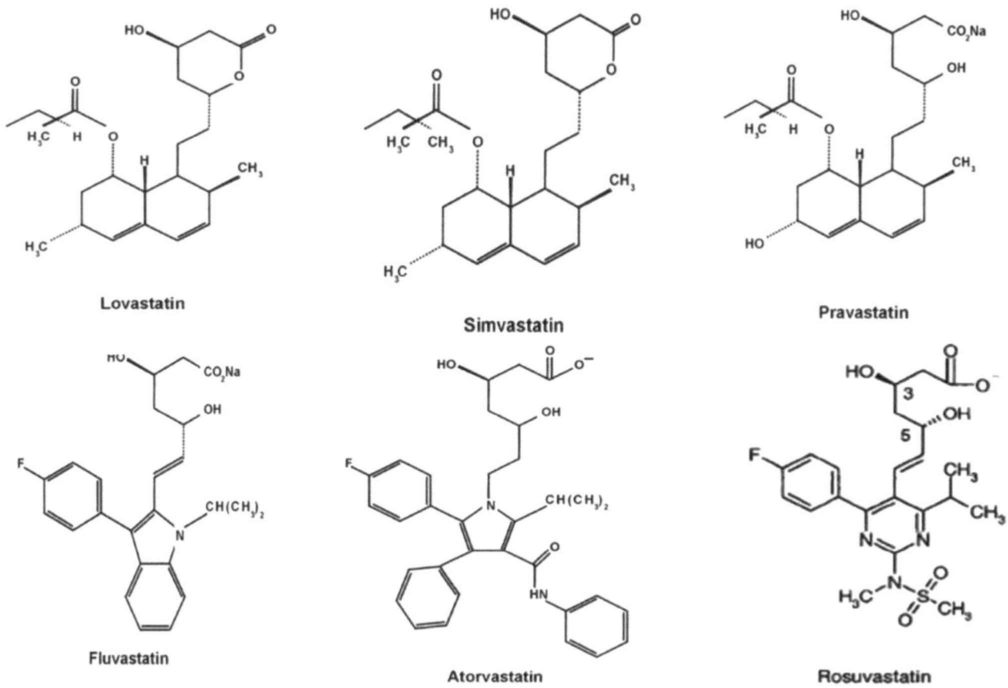

Figure 1. Chemical structure of statins [22, 30].

3. Pleiotropic effects of statins

However, the overall clinical benefits observed with statin therapy appear to be greater than what might be expected from changes in lipid profile alone, suggesting that the beneficial effects of statins may extend beyond their effects on serum cholesterol levels.

Statins reduce cardiovascular events in not only hypercholesterolemic but also normocholesterolemic patients. Because of the effects of lipid lowering on atherosclerosis, statins reduce morbidity and mortality in patients with ischemic heart failure. Statins also improve heart function and survival in patients with non-ischemic heart failure. Indeed, statins improve neurohormonal imbalance and idiopathic dilated cardiomyopathy. Thus, the improvements in heart function by statins might be owing to cholesterol-independent mechanisms [2, 5, 7, 11, 13, 19, 22, 24, 29, 30, 32].

Moreover, clinical trials and clinical benefits had shown that statins' effects involved other pharmacological activities and not only changes in lipid levels. Cholesterol-independent or "pleiotropic" effects of statins involve improving or restoring endothelial function, decreasing oxidative stress and vascular inflammation, enhancing the stability of atherosclerotic plaques, inhibiting the thrombogenic response, and lowering oxidative stress. Moreover, some works shows statins beneficial extrahepatic effects on the immune system, CNS, and bone.

Statins might exert cholesterol-independent or pleiotropic effects by inhibiting the conversion of HMG-CoA to L-mevalonic acid and, in this manner, prevent the synthesis of important isoprenoids, such as farnesylpyrophosphate (FPP), geranylgeranyl pyrophosphate (GGPP) and ubiquinone, which are precursors of cholesterol biosynthesis and of lipid attachments for intracellular signaling molecules. In particular, inhibition of small GTP-binding proteins, Rho, Ras, and Rac, whose proper membrane localization and function are dependent on isoprenylation, may play an important role in mediating the direct cellular effects of statins on the vascular wall. These isoprenylated proteins constitute approximately 2% of total cellular proteins, and isoprenylated proteins might control diverse cellular functions, as signal transduction, growth of vascular smooth muscle, apoptosis and in the regulation of the vascular activity of NAD(P) H oxidase.

Ras and Rho isoprenylation by statins, lead to increase of the amount to both compounds in the cytoplasm cells. As Rho is the more important target in the geranylgeranylation way, inhibition of Rho y de Rho-kinasa is an very important mechanism for the pleiotropic effects of statins at the vascular wall [8, 19, 25] (Figures 2 and 3).

Hypocholesterolemic effects of statins can be explained by hepatic HMG-CoA reductase inhibition, whereas the independent cholesterol effects can be found in all kinds of cells.

As isoprenylated proteins might control diverse cellular functions, we can explain that statins might have additional effects beyond lipid lowering [3, 4, 8, 17, 20, 23, 25, 37] (Li et al., 2002].

Indeed, recent studies suggest that statins might be involved in immunomodulation, neuroprotection, and cellular senescence [2, 5, 7, 11, 13, 18, 22, 24, 29, 30, 31, 32, 35].

Finally, statin therapy can be used for patients with autoimmune diseases, such as multiple sclerosis [26, 34, 35]. Furthermore, in a 6 month, randomized, double-blind placebo-controlled clinical trial, patients with rheumatoid arthritis who received atorvastatin showed a reduction in disease activity [21]. However, it is too early to predict whether these promising data can translate into clinical benefit by statins in patients with autoimmune disease.

The potential clinical implications of statin pleiotropy suggests that perhaps other biomarkers, in addition to lipid levels, should be used to gauge the full efficacy of statin therapy in patients with cardiovascular risks or that statin therapy may be effective in disease states, such as inflammatory conditions, ischemic stroke, or cancer, where elevated cholesterol levels have not been shown to be a strong epidemiological risk for these diseases [2, 5, 7, 8, 11, 12, 13, 19, 20, 22, 24, 25, 29, 30] (Vaughan et al., 2003).

Some clinical trials, such as MIRACL (Myocardial Ischemia Reduction with Aggressive Cholesterol Lowering), TNT (Treating to New Targets), PROVE IT-TIMI 22, and SPARCL (Stroke Prevention by Aggressive Reduction in Cholesterol Levels), have shown that statins, when used in high doses, can reduce vascular risks better than when used in low doses. Although high doses, adverse effects are relatively low, except atorvastatin 80-mg, that is associated with higher rates of elevated hepatic transaminase, and simvastatin 80-mg with higher rates of myopathy and rhabdomyolysis. A challenge today is to discover if high-dose statin therapy provides greater benefits due to lower cholesterol levels or due to statin pleiotropic effects [2, 5, 7, 11, 13, 18, 19, 22, 24, 29, 30, 31, 35] (Vaughan et al., 2003).

http://dx.doi.org/10.5772/59202

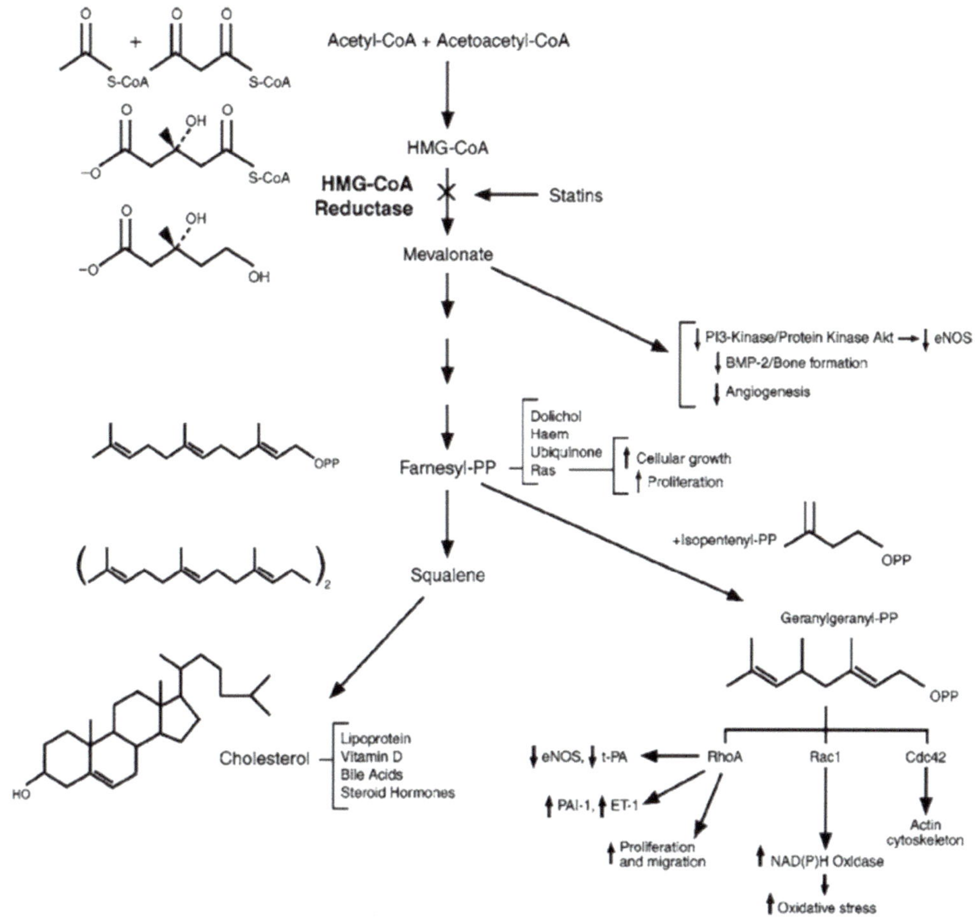

Figure 2. Biological actions of isoprenoids [19].

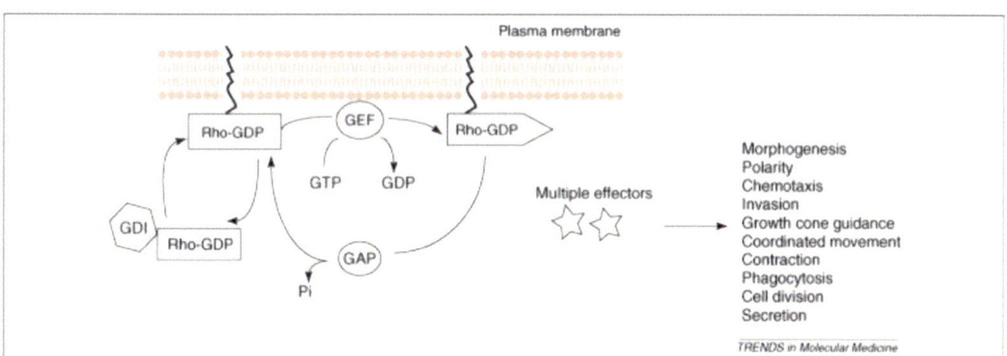

Figure 3. Regulation of the Rho GTPase cycle. Rho proteins cycle between a cytosolic, inactive GDP-bound state and a, membrane, active, GTP-bound state [35].

3.1. Improve or restore endothelial function

Hypercholesterolemia impairs endothelial function, and endothelial dysfunction is one of the earliest manifestations of atherosclerosis. When endothelial dysfunction appears, its principal sign is the impaired synthesis, release, and activity of endothelial-derived nitric oxide (NO). Endothelial NO inhibits several components of the atherogenic process, such as vascular relaxation and platelet aggregation, vascular smooth muscle proliferation, and endothelial-leukocyte interactions. [9, 15, 17, 19, 28, 38].

Statins could restore endothelial function, in part, by lowering serum cholesterol levels. Indeed, statins increase endothelial NO production by action over NO synthase (eNOS). Also, statins restore eNOS activity in hypoxia condition. Statins also inhibit the expression of endothelin-1, a potent vasoconstrictor and mitogen [6, 14].

3.2. Oxidative stress

Oxidative stress is defined as tissue injury resulting from a disturbance in theequilibrium between the production of reactive oxygen species (ROS) also known as free radicals and antioxidant defense mechanisms [3].

ROS have been implicated in many disease states, including neurodegenerative disease like Alzheimer and Parkinson disease, atherosclerosis, inflammatory conditions, certain cancers, diabetes mellitus (DM), cataract in the eye, pulmonary, renal, heart diseases, and the process of aging.

NADPH oxidase is an important signaling mediator in the signaling pathway mediated alpha-1-AR, stimulating hypertrophy in adult rat cardiac myocytes. Moreover, recently had been identified calmodulin, Ras and Raf-1 as the upstream signaling molecules in this pathway. In addition, the role of NAD (P) H oxidase in the development of cardiac hypertrophy has been demonstrated. This indicated an interesting new direction in the research of alpha-1-AR signaling mechanisms.

Polyunsaturated lipid acids (PUFAS) in plasma are susceptible to the oxidation process mediated by EROs. This leads to the transformation of the native LDL (LDLn) to oxidative LDL (oxLDL). The oxLDLs does not bind to the LDLn hosts; however oxLDLs bind to the scavenger hosts in monocytes / macrophagues, endothelium and vascular smooth muscle cells, with the consequence of the increase of these compounds and the intracellular generation of the foam cells, an important sign of early atherosclerotic damage [2, 4, 6, 8, 9, 14, 15, 17, 18, 28, 29, 33, 38].

The proliferation of vascular smooth muscle cells is a central event in the pathogenesis of vascular lesions, including post-angioplasty restenosis, transplant arteriosclerosis and veinous graft occlusion.

Statins possesses antioxidant properties by reducing lipid generation and its peroxidation and ROS production by the vascular NAD (P) H oxidase pathway, the susceptibility of lipoproteins to oxidation both in vitro and in vivo, i.e. they decrease the LDL oxidation, especially simvastatine, pravastatine, and lovastatine [4, 6, 9, 14, 15, 17, 24, 27, 28, 33, 36, 38, 39], decrease the pro-oxidant effects of Angiotensin II and of Endothelin-1 (peptides that stimulate vasoconstriction and increase of vascular smooth muscle cells), decreasing the NAD(P)H oxidase activity and the generation of superoxide anion as in vascular cells as in phagocytes, and increase the vascular synthesis of nitric oxide. Moreover statins inhibit vascular SMC proliferation by arresting cell cycle between the G1/S phase transition, decrease inflammatory cytokines, C-reactive protein C, and adhesion molecules, stimulate NO release, and stimulate activated hosts by PPAR, therefore decrease plasma lipid peroxidation products [4, 9, 14, 15, 17, 24, 27, 28, 33, 36, 38].

4. Statins and dementia

Recent epidemiological reports suggest that statins might be protective for Alzheimer's disease and for other types of dementia, as cerebrovascular disease. Alzheimer's disease is related to the effects of β-amyloid, and some experimental and clinical trials have shown that there is a pathophysiologic relation between β-amyloid and cholesterol levels. Statins, regardless of their brain availability, have been suggested to induce alterations in cellular cholesterol distribution in the brain. However, major studies are necessary to establish a relationship between statin therapy and Alzheimer disease [19].

5. Clinical trials relationed to pleiotropic effects of statins

HPS and ASCOT showed that the relative risk reduction by statin was independent of the treatment for lipid levels. Also, other studies suggest that the risk of myocardial infarctions in patients treated with statins is significantly lower compared to individuals with other cholesterol-lowering agents [18].

6. Conclusions

Statins reduce cardiovascular events in not only hypercholesterolemic but also normocholesterolemic patients. Moreover, clinical trials and clinical benefits have shown that statins' effects involved other pharmacological activities and not only changes in lipid levels. Cholesterol-independent or "pleiotropic" effects of statins involve improving or restoring endothelial function, decreasing oxidative stress and vascular inflammation, enhancing the stability of atherosclerotic plaques, inhibiting the thrombogenic response, and lowering oxidative stress. Moreover, some works show that statins have a beneficial extrahepatic effects on the immune system, CNS, and bone.

Statins might exert cholesterol-independent or pleiotropic effects by inhibiting the conversion of HMG-CoA to L-mevalonic acid and, in this manner, prevent the synthesis of important isoprenoids, which are precursors of cholesterol biosynthesis and of lipid attachments for intracellular signaling molecules. Inhibition of Rho GTPases in vascular cellwalls by statins improves expression of atheroprotective genes and inhibition of vascular SMC proliferation.

Author details

Sigrid Mennickent*

Address all correspondence to: smennick@udec.cl

Faculty of Pharmacy, University of Concepción, Concepción, Chile

References

[1] Acevedo, S., & Aguillon, R. (2004). Manejo de dislipidemias en pacientes diabéticos tipo 2. *Revista MedUNAB*, 6, 3.

[2] Arteaga, E., & Pollak, F. (2002). *Dislipidemias en la práctica clínica*, International Lipid Information Bureau, Santiago de Chile.

[3] Bendall, J.K., Cave, A.C., Heymes, C., Gall, N., & Shah, A.M. (2002). Pivotal role of gp91 (phox)-containing NADPH oxidase in angiotensin II-induced cardiac hypertrophy in mice. *Circulation*, 105, 293-296.

[4] Beltowski, J. (2005). Statins and Modulation of Oxidative Stress. *Toxicology Mechanism and Methods*, 15, 61.

[5] Brody, T., Larner, J., & Minulman, K. (1994). *Human Pharmacology. Molecular to Clinical*, 3ºEd., Mosby Year Book, St. Louis, USA.

[6] Carr, A.C., Mc Call, M.R., & Frei, B. (2000). Oxidation of LDL by mieloperoxidase and reactive nitrogen species: Reaction pathways and antioxidant protection. *Arterioscl. Throm. Vasc. Biol.*, 20, 1716-1723.

[7] Delgado, J., & Remers, W. (1998). *Wilson and Gisvolds. Textbook of Organic Medicinal and Pharmaceutical Chemistry*, Lippincott-Raven, Philadelphia, USA.

[8] Foncea, R., Carvajal, C., & Leighton, F. (2000). Endothelial cell oxidative stress and signal transduction. *Biological Research*, 33, 86-96.

[9] Fukumoto, Y., Libby, P., Rabkin, E., Hill, C.C., & Enomoto, M. (2001). Statins alter smooth muscle cell accumulation and collagen content in established atheroma of watanabe hyperlipidemic rabbits. *Circulation*, 103, 993-999.

[10] Garay, R., & Olivillo, M. (2003). Estatinas: Prevención Primaria y Secundaria de la Hipercolesterolemia. *Revista de Postgrado de la VI cátedra de medicina*, Universidad Nacional del Nordeste, Corrientes, Argentina, 125,15.

[11] Hardman, J., & Limbird, L. (2006). *Las Bases Farmacológicas de la Terapéutica,* Mc Graw-Hill, Mexico.

[12] Istvan, E.S., & Deisenhofer, J. (2001). Structural mechanism for statin inhibition of HMG-CoA reductase. *Science,* 292, 1160-1164.

[13] Katzung, B. (1999). *Farmacología Básica y Clínica,* Editorial El Manual Moderno, México.

[14] Kureishi, Y., Luo, Z., Shiojima, I., Bialik, A., & Fulton, D. (2000). The HMG-CoA reductase inhibitor simvastatin activates the protein kinase Akt and promotes angiogenesis in normocholesterolemic animals. *Nat. Med.,* 6, 1004-1010.

[15] Laufs, U., Gertz, H., Huang, P., Nickenig, G., & Bohm, M. (2000). Atorvastatin upregulates type III nitric oxide synthase in thrombocytes, decreases platelet activation, and protects from cerebral ischemia in normocholesterolemic mice. *Stroke,* 31, 2442-2449.

[16] Laufs, U., Wassmann, S., Schackmann, S., Haeschen, C., Bophm, M., & Nickening, G. (2004). Beneficial effects of statins in patients with non-ischemic heart faillure. *Z.Kardiol.,* 93,103-108.

[17] Lefer, A.M., Scalia, R., & Lefer, D.J. (2001). Vascular effects of HMG CoA-reductase inhibitors (statins) unrelated to cholesterol lowering: New concepts for cardiovascular disease. *Cardiovasc. Res.,* 49, 281-287.

[18] Liao, J.K. (2005). Clinical implications for statin pleiotropy. *Curr. Opin. Lipidol.,* 16(6), 624-629.

[19] Liao, J.K., & Laufs, U. (2005). Pleiotropic effects of statins. *Annu. Rev. Pharmacol. Toxicol.,* 45, 89-118.

[20] Maccarthy, P.A., Grieve, D.J., Li, M.J., Dunster, C., Kell, F.J., & Shah, A.M. (2001). Impaired endothelial regulation of ventricular relaxation in cardiac hypertrophy: Role of reactive oxygen species and NADPH oxidase. *Circulation,* 104, 2967-2974.

[21] Mc Carey, DW., et al. (2004). Trial of Atorvastatin in Rheumatoid Arthritis (TARA): Double-blind, randomised placebo-controlled trial. *Lancet,* 363, 2015-2021.

[22] Mc Evoy, G. (2012). *AHFS Drug Information,* 54ºEd., American Society of Health-System Pharmacists: Bethesda, USA.

[23] Nakagami, H., Takemoto, M., & Liao, J.K. (2003). NADPH oxidase-derived superoxide anion mediates angiotensin II-induced cardiac hypertrophy. *J.Mol.Cell Cardiol.,* 35, 851-859.

[24] Page, C., Curtis, N., Sutter, M., Walker, M., & Hoffman, B. (1998). *Farmacología Integrada,* Harcout, Madrid, Spain.

[25] Park, H.J., Kong, D., Iruela-Arispe, L., Begley, U., Tang, D., & Galper ,J.B. (2002). 3-hydroxy-3-methylglutaryl coenzyme A reductase inhibitors interfere with angiogenesis by inhibiting the geranylgeranylation of RhoA. *Circ. Res.*, 91, 143-150.

[26] Sena, A., et al. (2003). Therapeutic potential of lovastatin in multiple sclerosis. *J. Neurol.*, 250, 754-755.

[27] Silverman, R. (2004). *The organic Chemistry of Drug Design and Drug Action,* 2ºEd., Elsevier Academic Press, Amsterdam, Holland.

[28] Stalker, T.J., Lefer, A.M., & Scalia, R. (2001). A new HMG-CoA reductase inhibitor, rosuvastatin, exerts anti-inflammatory effects on the microvascular endothelium: The role of mvalonic acid. *Br.J. Pharmacol.*, 133, 406-412.

[29] Stryer, L. (1995). *Bioquímica,* 4ºEd., Editorial Reverté S.A., Barcelona, Spain.

[30] Sweetman, S. *Martindale, Guía Completa de Consulta Farmacoterapéutica,* 2ºEd., Pharma Editores S.L. Barcelona, España, 2006.

[31] Takemoto, M., & Liao, J.K. (2001). Pleiotropic effects of 3-hydroxy-3-methylglutaryl coenzyme: A reductase inhibitors. *Arterioscler. Thromb. Vasc. Biol.*, 21(11), 1712-1719.

[32] Vaughan, C.J., Gotto, A.M., & Basson, C.T. (2000). The envolving role of statins in the management of atherosclerosis. *J.Am.Coll.Cardiol.*, 31, 1-10.

[33] Vidal, F., Colome, C., Martinez-Gonzalez, J., & Badimon, L. (1998). Atherogenic concentrations of native low-density lipoproteins down-regulate nitric-oxide-synthase mRNA and protein levels in endothelial cells. *Eur. Biochem.*, 252, 378-384.

[34] Vollmer, T., et al. (2004). Oral simvastatin treatment in relapsing-remitting multiple sclerosis. *Lancet,* 363, 1607-1608.

[35] Wang, C.Y., Liu, P.Y., & Liao, J.K. (2008). Pleiotropic effects of statin therapy: molecular mechanisms and clinical results. *Trend Mol. Med.*, 14(1), 37-44.

[36] Woll, M. (1995). *Burger´s Medicinal Chemistry and Drug Discovery,* 5ºEd., John Wiley & Sons Inc., New York, USA.

[37] Xiao, L., Pimentel, D.R., Wang, J., Singh, K., Colucci, W.S., & Sawyer, D.B. (2002). Role of reactive oxygen species and NAD(P)H oxidase in alpha(1)-adrenoceptor signaling in adult rat cardiac myocytes. *Am. J. Physiol. Cell Physiol.*, 282, C926-934.

[38] Yang, Z., Kozai, T., Van Der, T., Loo, B., Viswambharan, H., & Lachat M. (2000). HMG-CoA reductase inhibition improves endothelial cell function and inhibits smooth muscle cell proliferation in human saphenous veins. *J.Am. Coll. Cardiol., 36, 1691-1697.*

[39] Yates,T., Mennickent, S., & Villegas, G. (2004). *Texto de Farmacoquímica. Aspectos Esructurales y Propiedades de los Medicamentos,* Editorial Universidad de Concepción, Concepción, Chile.

Chapter 10

Resistance of Statin Therapy, and Methods for its Influence

Lyudmila Georgieva Vladimirova-Kitova and
Spas Ivanov Kitov

Additional information is available at the end of the chapter

http://dx.doi.org/10.5772/60004

1. Introduction

Resistance happens when an individual has an incorrect response to the effectiveness of a drug as stated in the National Library of Medicine. It is difficult to give an accurate definition of statin resistance. Patients who fail to reach LDL-C target levels despite undergoing the best available therapy of the most highly tolerated dose of a more potent statin, are considered to be statin-resistant. Many individuals do not reach LDL-C target levels, even when compliance is taken into consideration. The reduction of LDL-C in response to statin therapy can vary from 5-70 %. This can be influenced by many factors. For instance,racial andestry, with attenuated responses in blacks compared to whites. A study comparing statin resistance patients to patients who show no resistance to statin has yet to appear.

The resistance to statins can be related to differences in drug absorption, drug transport, intrahepatic drug metabolism, drug metabolism within other organs, and drug excretion mechanisms. The same can occur due to differences in the level of the various target pathways that are unrelated to pharmacokinetics, including HMG-CoA reductase, as well as various points along the cholesterol biosynthesis and lipoprotein metabolic pathways.

2. Possible causes of statin resistance

According to Herman and Moncada the process of atherogenesis includes 28 stages. [48] Key points in this process are two - oxygenated LDL-cholesterol and endogenous nitric oxide synthase. Statin reistance may exist in both directions:

2.1. Failed targeting LDL cholesterol

It seems that not only genetic but environmental factors can influence the LDL-C response to statins. Studies have found that patients with hypertension have a smaller decrease than those without hypertension. Furthermore, smokers have smaller statin-induced LDL-C decrease compared with nonsmokers[47]. It also seems that inflammation might cause statin resistance. Namely, it has been shown that inflammatory cytokines, in particular IL-1b which affects sterol regulatory element binding protein cleavage-activating protein, cause statin resistance due to the disruption of LDL-R feedback regulation. Therefore, it has been suggested that in inflammatory states, higher concentrations of statin may be required to achieve the appropriate LDL-C lowering [107]. Particularly interesting are observations concerning certain subpopulations of patients who might be resistant to statin treatment. Some studies have shown statins to be less effective in individuals with HIV infection. [22]. Other studies have a contraversal perspective. [55]. The role of concomitant amiodarone treatment in statin resistance was also suspected. Both amiodarone and amiodarone induced hypothyroidism influence the synthesis of LDLR, which may explain the lack of statin effect. Thyroid hormone is one of several hormones that control gene expression of the LDLR and hypothyroidism is a wellknown cause of secondary dyslipidemia characterized by elevated LDL-C levels. Similar to hypothyroidism, administration of amiodarone also increases LDL-C levels, which is the result of a decreased expression of the LDLR gene [1].

More recently, an approach was published which used metabolomics to identify markers indicative of mechanisms that contribute to differences in LDL-C response to statin. Metabolic changes were shown to be more comprehensive in responders to statin treatment than those seen in nonresponders. The baseline cholesterol ester and phospholipid metabolites correlated with LDL-C response to treatment [56]. It has also been suggested that clusters of metabolites involved in multiple pathways not directly connected with cholesterol metabolism might as well play a role in modulating the response to statin therapy - influence statin resistance [90].

Insufficient LDL-C response to statin treatment is probably the result of pseudo-resistance, which could be caused by nonadherence or nonpersistence in real life circumstances. [68].

3. Lack of effect on the endothelium-dependent vasodilation after targeting LDL-C

There is a lot of evidence that the endothelium plays a crucial role in the maintenance of vascular tone and structure. [39; 40, 41; 38; 5; 51; 9]. One of the major endothelium-derived vasoactive mediators was shown to be nitric oxide (NO). [38; 74; 51; 67]. Multifactional are the mechanism by which NO activity is reduced: reduced NO release, NO inactivation by superoxide anion, or reduced NO production by NO synthase (NOS). [91] Decrease in NOS expression by oxidized low-density lipoprotein (LDL) can cause impaired NO production [77; 91], or by the presence of asymmetric dimethylarginine (ADMA). [72; 16 ;29]

According to Herman and Moncada the basis of atherogenesis remain oxygenated LDL and eNOS. Lipid-regulating effects of statins in terms of LDL-cholesterol are undeniable, but the pleiotropic discussioncy is a particularly relevant issue of resistance of statin therapy in patients with high levels of ADMA - endogenous inhibitor of eNOS. Research of statin influence on flow-mediated vasodilation (FMD) reveals controversial results. Some studies indicate that there is an effect, whereas others document the opposite tendency [18]. There is a number of studies on simvastatin and likewise they demonstrate controversial findings. These controversies can be dismissed by studing ADMA levels.(18 ;16;6). It has been suggested that ADMA could modify the effect of statins on myocardial blood flow and on FMD% (53).

In our subsequent studies found in a logical sequence following facts. This facts determinate ADMA as a basic factor for statin`s resistans.

International recommendations underline the importance of diagnosis and treatment of asymptomatic individuals with high absolute cardiovascular risk [10; 37; 8], as individuals with severe hypercholesterolemia. [47; 45; 58] the levels of ADMA in patients with severe hypercholesterolemia in our study are higher than those cited in the literature in the same population patients. [13].

1. A good marker of endothelial dysfunction is considered to be ADMA, as indicated by recent publications. [16]. Subjects with cardiovascular risk – hypercholesterolemia, hyperhomocysteinemia, diabetes mellitus, hypertension, smoking, erectile dysfunction having increased ADMA levels. [67; 11; 16,17]. Plasma levels of ADMA have been shown to be elevated in hypercholesterolemic rabbits [108]. The elevation of ADMA is associated with reduced activity of NOS in animal models, as well as in young asymptomatic hypercholesterolemic adults [13]. The mechanism of increased ADMA in hypercholesterolemia is not very clear - LDL cholesterol increases the expression of ADMA precursor protein and reduces the activity of the enzyme dimethyl arginine dimethyl amino hydrolase. [52; 15] Increased ADMA are associated with reduced NO synthesis and this assessed by impaired endothelium-dependent vasodilatation. Flow-mediated dilatation (FMD) - shear stress during hyperemia activates receptors on the endothelial cell surface and causes influx of intracellular calcium, which activates eNOS and NO release [54; 24; 80; 60]. The main effect that dilatation has in respons to shear stress during FMD is influenced by NO and to a smaller extent on prostaglandins and endothelial-dependent hyperpolarizing factors [78; 54; 31; 30; 73]. Ultrasound determination of flow-mediated dilatation of the brachial artery as a method has many advantages – it is non-invasive, with good reproducibility and reliable. [3; 28; 31; 36; 61]. There is convincing evidence that reduced percentage of FMD (FMD%) is a marker of coronary endothelial dysfunction [3].

Several studies have associated hypercholesterolemia with reduced FMD% and this effect can be reversed by L-arginine [34; 26; 32; 33]. However, L-arginine does not lead to the improvement of endothelial dependent vasodilatation in normocholesterolemic individuals. In this condition indicate the main role of endogenous ADMA. [11; 44] Furthermore, a recent publication demonstrated that improvement of FMD% under statin treatment depends on the ADMA levels [53; 12]. Little is know about the relationship between ADMA, and FMD%. In a small number of hypercholesterolemic patients ADMA was shown to be positively correlated with FMD% in mild hypercholesterolemia [13]. A recent paper demonstrated that low cardiovascular risk subjects have increased ADMA level. [6]. No data exist about the relationship between ADMA and FMD% in severe hypercholesterolemia patients. In our study

"Relationship of asymmetric dimethylarginine with flow-mediated dilatation in subjects with newly detected severe hypercholesterolemia" was the evaluation of the relationship between ADMA and FMD, also that of ADMA and lipid parameters as well as other endothelial dysfunction in newly detected subjects with severe hypercholesterolemia. The major findings of the present study are that: (1) plasma levels of ADMA, are increased in severe hypercholesterolemia; (2) there is a significant link between ADMA and age, Apo-B, Apo-B / Apo-A_1 and tHcy; (3) newly detected severe hypercholesterolemia has reduced flow-mediated endothelial dependent vasodilatation, there is a correlation between plasma levels of FMD% and age, Apo-B, Apo-B/Apo-A1 and tHcy; and (4) homocystein levels has no contribution to the atherogenic risk in the patients.

Newly detected severe hypercholesterolemia is associated with elevated ADMA, and to the proportional increase in total cholesterol. The ADMA correlates with age, Apolipoprotein-B, Apo-B/Apo-A_1 and tHcy. Apo-B was found to indicate elevated ADMA in these patients. FMD % correlates most strongly with age, Apolipoprotein-B, index Apo-B / Apo-A_1 and tHcy. In multiple regression analysis, ADMA is the strongest predictor for FMD%. ADMA is the main modulator of FMD% - among the investigated biomarkers in newly detected severe hypercholesterolemia. Serious functional changes in the vascular wall are cause by increased level of ADMA. At the same time, ADMA is found to be a predictor of flow-modulated vasodilation of the brachial artery which also makes a probable marker for endothelial dysfunction. Therefore, measuring ADMA levels in newly detected severe hypercholesterolemia is of great importance when FMD% changes need to be clarified.

2. In the next study we investigated intima-media complex of carotid artery. The intima-media thickness (IMT) of the CCA is one of the validated measurements of subclinical atherosclerosis, as early as structural vascular abnormalities [85]. Intima-media thickening of the CCA correlates with the coronary risk factors [80] and with associated with the degree of coronary atherosclerosis. It serves as a predictor of coronary and vascular events in different patients' populations. Intima-media thickening reflects both intimal atherosclerosis and medial hypertrophy. It is used to evaluate the luminal and wall characteristics of the carotid artery. In the literature, hypercholesterolemia has an important role in early-onset IMT changes in the CCA However, there is not a lot of data about asymptomatic subjects with newly detected severe hypercholesterolemia.[72]. In the literature, data on the IMT of CCA predictors is controversial. There are a few studies of the endothelium-related biomarkers (ADMA, tHcy, soluble cell adhesion molecules), especially in asymptomatic subjects with newly detected severe hypercholesterolemia [72].

The research "Predictors of the intima-media thickness of carotid artery in asymptomatic newly detected severe hypercholesterolemic patients" age and Apo-B were established as the most important statistically significant factors related to IMT mean of CCA. This fact illustrates that they determine the slow progressive structural changes in the vascular wall. The Apo-B is a better biomarker of the total number of atherogenic particles. It might be concluded that Apo-B is a better factor for assessment of risk, as LDL cholesterol underestimates the risk in asymptomatic subjects with newly detected severe hypercholesterolemia.

http://dx.doi.org/10.5772/60004

In the study "Intima-Media Thickness and Flow-Mediated Vasodilation in Asymptomatic Subjects with Newly Detected Severe Hypercholesterolemia", our results show a significant correlation between IMT mean and FMD%. The correlation is still present when separating IMT on the basis of the level of thickening. This supports the idea that the two noninvasive methods complete each other. It is important with regard to building a diagnostic algorithm. These methods show early subclinical atherosclerosis but by different trigger mechanisms.

3. After establishing who is a predictor of FMV - ADMA, the next study proved that ADMA is the main determinant of the effect of simvastatin on FMV in severe hypercholesterolemia - "Asymmetric dimewthylarginine determines the effect of simvastatin on endothelium-dependent vasodilation in severe hypercholesterolemia" Future Medicine Clinical Lipidology 2010. With respect to their total cholesterol, LDL-cholesterol and FMD% the two groups of hypercholesterolemic patients (according to the plasma ADMA levels) differ significantly. ADMA, cell adhesion molecules or total homocysteine levels are not affected by Simvastatin in moderate dose [40 mg). Higher baseline levels of ADMA affect the ability of statins to improve endothelium-dependent vasodilation by diminishing it. Subjects from the same population, but with lower baseline levels of ADMA experience the same effect of simvastatin. Therefore, ADMA seems to be a pathophysiologycal modulator of the statin therapeutic response. The present study has been confirm by studies that there is a connection between ADMA and FMD% response to statins found by Böger et al. The different is that in our study is in the larger group of the patients.

In terms of non-randmized study "Effect of Moderate and High-Dose Simvastatin on Asymmetric-Homocysteine Metabolic Pathways in Patients with Newly Detected Severe Hypercholesterolemia" was demonstrated dose-dependent effect of simvastatin on the levels of ADMA.The 40 mg simvastatin has no effect on ADMA and homocysteine level in contrast to 80 mg, after target LDL-levels are reached ≤2.6 mmol/L. It is likely that statin-pleiotropic effects on ADMA-homocysteine metabolic pathways are independent of their lipid-regulating properties.

In another of our observation "Asymmetric dimethylarginine-a determinant of the effect of the high dose Simvastatin confirmed this dose-dependent effect". The two groups of patients (according to the plasma ADMA levels) differ significantly with respect to their total cholesterol, LDL-cholesterol and FMD%. Simvastatin in moderate dose (40 mg) does no affect ADMA, cell adhesion molecules and total homocysteine levels. The higher levels of ADMA change the ability of statins to improve the endothelium-dependent vasodilatation, by diminishing it. This shows that ADMA is a pathophysiological modulator of the statin therapeutic response. This study confirms that, for the first time, there is a correlation between ADMA levels and FMD% response to statins, found by Böger et al., but in the larger group of patients with severe hypercholesterolemia and with higher dose simvastatin. Obviously, these mechanisms require further investigation

To give a more precise answer to the question of dose-dependent manner for avoidable statin resistance subsequently conducted a randomized, placebo-controlled study "The effect of simvastatin on asymmetric dimethylarginine and flow-mediated vasodilation after optimizing the LDL level — A randomized, placebo-controlled study" The major findings of the present study are 1. Significantly higher ADMA and tHcy were seen in patients with severe hypercholesterolemia compared to the control group. 2. Administration of 40 mg simvastatin for one month results in no variation in ADMA, tHcy plasma levels and FMD%, following optimizing of the LDL. 3. Administration of 80 mg simvastatin for a month leads to a variation of ADMA and tHcy plasma levels and FMD% after optimizing the LDL. FMD%-changes can be predicted with ADMA levels and ApoB%-changes is a predictor of LDL-changes% in patients on 80 mg simvastatin (for one month) following the optimization of the LDL-C.

This study gives evidence that in experimental models and in humans (59), higher ADMA levels have a harmful effect on the coronary endothelium. On the other hand, the experimental model shows that statins have no protective effect against that harmful effect of ADMA on the endothelium. This provokes a discussion as to whether ADMA is the pathophysiological modulator of the therapeutic response of statins in hypercholesterolemia.

The ADMA in severe hypercholesterolemia are higher compared to those in patients in similar research protocols (13), and are similar to those in our previous research studies. Applying various laboratory methods(ELISA in the present study, high-pressure liquid chromatography in other studies) does not allow for the mean levels of ADMA to be compared directly. Using ELISA to differentiate the sample groups is less reliable than LC-MS.This is caused by the fac that the higher coefficient of variation and to the fact that the matrix dependence is likely to cloud or mimic the differences The ADMA ELISA method can be used for clinical investigations in which groups of samples are compared and the result is the shift of the ADMA concentration in response to an intervention. The application of ELISA analysis in our study is the likely ex- planation of the higher levels of ADMA, in comparison with other studies (13). On the other hand, this is likely due to the higher levels of total cholesterol > 7.5 mmol/l and LDL-C > 4.9 mmol/l. The difference in L-arginine substitution in hypercholesterolic patients and normo-cholesterolic patients is explained by the higher levels of ADMA in hypercholesterolic petients in comparison with controls with controls (11; 44).

The mechanism of an increased ADMA level in hypercholesterolemia is not clear enough. An association between ADMA and hypercholesterolemia has been previously observed [13]. Laufs et al. (1998) demonstrated that simvastatin reverse, in a dose-dependent manner, the inhibitory effect of oxidized LDL on NO production. It has been suggested that LDL- cholesterol increases the expression of ADMA precursor protein. This reduces the activity of the enzyme dimethylarginine dimethylaminohydrolase, which breaks down ADMA [52]. This is why, by decreasing cholesterol levels with statin therapy, ADMA plasma levels will decrease as well. The therapeutic hypothesis that the decrease of circulating ADMA levels can be achieved by lowering plasma cholesterol levels is the main idea in this publication.

In randomized, placebo-controlled research, a statistically significant reduction of ADMA plasma levels has been established following a one-month therapy with 80 mg simvastatin, yet the 40 mg simvastatin dose does not result in achieving the LDL target levels. The study showed that a 40 mg simvastatin therapy for 3 months does not produce the desired effect. Therefore, it is likely that the pleiotropic effect of the statins (respectively ADMA and tHcy) is independent from the lipid-regulation in a short-term and long-term plan. The lack of effect on 40 mg simvastatin coincides with the results presented in other studies but there is no optimizing of LDL-C level. The research in similar articles regarding the effect of 80 mg simvastatin on ADMA levels is scant. Most research works have documented a negative effect in hypercholesterolemia. However, these studies have tested a considerably smaller number of patients (64). The present study comprises 85 patients and LDL target levels have been optimized regarding the risk category. The established statistically significant therapeutic effect of 80 mg simvastatin on ADMA is comparable to the results from a recently published study — an experimental model of the effect of simvastatin on ADMA tissue levels (64). This recent experimental data shows that simvastatin regulates dimethylarginine dimethylamino-hydrolase transcription via the transcription factor Sterol Regulatory Element Binding Protein. The latter is activated by statins due to a reduction of plasma membrane cholesterol. These experimental models suggest that the level of asymmetric dimethylarginine will be decreased by statin therapy. Almost all other clinical studies (of smaller sample size and shorter duration) showed no effect of statins on ADMA (positive effect only 10 mg rosuvastatin and 80 mg fluvastatin). It is unclear whether the higher plasma levels of ADMA in human disease states correlate with a higher intracellular level. Studies testing the statin effect in vivo have reported endothelial protection without overly affecting plasma ADMA levels, however in these studies the tissue levels of ADMA have not been taken into consideration. It is likely that in the present study achieving the LDL-C target level substitutes for the LDL-cholesterol tissue levels. Similar titrations have not been carried out in any other related articles so far. The results of the present study provide further clinical evidence to the experimental model of the Ivashchenko et al., that simvastatin regulates dimethylarginine dimethylaminohydrolase transcription via the transcription factor Sterol Regulatory Element Binding Protein.

The present study shows a statistically significant increase in FMD% in patients on 80 mg simvastatin therapy for one month in the presence of controversial results in related materials on this issue. The mechanism of this improvement is proved to be related to the enhancement of gene expression of eNOS (64). On the other hand, the FMD%-changes correlate (correlations with all biomarkers at a baseline level and the %-changes have been tested) significantly only with the baseline level of ApoB, ADMA, and tHcy. Interestingly enough,patients with ADMA levels greater than 1 μmol/l, following statin therapy, appear to have only small or no FMD% changes. A likely explanation of this finding is that in patients with ADMA greater than 1 μmol/l, competes with L-arginine as a substrate for eNOS and thus decreases the production and availability of endothelium-derived NO. For this reason, in such patients, there are no FMD% changes following statin therapy. In patients with documented small FMD% changes, the most likely explanation is the action of other mediators (endothelium-derived hyperpola-rizing factor or prostaglandins) that lead to vasodilation through calcium-activated potassium channels simvastatin (80 mg daily).

The high simvastatin doses should be done with caution. According to the Food and Drug Administration monitoring are also important every 3 and 6 months during the course of therapy.

In the multifactor regressive analysis only the initial ADMA levels remain predictors of an FMD%-change. For the first time, in 2007 Böger GI et al. established that ADMA determines FMD%- changes in a small hypercholesterolemic patients group (treated with a smaller simvastatin dose — 40 mg (12). Further clinical studies can be based off of this study, in order to achieve LDL-target levels and to optimize the effect of different doses statins on ADMA. Other statins are better tolerated at a high dose (atorvastatin, pravastatin, fluvastatin, lovastatin). There is only one study testing the effect of 80 mg fluvastatin treatment in hypercholesteromic patients with metabolic syndrome, which demonstrated decrease in plasma ADMA level at 6 weeks.

What is interesting is that the established fact that the Apo-B%-change (not the LDL%-change) is a predictor of the changes in the plasma levels of ADMA (ADMA%-change) in the linear regression model. It's very likely that this is due to the level of the smallest atherogenic and dense particles are reflected my ApoB. The fact that ApoB is a predictor of the ADMA%-change presumably is due to the higher proportion of patients with family Apo B defect (previously reported in patients with hypercholesterolemia in our previous studies.

Statins vary in their pharmacokinetics and pharmacodynamics. There is a difference in their lipid regulating and pleiotropic effect. Therefore, the data on simvastatin could not be referred to other statins. There is no other therapeutic option in cases with high ADMA levels in hypersholesterolic ptients,apart from 80 mg simvastatin. The clinical significance of our study is that high-risk patients with severe hypercholesterolemia, a family history of premature atherosclerosis and a high level of plasma ADMA, the high dose of Simvastatin is a possible therapeutic option. Substituting with L-arginine is another possible approach (11; 44; 92). These two hypotheses complete one another.

A number of factors are the cause of controversial results on the effects of statins on the endothelial-dependent vasolidation. 1. The clinical studies, testing the effect of statins on ADMA and FMD% involve only a small number of patients for a short period of time. 2. LDL levels are not optimized in accordance with the risk category of hypercholesterolemic patients (the pleiotropic effects of statins are partly connected to lipid regulating ones). 3. The improvement of FMD% via increasing the activity of NO with the statin therapy is connected additionally to the effect on other inhibitors of eNOS apart from ADMA. 4. In most studies there is no testing of ADMA tissue levels.

The present study established patients with severe hypercholesterolemia have high ADMA levels in comparison with the control group. One-month treatment with 80 mg simvastatin, aimed at achieving LDL target levels of ≤ 2.6 mmol/l in high-risk contingents with severe hypercholesterolemia leads to a statistically significant reduction of ADMA and an increase of FMD% in contrast with 40 mg simvastatin therapy. The FMD%-changes correlate in a statistically significant way with the initial ApoB, ADMA and tHcy levels. The baseline ADMA levels are a predictor of FMD% changes and Apo-B%-changes is a predictor of ADMA%-changes at baseline and post one-month therapy with 80 mg simvastatin. In case of optimized LDL target levels it appears that ADMA is a major modulator of FMD%-change.

4. The impact of genetic factors on statin resistance

The same dose of the same statin in different individuals produces different LDLC decreases. The time to reach maximum LDL-C decrease differs significantly between individuals. [81;

82] Such a wide interindividual variation as the response to statins is more and more attributed, at least partly, to the polymorphisms in genes affecting statin pharmacodynamics and pharmacokinetics. The resistance to statins has been associated with polymorphisms in the HMG-CoA-R, ABCB1, ABCG2, ABCC1, ABCC2, OATP1B1, OATP2B1, RHOA, NPC1L1, FXR, CYP7A1, ApoE, PCSK9, LDLR, LPA, CETP, and TNF-a genes. However, currently, there is still not enough evidence to advocate pharmacogenetic testing before initiating therapy with statins.

Pharmacogenetics seeks to determine the role of genetic factors in variation of statin response. However, today the origins of the notable interindividual variation in response to statins are still poorly understood. In a number of studies, genetic variability has been shown to affect statin responsiveness thus influencing statin resistance. These studies have identified numerous candidate genes (>50) and dozens of single-nucleotide polymorphisms (SNPs). It have been reported to be associated with differing aspects of statin response - pharmacokinetics and pharmacodynamics of statins being potential determinants of drug responsiveness in terms of LDL-C lowering. Although genes are supposed to be associated with statin cholesterol-lowering efficacy, the magnitude of variation in statin response that could be explained by these associations is still questionable. [62; 89; 35; 79; 71]

The association between SNPs in genes involved in lipid metabolism and total cholesterol and LDL-C response to statin therapy is of particular interest. The 3-hydroxyl-3- methylglutaryl coenzyme A reductase (HMG-CoA-R) gene encoding the enzyme HMG-CoA-R, which is the principal target of statins, because the foremost pharmacological action of these drugs is exactly the competitive inhibition of HMG-CoA-R. The last one might be one of the candidate genes when analyzing the SNPs as a possible cause of diminished statin responsiveness. When SNPs and the common haplotypes inferred from them were tested for association with plasma LDL-C levels and LDL-C response to statin treatment, it has been shown that HMG-CoA-R gene polymorphisms are associated with reduced plasma LDL-C levels and LDL-C response to simvastatin. [104; 42; 75; 84; 88; 49; 50]

Therefore, although it was considered that genome-wide association studies may yield a more comprehensive set of markers for predicting statin efficacy and/or resistance, this has not been proven so far and the results of these studies cannot be translated into clinical practice yet. We need future pharmacogenetic research [93].

5. Conclusion

It is difficult to give an accurate definition of statin resistance. The patients who fail to reach LDL-C target values despite the best available therapy, mostly a highest tolerable dose of a more potent statin, are considered to be statin-resistant. Resistance to statins can be related to differences in drug absorption, transport, intrahepatic drug metabolism, drug metabolism within other organs, and drug excretion mechanisms. Possible causes of statin resistance: **1.Failed targeting LDL cholesterol** - smokers have smaller statin-induced LDL-C decrease compared with nonsmokers and the patients with hypertension have smaller decrease than those without hypertension, inflammation might cause statin resistance. The role of concomitant amiodarone treatment in statin resistance was also suspected. It has also been suggested that clusters of metabolites involved in multiple pathways not directly connected with cholesterol metabolism might as well play a role in modulating the response to statin therapy and therefore influence statin resistance. **2.Lack of effect on the endothelium-dependent vasodilation after targeting LDL-C.** There is much evidence that improvement of endothelium-dependent vasodilation under statin treatment depends on the ADMA levels. At this stage of knowledge, there are two options for the management of this type of statin resistance - the use of a high dose of a statin, or the addition of L-Arginine to the statin. These two strategies are not contradictory, but complementary. 3. **The impact of genetic factors on statin resistance.** The resistance to statins has been associated with polymorphisms in the HMG-CoA-R, ABCB1, ABCG2, ABCC1, ABCC2, OATP1B1, OATP2B1, RHOA, NPC1L1, FXR, CYP7A1, ApoE, PCSK9, LDLR, LPA, CETP, and TNF-a genes. However, currently, there is still not enough evidence to advocate pharmacogenetic testing before initiating therapy with statins.

Author details

Lyudmila Georgieva Vladimirova-Kitova* and Spas Ivanov Kitov

*Address all correspondence to: kitov@vip.bg

Medical University, Plovdiv, Bulgaria

References

[1] Al-Sarraf A, Li M, Frohlich J. Statin resistant dyslipidemia in a patient treated with amiodarone. BMJ Case Rep 2011. http://dx.doi.org/10.1136/bcr.08.2011.4620

[2] Andel M. Hyperlipoproteinemia impairs endothelium-dependent vasodilatation. Physiol Res [2004]; 53: 471–480

[3] Anderson TJ. Assessment and treatment of endothelial dysfunction humans. J Am Coll Cardiol [1999]; 34: 631–638

[4] Anderson TJ, Mark AL. Flow-mediated and reflex changes in large peripherial artery tone in humans. Circulation [1989]; 79: 93–100

[5] Anderson TJ, Uehata A, Gerhard MD, Meredith IT, Knab S, Delagrange D, Lieberman EH, Ganz P, Creager MA, Yeung AC, Selwyn AP. Close relation of endothelial function in the human coronary and peripheral circulation. J Am Coll Cardiol [1995]; 26: 1235–1241

[6] Ardigo D, Stüehlinger M, Franzini L, Valtueña S, Piatti PM, Pachinger O, Reaven GM, Zavaroni I. ADMA is independently related to flow- mediated vasodilation in subjects at low cardiovascular risk. Eur J Clin Invest [2007]; 37: 263–269

[7] Arnesen E, Refsum H, Bonaa KH, Ueland PM, Forde OH, Nordrehaug JE. Serum total homocysteine and coronary heart disease. Int J Epidemiol [1995]; 24: 704–709

[8] Ballantyne CM. Changing lipid-lowering guidelines: whom to treat and how low to go. Eur Heart J [2005]; 7(Suppl. A): A12–A19

[9] Behrendt D, Ganz P. Endothelial function: from vascular biology to clinical applications. Am J Cardiol [2002]; 90(Suppl. 3]: 40L–48L

[10] Betteridge DJ, Morrell JM. Clinicans' Guide to Lipids and Coronary Heart Disease, 2nd edn [2003]. A Hodder Arnold Publication, London, UK, pp. 275–278. Bhagat K, Hingorani A, Vallance P. Flow-associated or flow-mediated?More than just semantics. BMJ [1997]; 78: 7–8.

[11] Böger GI, Maas R, Schwedhelm E, Bierend A, Benndorf R, Kastner M, Steenpaß A, Böger RH. Improvement of endothelium-dependent vasodilation by simvastatin is potentiated by combination with L-arginine in patients with elevated asymmetric dimethylarginine levels. J Am Coll Cardiol [2004]; 43(Suppl.): 525A

[12] Böger GI, Rudolf TK, Renke M, Schwedhelm E, Dumbadze E, Bierend A, Benndorf RA, Böger RH. Asymmetric dimethylarginine determines the improvement of endothelium-dependent vasodilatation by Sim- vastatin. J Am Coll Cardiol [2007]; 49: 2274–2282

[13] Böger RH, Bode-Böger SM, Szuba A, Tsao PS, Chan JR, Tangphao O, Blaschke TF, Cooke JP. Asymmetric dimethylagrinine (ADMA): a novel risk factor for endothelial dysfunction. It's role in hypercho- lesterolemia. Circulation [1998]; 98: 1842–1847

[14] Böger RH, Bode-Böger SM. The clinical pharmacology of L-arginine. Annu Rev Pharmacol Toxicol [2001]; 41: 79–99

[15] Böger RH, Sydow K, Borlak J, Thum T, Lenzen H, Schubert B, Tsikas D, Bode-Böger SM. LDL cholesterol upregulates synthesis of asymmetrical dimethylarginine in human endothelial cells. Circ Res [2000]; 87: 99–105.

[16] Böger RH, Vallance P, Cooke JP. Asymmetric dimethylarginine (ADMA):a key regulator of nitric oxide synthase. Atherosclerosis [2003]; 4(Suppl. 4]: 1–3

[17] Böger RH. Association of asymmetric dimethylarginine and endothelial dysfunction. Clin Chem Lab Med [2003a); 41: 1467–1472

[18] Böger RH. Asymmetric dimethylarginine (ADMA) and cardiovascular disease: insights from prospective clinical trials. Vasc Med [2005]; 10(Suppl. 1]: S19–S25

[19] Böger RH. Asymmetric dimethylarginine (ADMA) modulates endothelial function-therapeutic implications. Vasc Med [2003b); 8: 149–151

[20] Böger RH. Asymmetric dimethylarginine (ADMA) modulates endothelial function – therapeutic implications. Vasc Med [2003c); 8: 149–151

[21] Böger RH. Asymmetric dimethylarginine, an endogenous inhibitor of nitric oxide synthase, explain the ''L-arginine paradox'' and acts as a novel cardiovascular risk factor. J Nutr [2004]; 134: 2842S–2847S

[22] Boccara F, Simon T, Lacombe K, Cohen A, Laloux B, Bozec E, et al. Influence of pravastatin on carotid artery structure and function in dyslipidemic HIV-infected patients receiving antiretroviral therapy. AIDS 2006;20:2395e8

[23] Bode-Böger SM, Böger SM, Kienke S, Junker W, Fro°lich JC. Elevated L- arginine/dimethylarginine ratio contributes to enhanced systemic NO production by dietary L-arginine in hypercholesterolemic rabbits. Biochem Biophys Res Commun [1996]; 219: 598–603

[24] Celermajer DS. Noninvasive detection of atherosclerosis. N Engl J Med[1998]; 339: 2014–2015

[25] Celermajer DS, Sorensen KE, Gooch VM, Spiegelhalter DJ, Miller OI, Sullivan ID, Lloyd JK, Deanfield JE. Non-invasive detection of endo- thelial dysfunction in children and adulst at risk of atherosclerosis. Lancet [1992]; 340: 1111–1115

[26] Chowienczyk PJ, Watts GF, Cockroft JR, Ritter JM. Impaired endothe- lium-dependent vasodilatation of forearm resistans vessels in hypercholesterolemia. Lancet [1992]; 340: 1430–1432

[27] Christen WG, Ajani UA, Glynn RJ, Hennekens CH. Blood levels of homocysteine and increased risks of cardiovascular disease: causal or casual? Arch Intern Med [2000]; 160: 422–434

[28] Cooke JP, Rossitch E Jr, Andon NA, Loscalzo J, Dzau VJ. Flow activates an endothelial potassium channel to release an endogenous nitrovaso- dilatator. J Clin Invest [1991]; 88: 1663–1671

[29] Cooke JP. Asymmetric dimethylarginine The Über marker? Circulation [2004]; 109: 1813–1819

[30] Corretti MC, Anderson TJ, Benjamin EJ, Celermajer D, Charbonneau F, Creager MA, Drexler H, Gerhard-Herman M, Herrington D, Vallance P, Vogel R. Guidelines for the ultrasound assessment of endothelial- dependent flow-mediated vasodilatation of the brachial artery. J Am Coll Cardiol [2002]; 39: 257–265

[31] Corson MA, James NL, Latta SSE, Nerem RM, Berck BC, Harrison DG. Phosphorylation of endothelial nitric oxide synthase in response to fluid shear stress. Circ Res [1996]; 79: 984–991

[32] Creager MA, Cooke JP, Mendelsohn ME, Gallagher SJ, Coleman SM, Loscalzo J, Dzau VJ. Impaired vasodilatation of forearm resistens vessels in hypercholesterolemic humans. J Clin Invest [1990]; 86: 228–234

[33] Creager MA, Gallagher SJ, Girerd XJ, Coleman SM, Dzau VJ, Cooke JP. L-arginine improve endothelium-dependent vasodilatation in hyper- cholesterolemic humans. J Clin Invest [1992]; 90: 1248–1953

[34] Davies PF, Rothblat GH, Wilensky RL, Yun Fang IL, Mohler ER, Hsieh IE, Osman H, Hashemi SM. Endothelium in vitro and in vivo hyper- cholesterolemia suppresses inwardly rectifying K+ channels in aortic. Circ Res [2006]; 98: 1064–1071

[35] Donnelly LA, Doney AS, Dannfald J, Whitley AL, Lang CC, Morris AD, et al. A paucimorphic variant in the HMG-CoA reductase gene is associated with lipid-lowering response to statin treatment in diabetes: a GoDARTS study. Pharmacogenet Genomics 2008;18:1021e6

[36] Faulx MD, Wright AT, Hoit BD. Detection of endothelial dysfunction with brachial artery ultrasound scanning. Am Heart J [2003]; 145: 943–951

[37] Favre A, Monpere C, Voyer C, Mirguetn C, Quilliet-Thebaud N, Vern- ochet P, Brochier M. How to improve primary prevention in asymptomatic high risk subjects. Eur Heart J [2004]; 6(Suppl. J): j59–j63

[38] Furchgott RF. Endothelium-derived relaxing factor: discovery, early studies, and identification as nitric oxide. Biosci Rep [1999]; 19: 235–251. Furchgott RF, Jothianandan D. Endothelium-dependent and -indepen- dent vasodilation involving cyclic GMP: relaxation induced by nitric oxide, carbon monoxide and light. Blood Vessels [1991]; 28: 52–61

[39] Furchgott RF, Zawadzki JV. The obligatory role of the endothelium in the relaxation of arterial smooth muscle by acetylcholine. Nature [1980]; 288: 373–376

[40] Furchgott RF. Role of endothelium in responses of vascular smooth muscle. Circulation Res [1983]; 53: 557–573

[41] Furchgott RF. Studies on Relaxation of Rabbit Aorta by Sodium Nitrite: The Basis for the Proposal that the Acid-Activatable Inhibitory Factor from Retractor Penis is Inorganic Nitrite and the Endothelium-Derived Relaxing Factor is Nitric Oxide. In Vasodilation: Vascular Smooth Muscle, Peptides, and Endothelium. [1988], pp. 401–414. Raven Press, New York.

[42] Generaux GT, Bonomo FM, Johnson M, Doan KM. Impact of SLCO1B1 (OATP1B1] and ABCG2 (BCRP) genetic polymorphisms and inhibition on LDL-C lowering and myopathy of statins. Xenobiotica 2011;41:639e51

[43] Genest JJ, McNamara JR, Upson B, Salem DN, Ordovas JM, Schaefer EJ. Prevalence of familial hyperhomocyst(e)inemia in men with prema- ture coronary disease. Arterioscler Thromb [1991]; 11: 1129–3635

[44] Gornic HL, Creager MA. Arginine and endothelial and vascular health. J Nutr [2004]; 134: 2880S–2887S.

[45] Gotto AM. Management of dyslipidemia. Am J Med [2002]; 112(Suppl. 8A): 10S–18S

[46] Greenland P, Abrams J, Aurigemma GP, Bond MG, Clark LT, Criqui MH, Crouse JR, Friedman L, Fuster V, Herrington DM, Kuller LH, Ridker PM, Roberts WC, Stanford W, Stone N, Swan HJ, Taubert KA, Wexler

[47] Greenland P, Abrams J, Aurigemma GP, et al.Prevention conference V: beyond secondary prevention: identifying the high-risk patient for primary prevention: noninvasive tests of atherosclerotic burden: writing group III. Circulation [2000]; 101: e16–e22

[48] Herman AG, Moncada S. Therapeutic potential of nitric oxide donors in the prevention and treatment of atherosclerosis European Heart Journal [2005] 26, 1945–1955

[49] Hu M, Lui SS, Tam LS, Li EK, Tomlinson B. The farnesoid X receptor -1G>T polymorphism influences the lipid response to rosuvastatin. J Lipid Res 2012;53:1384e9

[50] Hubacek JA, Vrablik M. Effect of apolipoprotein E polymorphism on statin-induced decreases in plasma lipids and cardiovascular events. Drug Metabol Drug Interact 2011;26:13e20

[51] Ignarro LJ. Nitric Oxide: Biology and Pathobiology [2000], pp. 547–568. Academic Press, London

[52] Ito A, Tsao PS, Adimoolam S, Kimoto M, Ogawa T, Cooke JP. Novel mechanism for endothelial dysfunction: dysregulation of dimethy- larginine dimethyl amino hydrolase. Circulation [1999]; 99: 3092–3095

[53] Janatuinen T, Laakso J, Laaksonen R, Nuutila P, Lehtimaki T, Raitakari OT, Knuuti J. Plasma asymmetric dimethylarginine modifies the effect of pravastatin on myocardial blood flow in young adults. Vasc Med [2003]; 8: 185–189

[54] Joannides R, Haefeli WE, Linder L, Vincent R, Bakkali EH, Thuillez C, Lu° scher TF. Nitric oxide responsible for flow-dependent dilatation of human peripherial Conduit arteries in vivo. Circulation [1995]; 91: 1314–1319.

[55] Johns KW, Bennett MT, Bondy GP. Are HIV positive patients resistant to statin therapy? Lipids Health Dis 2007;6:27

[56] Kaddurah-Daouk R, Baillie RA, Zhu H, Zeng ZB, Wiest MM, Nguyen UT, et al. Lipidomic analysis of variation in response to simvastatin in the Cholesterol and Pharmacogenetics Study.Metabolomics 2010;6:191e201

[57] Kang SS, Wong PW, Cook HY, Norusis M, Messer JV. Protein-bound- homocyst(e)ine. A possible risk factor for coronary artery disease. J Clin Invest [1986]; 77: 1482–1486

[58] Kastelein JJP. The realities of dyslipidaemia: what do the studies tell us? Eur Heart J [2005]; 7(Suppl. F): F27–F33

[59] Kielstein JT, Cooke JP. Should we measure asymmetric dimethylarginine in patients with coronary artery disease? Clin Chem [2007]; 53: 161– 163

[60] Kitamoto Sh, Egashira K. Endothelial dysfunction and coronary atherosclerosis. Curr Drug Targets Cardiovas Haematol Disord [2004]; 4: 13–22. Knekt P, Reunanen A, Alfthan G, Heliövaara M, Harri Rissanen H,

[61] Kobayashi K, Akishita M, Yu W, Hashimoto M, Ohni M, Toba K. Interrelationship between non-invasive measuments of atherosclero- sis: flow-mediated dilatation of brachial artery, carotid intima-media thickness and pulse wave velocity. Atherosclerosis [2004]; 173: 13–18

[62] Krauss RM, Mangravite LM, Smith JD, Medina MW, Wang D, Guo X, et al. Variation in the 3-hydroxyl-3-methylglutaryl coenzyme a reductase gene is associated with racial differences in low-density lipoprotein cholesterol response to simvastatin treatment. Circulation 2008;117:1537e44

[63] Landmesser ULF, Hornig B, Drexler H. Endothelial dysfunction in hypercholesterolemia: mechanism, pathophysiological importans and therapeutic interventions. Semin Thromb Hemost [2000]; 26: 529–537

[64] Laufs U, La F, Plutzky J, Liao JK. Upregulation of endothelial nitric oxide synthase by HMG CoA reductase inhibitors. Circulation [1998]; 97:1129–1135

[65] Lentz SR, Radionov RN, Dayal S. Hyperhomocysteinemia, endothelial dysfunction, and cardiovascular risk: the potential role of ADMA. Atherosclerosis [2003]; 4(Suppl. 4]: 61–65

[66] Lim S, Seon KM, Soo PK, Ho LJ, Hee AG, Ja YM *et al.* Correlation of plasma homocysteine and mitochondrial DNAcontent in peripheral blood in healthy women. Atherosclerosis [2001]; 158: 399–405

[67] Lin K, Lin SC. A tale of two molecules: nitric oxide and asymmetric dimethylarginine. Acta Cardiol Sin [2004]; 20: 201–211

[68] Mann DM, Woodward M, Muntner P, Falzon L, Kronish I. Predictors of nonadherence to statins: a systematic review and meta-analysis. Ann Pharmacother 2010;44:1410e21

[69] Marniemi J, Aromaa A. Hyperhomocystinemia a risk factor or a consequence of coronary heart disease? Arch Intern Med [2001]; 161: 1589–1594

[70] Medina MW, Theusch E, Naidoo D, Bauzon F, Stevens K, Mangravite LM, et al. RHOA is a modulator of the cholesterollowering effects of statin. PLoS Genet 2012;8:e1003058

[71] Mega JL, Morrow DA, Brown A, Cannon CP, Sabatine MS. Identification of genetic variants associated with response to statin therapy. Arterioscler Thromb Vasc Biol 2009;29:1310e5

[72] Miyazaki H, Matsuoka H, Cooke J, Usui M, Ueda S, Okuda S, Imaizuma T. Endogenous nitric oxide synthase inhibitor. Circulation [1999]; 99: 1141–1146

[73] Moens AL, Goovaerts I, Claeys MJ, Vrints CJ. Flow-mediated vasodila- tion: a diagnostic instrument, or an experimental tool? Chest [2005]; 127: 2254–2263

[74] Murad F. Discovery of some of the biological effects of nitric oxide and its role in cell signaling. Biosci Rep [1999]; 19: 133–154

[75] Niemi M, Schaeffeler E, Lang T, Fromm MF, Neuvonen M, Kyrklund C, et al. High plasma pravastatin concentrations are associated with single nucleotide polymorphisms and haplotypes of organic anion transporting polypeptide-C (OATP-C, SLCO1B1]. Pharmacogenetics 2004;14:429e40

[76] Nygard O, Vollset SE, Refsum H *et al.* Total plasma homo-cysteineand cardiovascular risk profile. The Hordaland Homocysteine Study. JAMA [1995]; 274: 1526–1533

[77] Oemar BS, Tschudi MR, Godoy N, Brovkovich V, Malinski T,Lüscher TF. Reduced endothelial nitric oxide synthase expression and production in human atherosclerosis. Circulation [1998]; 97: 2494–2498

[78] Pohl U, Holtz J, Busse R, Bassenge E. Crucial role of the endothelium in the vasodilator response to flow in vivo. Hypertension [1985]; 8: 37–44

[79] Polisecki E, Muallem H, Maeda N, Peter I, Robertson M, McMahon AD, et al. Genetic variation at the LDL receptor and HMG-CoA reductase gene loci, lipid levels, statin response, and cardiovascular disease incidence in PROSPER. Atherosclerosis 2008;200:109e14

[80] Raitakari OT, Celermajer DS. Testing for endothelial function. Ann Med [2000]; 32: 293–304

[81] Reiner Z, De Bacquer D, Kotseva K, Prugger C, De Backer G, Wood D. EUROASPIRE III study group. Treatment potential for dyslipidaemia management in patients with coronary heart disease across Europe: findings from the EUROASPIRE III survey. Atherosclerosis 2013;231:300e7

[82] Reiner Z, Tedeschi-Reiner E. Prevalence and types of persistent dyslipidemia in patients treated with statins. Croat Med J 2013;54:339e45

[83] Ridker PM, Manson JE, Buring JE, Shih J, Matias M, Hennekens H. Homocysteine and risk of cardiovascular disease among postmeno- pausal women. JAMA [1999]; 281: 1817–1821

[84] Rodrigues AC, Perin PM, Purim SG, Silbiger VN, Genvigir FD, Willrich MA, et al. Pharmacogenetics of OATP transporters reveals that SLCO1B1 c.388A>G variant is determinant of increased atorvastatin response. Int J Mol Sci 2011;12:5815e27

[85] Simon JA, Lin F, Hulley SB, Blanche PJ, Waters D, Shiboski S, et al. Phenotypic predictors of response to simvastatin therapy among African-Americans and Caucasians: the cholesterol and pharmacogenetics (CAP) Study. Am J Cardiol 2006;97:843e50

[86] Stühlinger M, Stanger Ol. Asymmetric dimethylarginine (ADMA): a possible link between homocystein and endothelial dysfunction. Current Drug Metabolism [2005]; 6: 3–14

[87] Stühlinger M, Tsao Ph, Her J, Kimoto M, Balint R, Cooke J. Homocysteine impairs the nitric oxide synthase pathway:role of asymmetric dimethylarginine. Circulation [2001]; 104: 2569–2575

[88] Takane H, Miyata M, Burioka N, Shigemasa C, Shimizu E, Otsubo K, et al. Pharmacogenetic determinants of variability in lipid-lowering response to pravastatin therapy. J Hum Genet 2006;51:822e6

[89] Thompson JF, Hyde CL, Wood LS, Paciga SA, Hinds DA, Cox DR, et al. Comprehensive whole-genome and candidate gene analysis for response to statin therapy in the treating to new targets (TNT) cohort. Circ Cardiovasc Genet 2009;2:173e81

[90] Trupp M, Zhu H, Wikoff WR, Baillie RA, Zeng ZB, Karp PD, et al.Metabolomics reveals amino acids contribute to variation in response to simvastatin treatment. PLoS One 2012;7:e38386

[91] Tsao Ph, Cooke JP. Endothelial alteration in hypercholesterolemia: more than simply vasodilatator dysfunction. J Cardiovasc Pharmacol [1998]; 32(Suppl. 3]: S48–S53

[92] Tsikas D, Böger RH, Sandmann J, Bode-Böger SM, Flo°lich JC. Endoge- nous nitric oxide synthase inhibitors are responsible for the L-arginine paradox. FEBS Lett [2000]; 478: 1–3

[93] van der Baan FH, Knol MJ, Maitland-van der Zee AH, Regieli JJ, van Iperen EP, Egberts AC, et al. Added value of pharmacogenetic testing in predicting statin response: results from the REGRESS trial. Pharmacogenomics J 2013;13:318e24

[94] Veerkamp MJ, de Graaf J, den Heijer M, Blom HJ, Stalenhoef AFH. Plasma homocystein in subjects with familial combined hyperlipid- emia. Atherosclerosis [2003]; 166: 111–117

[95] *Vladimirova-Kitova L,* D. Terzieva, F. Nikolov. Asymmetric dimewthylarginine determines the effect of simvastatin on endothelium-dependent vasodilation in severe hypercholesterolemia Future Medicine Clinical Lipidology 2010: 5 [1]; 29-41

[96] Vladimirova-Kitova L, D. Terzieva. Intima-media thickness and flow mediated vasodilation in asymptomatic subjects with newly detected severe hypercholesterolemia Echocardiography 2009; 26 [9]: 1060-1068

[97] *Vladimirova-Kitova L,* Deneva T, Marinov B. Predictors of the intima-media thickness of carotid artery in asymptomatic newly detected severe hypercholesterolemic patients. Clin Physiol Funct Imaging. 2010; 30 [4]: 250-259

[98] *Vladimirova-Kitova L,* Deneva-Koycheva T. Asymmetric dimethylarginine- a determinant of effect of the high dose simvastatin. Clinical biochemistry. 2010 [43]: 843-850

[99] *Vladimirova-Kitova LG,* Deneva T. I, Marinov B. Effect of Moderate and High-Dose Simvastatin on Asymmetric Dimethylarginine-Homocysteine Metabolic Pathways in Patients with Newly Detected Severe Hypercholesterolemia. Cardiovasc Therapeutics 2011 [29] : 340-348

[100] *Vladimirova-Kitova LG,* Deneva TI. Simvastatin and asymmetric dimethylarginine-homocysteine metabolic pathways in patients with newly detected severe hypercholesterolemia. Clin Lab. 2010; 56 [7-8]: 291-302

[101] *Vladimirova-Kitova LG,* Deneva-Koicheva TI The effect of simvastatin on Asymmetric Dimethylarginine after optimizing the LDL – a randomized, placebo-controlled study. Vascular Pharmacology. 2012, 56 [3-4]: 122-130

[102] *Vladimirova-Kitova LG,* Deneva-Koycheva T.I. Increased intima-media thickness in carriers of the LDL-receptor defective gene versus noncarriers with newly detected asymptomatic severe hypercholesterolemia. Echocardiography. 2011 28, [2], 223–234

[103] Vladimirova-Kitova, L.G., Deneva, T., Angelova E.,. Nikolov, F., Marinov B., Mateva, N. Relationship of asymmetric dimethylarginine with flow-mediated dilation in subjects with newly detected severe hypercholesterolemia. Clinical Physiology and Functional Imaging 2008 28[6], 417-425

[104] Voora D, Shah SH, Reed CR, Zhai J, Crosslin DR, Messer C, et al. Pharmacogenetic predictors of statin-mediated low-density lipoprotein Cholesterol Reduction and Dose Response Circ Cardiovasc Genet. Dec 2008; 1[2]: 100–106

[105] Whinchup PH, Refsum H, Perry IJ. Serum total homocysteine and coronary heart disease: prospective study in middle aged men. Heart [1999]; 82: 448–454

[106] Wu LL, Wu J, Hunt SC, James BC, Vincent GM, Williams RR *et al.* Plasma homocyst(e)ine as a risk factor for early familial coronary artery disease. Clin Chem [1994]; 40: 552–561

[107] Y1 Chen, Ku H, Zhao L, Wheeler DC, Li LC, Li Q, et al. Inflammatory stress induces statin resistance by disrupting 3-hydroxy-3-methylglutaryl-CoA reductase feedback regulation. Arterioscler Thromb Vasc Biol 2014;34:365e76

[108] Yu X, Li Y, Xiong Y. Increase of a endogenous inhibotor of nitric oxide synthesis in serum of high cholesterol fed rabbits. Life Sci [1994]; 54: 753–758

Chapter 11

Interaction Studies of ACE Inhibitors with Statins

Safila Naveed

Additional information is available at the end of the chapter

http://dx.doi.org/10.5772/59491

1. Introduction

1.1. Angiotensin-Converting Enzyme Inhibitors

1.1.1. History

In the 1950s, it was discovered that angiotensin exists as both an inactive decapeptide angiotensin I and an active octapeptide angiotensin II. Human angiotensin-converting enzyme contains 277 amino-acid residues and has two homologous domains, each with a catalytic site and a region for binding Zn^{+2} [1, 2]. The degradation of bradykinin to inactive peptides occurs via action of ACE; ACE thus not only produces a potent vasoconstriction but also inactivates a potent vasodilator. In 1965, Ferreira [3] studied the physiological effects of snake poisoning and discovered a specific component from the venom of the pit viper, Bothrops jararaca, which inhibits degradation of the peptide bradykinin and potentiate hypotensive action of bradykinin potentiating factors (BPFs), basically amino-acid-containing peptides. Bakhle [4] reported that these same peptides had an inhibitory activity on ACE of dog lung homogenate and inhibited the enzymatic conversion of angiotensin I to angiotensin II. Brunner and Laragh [5] administered them to hypertensive patients and found them to be extremely effective in lowering blood pressure. The structural requirements for substrates of angiotensin-converting enzyme to cleave a substrate are found to be similar to those observed with carboxypeptidase A of bovine pancreas [6, 7].

The molecule ACE is a zinc metallopeptidase and has a similar mode of action to carboxypeptidase [8]. In 1970, the Bradykinin-potentiating pentapeptide BPP5a was isolated, which inhibited enzyme angiotensin and decreased blood pressure [9]. The significance of ACE in the pathogenesis of hypertension was not fully appreciated until 1977, when Ondetti [10] first isolated and then synthesized the naturally occurring non-peptide, teprotide. He proposed a hypothetical model of the active site of ACE and used it to predict and design compounds that would occupy the carboxy-terminal binding site of the enzyme captopril, a specific potent inhibitor of ACE. Clinical trials showed excellent anti-hypertensive properties and these results had a major impact on the treatment of cardiovascular disease [11]. The first demonstration of an orally active ACE inhibitor was made on 31 March 1975, when the succinyl group was replaced with a derivative of cysteine, increasing inhibitory potency about 2,000-fold because sulphhydryl of cysteine bound with zinc more tightly than the carboxyl of succinyl. This resulted in captopril, with a dramatic effect on renal function and on hypertension [12]. Enalapril is basically a first derivative of ACE inhibitor, which was developed to overcome the limitations of captopril. Lisinopril is a lysine analogue of enalaprilat (the active metabolite of enalapril). *In vitro* lisinopril is slightly more potent than enalaprilat. It is a non-sulphhydryl angiotensin-converting-enzyme (ACE) inhibitor active without metabolism and is absorbed in its active form.

1.1.2. Chemistry

Angiotensin enzyme inhibitors are basically ester-containing drugs that show 100-1000 times less activity than their active form; these inhibitors are synthetic in nature and can be classified on the basis of their chemical structure. They can be grouped as sulphhydral-containing (fentiapril, pivalopril, zofenopril, alacepril, etc.), dicarboxyl-containing (lisinopril, benazepril, quinapirl, perindopril, indopril, pentopril, indalapril, alazapril, moexipril, romipril, spirapril, etc.), phosphorous-containing (fosinopril) [13] and naturally occurring lactokinins and casokinins. [14]

Drug	Nomenclature	Structure	Ref
Enalapril	(S)-1-[N-[1-(ethoxycarbonyl)-3-phenyl propyl]-L-alanyl]-L-proline,(Z)-2-butenedioate salt	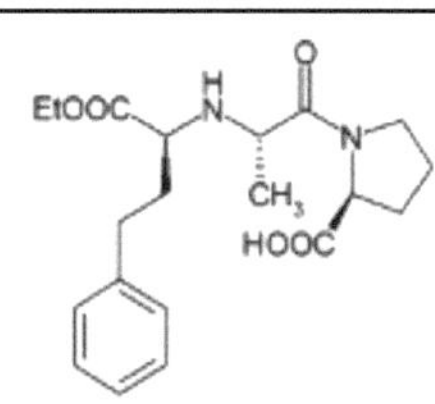	[15]
Captopril	1-(3-mercapto-2-dmethyl-1-oxopropyl)-1-proline (S,S)	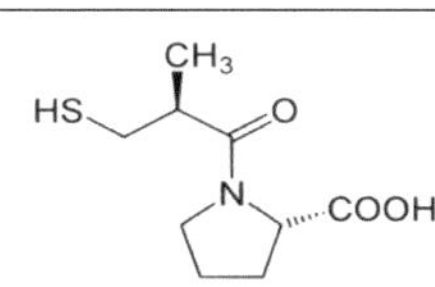	[16]
Lisinopril	((S)-1-[N2-(1-carboxy-3-phenylpropyl)-1-lysyl]-1-proline dehydrate	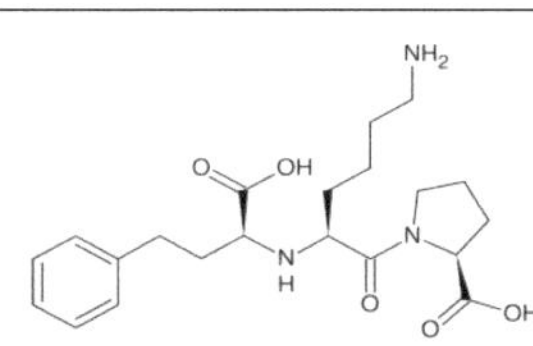	[16]

Table 1. ACE Inhibitors with structure and nomenclature

In general we can say that all ACE inhibitors differ by three properties: potency, conversion from pro-drug to active form, and pharmacokinetics (i.e., ADME). They also differ in terms of tissue distribution. All ACE inhibitors have a similar antihypertensive efficacy – they effectively block the conversion of angiotensin 1 to angiotensin II – and all have similar therapeutic indications, adverse effect profiles and contraindications.

1.1.3. Mechanism of action

These inhibitors block the converting enzyme of angiotensin, which is responsible for cleavage from angiotensin I, which is decapeptide, to angiotensin II, which is octapeptide [17, 18], and lower the BP by reducing PVR (peripheral vascular resistance). They also decrease aldosterone secretion and the resulting sodium and water retention.

1.1.4. Pharmacokinetics

The oral bioavailability of ACE inhibitors ranges from 13% to 95% [19, 20]. Most ACE inhibitors are administered as pro-drugs that remain inactive until esterified in the liver [21]. Pharmakokinetic characteristics of different ACE inhibitors are given in Table 2

Drug	Oral resorption %	Protein binding %	Elimination half-life hr	Metabolism	Usual dose (mgd^{-1})
Enalapril	60	<08	11	Partly converted enalaprilate	5-20
Captopril	>25	30	1.7	Partly metabolized	25-50
Lisinopril	25	0	41	Non metabolized	5-20

Table 2. Pharmacokinetic of ACE Inhibitors

1.1.5. Therapeutic use

ACE inhibitors are effective in patients with mild to moderately severe hypertension, normal or low plasma renin activity, collagen vascular disease and cardiovascular disease [22, 23]. They are also used in the prevention and treatment of myocardial infarction [24, 25] and in the management of cardiac arrhythmias [26]. They can decrease the progression of atherosclerosis, microalbuminuria and diabetic retinopathy, and produce a beneficial effect in patients with Bartter's syndrome [27].

1.1.6. Adverse effects

ACE inhibitors have a relatively low incidence of side effects and are well tolerated; however, dry cough is common, appearing in 10-30% of patients. This appears to be related to the elevation in bradykinin [28-30]. Hypotension is seen especially in patients with heart failure [31], angiooedema (life-threatening airway swelling and obstruction; 0.1-0.2% of patients) and hyperkalaemia. ACE inhibitors are contraindicated in pregnancy, in the first trimester associated with a risk of major congenital malformations, particularly affecting the cardiovascular and central nervous systems [32]. The most common (≥1% of patients) adverse effects include hypotension, fatigue, dizziness, headache, nausea and other gastrointestinal disturbances, dry cough, hyperkalaemia and renal impairment. Rash and taste disturbances are more prevalent with captopril and are attributed to its sulphhydryl moiety; eosinophilia has also been reported. Most of the adverse effects are reversible on withdrawing therapy [33]. Treatment with ACE inhibitor has been associated with the development of anaphylactoid reaction [34].

1.1.7. Drug interactions

Hypotensive effect of ACE inhibitors decreased when given in combination with non-steroidal anti-inflammatory drugs [35], but this effect was enhanced with calcium-channel blockers and beta-blockers [36]. Granulocytopaenia occurs after combined therapy of ACE inhibitors and interferones [37]. ACE inhibitors interact with different drugs, like NSAIDs [38]. Cytokines antagonize the hypotensive effect of ACE inhibitors [39]; severe hypokalaemia occurs with potassium-depleting diuretics [40] and potassium-sparing diuretics produce hyperkalaemia [41, 42]. ACE inhibitors were shown to increase potassium levels in the body [43]. Alpha-blockers enhance the hypotensive effect of ACE inhibitors [44]. Iron supplementation successfully decreases cough induced by ACE inhibitors [45] and can interfere with the absorption of ACE inhibitors [46]. Hypoglycaemic effect is enhanced with anti-diabetics and insulin [47, 48]. Combination of azathioprine and ACE inhibitors is associated with anaemia [49]. The risk of bone marrow depression is increased in patients taking concomitant therapy of ACE inhibitors and immunosuppressive agents.

1.2. HMG-CoA reductase inhibitors (statins)

3-hydroxy-3-methylglutaryl coenzyme A (HMG-CoA) reductase inhibitors (statins) are the most effective among all hypolipidaemic agents [50]. These lipid-lowering drugs are increasingly used for primary and secondary hindrance of cardiovascular disease [51]; they have only been recognized for treatment of hyperlipidaemia. In clinical studies, statins are highly effective in enhancing HDL levels while reducing total cholesterol, LDL cholesterol, apolipoprotein B and triglyceride levels.

The normal treatment regimen for these drugs involves daily exposure over a period of many years [52, 53]. They have also been examined in combination with cures of multiple sclerosis, osteoporosis, Alzheimer's disease and dropping the superfluous increased occurrence in CHD in women on HRT treatment [54]. They have anti-thrombogenic, anti-inflammatory and anticoagulant properties [55, 56]. These therapeutic properties are independent of lipid lowering [57], and the benefits of statins appear to be independent of baseline cholesterol [58]. They can be classified into subclasses: the naturally or fungi-derived first generation, and the synthetic second generation. The first generation includes simvastatin, lovastatin and pravastatin, and the second atorvastatin and rosuvastatin. They can be further divided into the lipophilic group (simvastatin, lovastatin and atorvastatin) and the OH hydrophilic group (pravastatin and rosuvastatin) [59].

Statin	Nomenclature	Structure
Rosuvastatin	(3*R*,5*S*,6*E*)-7- [4-(4-fluorophenyl)-2- (*N* methyl-methanesulphonamido)-6-(propan-2-yl) pyrimidin -5-yl]-3,5-dihydroxyhept- 6-enoic acid	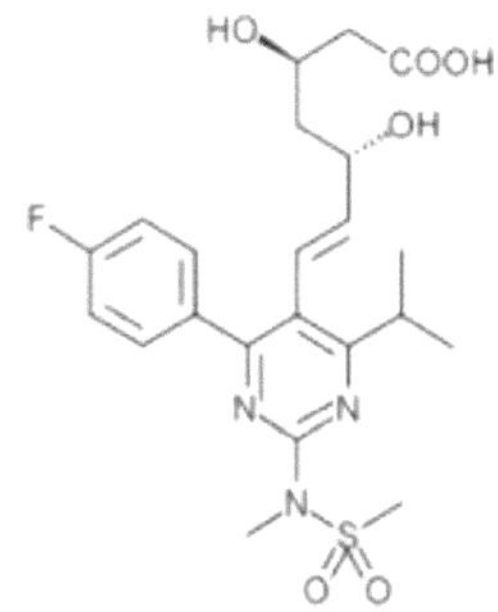
Atorvastatin	[R-(R*,R*)]-2-(4-fluorophenyl)-β,δ-dihydroxy-5- (1-methylethyl)-3-phenyl-4[(phenylamino) carbonyl]-1 H - pyrrole-1-heptanoic acid	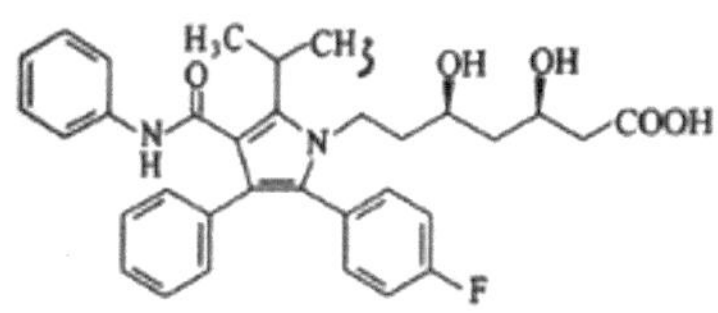
Simvastatin	[1S-[1α,3α,7β,8β(2S*,4S*), 8aβ]]-2,2-dimethyl-butanoic acid1,2,3,7,8, 8a-hexahydro-3,7-dimethyl -8- [2-(tetrahydro-4-hydroxy-6-oxo- 2H-pyran-2-yl ethyl]-1- naphthalenyl ester	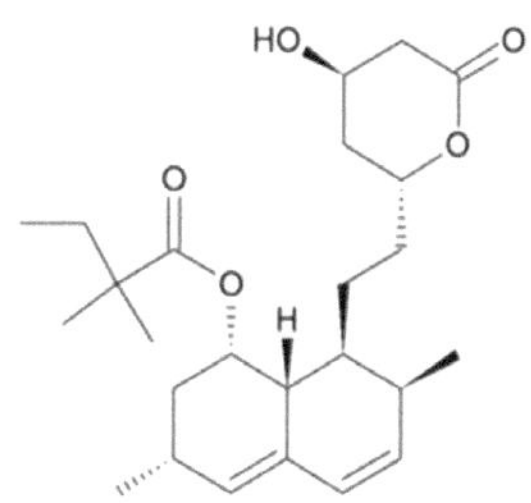
Pravastatin	[1 S- [1alpha(beta S*, delta S*), 2, 6alpha ,8beta(R*):8]]-1,2,6,7,8,8a-hexahydro-beta, delta,[6-trihydroxy-2-methyl-8- [2-methyl-1-oxobutoxy]-1- phthaleneheptanoic acid salt	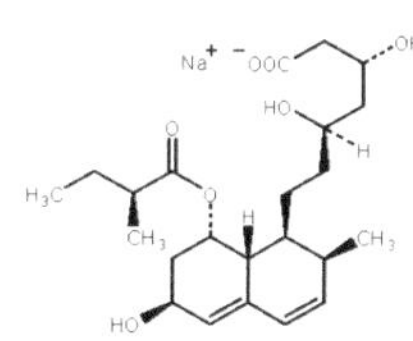

Table 3. Statins with structure and chemical name

2. Experiment

2.1. Materials

Raw materials used were of pharmaceutical purity and were obtained from different pharmaceutical companies (Table 4). Tablets were purchased from a local pharmacy; each product was labelled with an expiry date not earlier than two years from the time of these studies.

Class	Drugs	Brands	Potency (mg)	Pharmaceutical industry
ACE inhibitors	Enalapril	Renitec	10	MSD
	Captopril	Capoten	25	Bristol Meyers (Pvt.) Ltd.
	Lisinopril	Lisinopril	5	Atco Laboratories Ltd.
Statins	Rosuvastatin	X-plended	20	Pharm Evo (Pvt.) Ltd.
	Atorvastatin	Atopitar	10	Atco Pharma (Pvt.) Ltd.
	Pravastatin	Pravachol	20	Bristol Meyers (Pvt.) Ltd.
	Simvastatin	Atcol	10	Geofman Pharma (Pvt.) Ltd.

Table 4. Drugs, brands and manufacturers

2.1.1. Reagents

Analytical-grade solutions were used for the performance of the experiment. Methanol and acetonitrile were of HPLC grade and other reagents included HCl, sodium hydroxide (NaOH), sodium chloride (NaCl), disodium hydrogen orthophosphate, potassium dihydrogen orthophosphate, ammonium chloride, NH_3 solution (10%), phosphoric acid (8%) (Merck Germany). Organic solvents used were methanol, ethanol, ethyl acetate, chloroform, acetronitrile, triethylamine and DMSO (Merck HPLC Grade Germany).

2.1.2. Equipment

A UV-visible spectrophotometer (Shimadzu Model 1601, Japan) with 10-mm path length was connected to a computer with UVPC version 3.9 software. A Stedec CSW-300 was used for deionization of water. Dissolution was accomplished using BP 2009 standards. Chromatographic studies were carried out by using two Shimadzu HPLC systems, one equipped with an LC-10 AT VP pump (SPD-10 A VP), and the second with an LC-20AT UV/VIS detector utilizing Hypersil, ODS, C18 (150×4.6 mm, 5 micron) and a Purospher® STAR RP-18 column. Chromatographic data peaks were analysed using Shimadzu Japan CBM-102, class GC 10 software.

Infrared studies were performed using Shimadzu FTIR Prestige-21. Spectral analysis was performed using Shimadzu software. The proton H^1-NMR spectra were calculated on a Bruker (AMX 500 MHz) spectrometer using TMS as an internal standard. Melting points were recorded using Gallen kamp melting-point apparatus Minnesota Mining And Manufacturing Company.

2.2. Methods

2.2.1. Preparation of simulated gastric juice and buffers

0.1 N HCl was prepared by using 9 mL HCl (11 N) in a volumetric flask; the volume was made up with de-ionized water. Chloride buffer at pH 4 was prepared by dissolving 3.725 g of KCl (potassium chloride) in deionized water and 0.1N HCl was used for pH adjustment. For preparation of PO_4 (phosphate buffer pH 7.4) 0.6 gm of potassium dihydrogen orthophosphate was used, plus 6.4 g of disodium hydrogen orthophosphate and 5.85 g of NaCl (sodium chloride), and the pH was adjusted. Preparation of NH_3 ammonia buffer at pH 9 was done using 4.98 g of NH4Cl ammonium chloride and pH-adjusted with 10% ammonia.

2.2.2. *Construction of the calibration curve of drugs*

The above standard solutions of all drugs were scanned in the region 200-700 nm against the reagent blank, and absorbance maxima were recorded as shown in Table 5. Calibration curves were constructed between concentration and absorbance. Epsilon values and linear coefficients were calculated in each case at all the above-described pH values. Beer Lambert's law was obeyed at all concentrations and pHs.

Class of drugs	Analytes	Wavelength (nm)	Conc. range (m Mole)
ACE inhibitors	Enalapril	203, 206, 207, 208	1-9 x 10^{-5}
	Captopril	203, 204, 206	5 -14 x 10^{-7}
	Lisinopril	206	1-10 x 10^{-5}
Statins	Atorvastatin	241	0.5-4.5 × 10^{-2}
	Rosuvastatin	240	1-5 × 10^{-5}
	Simvastatin	231, 238, 246	1-9 × 10^{-5}
	Pravastatin	235	1-9 × 10^{-5}

Table 5. Please Add Caption

2.2.3. *Monitoring of drug interactions of enalapril, captopril and lisinopril by high-performance liquid chromatography*

HPLC methods for simultaneous determination of enalapril, captopril and lisinopril with statins in raw materials, pharmaceutical dosage forms or in human serum were developed and validated according to ICH guidelines. These methods were then applied to drug-drug, drug-metals and drug-antacid interaction studies.

2.2.4. *Chromatographic conditions*

Isocratic elution was performed at ambient temperature with two different types of column. Hypersil, ODS, C18 (150×4.6 mm, 5 micron) and Purospher® STAR RP-18, for assay of enalapril, captopril and lisinopril and simultaneous determination of these drugs with interacting drugs, respectively. The mobile phase, flow rate, wavelength and UV detection were varied as shown in Table 6. A sample volume of 20 μL was injected in triplicate onto the HPLC column and the elute was monitored at different wavelengths.

2.2.5. Preparation of standard solutions

Stock reference standard solutions of all drugs were prepared daily by dissolving appropriate amounts of each drug in mobile phase to yield final concentration of 300 μgmL^{-1}. For the calibration standards, calibrators of each drug were prepared by making serial dilutions from stock solutions. All solutions were filtered through 0.45 μm filter and degassed using sonicator.

2.2.6. Preparation of pharmaceutical dosage from samples

Pharmaceutical formulations of the respective brands commercially available in Pakistan were evaluated. In each case, groups of 20 tablets were individually weighed and finely ground in a mortar. The portion of the powder equivalent to the amount of drug was transferred into a volumetric flask and completely dissolved in mobile phase, and then diluted with this solvent up to the mark. After filtration using a 0.45 micrometre μm filter this was then injected.

2.2.7. Preparation of standard plasma solutions

Samples of blood used were collected then centrifuged at 3000 rpm for at least ten minutes, Supernatant solution was stored at –20°C. The solution serum was deprotinated by using (ACN) acetonitrile, and this solution was spiked daily with working solutions for required concentrations of ACE inhibitors and interacting drugs (statins). 10 μL of sample was injected and chromatographed under the above conditions.

Drug	Mobile phase			pH	Flow rate	Detection
	MeOH	ACN	H_2O		mLmin^{-1}	nm
Enalapril assay	70	-	30	3.5	1	215
Enalapril + statins		60	40	3	1.8	230
Captopril	50	-	50	2.9	1	220
Captopril + statins	-	60	40	2.9	1.5	230
Lisinopril	80	2.5	17.5	3	1	225
Lisinopril + statins	-	60	40	3	1	225

Table 6. Chromatographic conditions of HPLC methods

2.2.8. Method development and optimization

HPLC methods were developed and optimized for certain parameters before method validation. The optimization of the analytical procedure was carried out by varying the mobile-phase composition, flow rate, pH of the mobile phase, diluent of solutions and wavelength of analytes in order to achieve symmetrical peaks with good resolution at reasonable retention time.

2.2.9. Method validation

All validation parameters were established according to the guidelines given by ICH: system suitability, linearity, selectivity of drugs, specificity, (concentration-detector response relationship), accuracy or precision and sensitivity with systems, i.e., D and Q (detection and quantification) limit.

Specificity and linearity

The drugs were spiked with pharmaceutical formulations containing different excepients. The linearity of the proposed method was checked at different levels of concentration with different groups. Correlation coefficient was linear; intercept and slope values were also calculated.

Suitability of system

The system suitability of the method was evaluated by analysing five replicate analyses of the drug at a specific concentration for repeatability, (peaks) symmetry factor, theoretical plates for columns, resolution of peaks between interacting drugs, and relative retention of drugs.

Accuracy and precision

Accuracy was calculated at three different levels of concentration (80±20%) by spiking a known amount of the drug. Three or four injections of each drug were injected into the system and the percentage recovery was calculated.

For precision, six replicates of each level were injected into the system on two different non-consecutive days in each case, and the %RSD was calculated.

Limit of detection and quantification

The detection limit (LOD) of the method was calculated by the formula LOD = 3.3 SD/slope. The quantitation limit (LOQ) – the lowest level of analyte that is accurately measured – was set at ten times the noise level (LOQ = 10σ/S, where σ is the standard deviation of the lowest standard concentration and S is the slope of the standard curve).

Robustness

Robustness was established by changing the concentration of mobile phase (water, methanol and acetonitrile), wave length, flow rate and pH. At least five repeated solutions were used with small variations of different parameters. Parameters that were changed mainly had a small deviation: ± 0.2% flow rate/pH, and ±5% for wave length.

Ruggedness

Ruggedness was determined in different labs. Lab 1 was the (RIPS) Research Institute of Pharmaceutical Sciences, Faculty of Pharmacy, Karachi University, and the other at the same university in the Department of Chemistry. Two different instruments (LC 10/LC 20) and two different columns (Purospher STAR C_{18}/Hypersil ODS) were used.

2.2.10. Interaction studies by HPLC

Enalapril solution was mixed with a solution of the interacting drug (statins), which gave a final concentration of 100 μgmL^{-1} for each constituent). These solutions were kept in a water bath at 37 °C for three hours. An aliquot of 5 mL was withdrawn at 30-minute intervals; after making appropriate dilutions it was filtered through 0.45 μ filter paper and three replicates were injected into the HPLC system. The concentration of each drug was determined and the percentage recovery was calculated; the same procedure was applied for captopril and lisinopril.

2.3. Synthesis of ACE inhibitors and interacting-drugs complexes

Complexes of enalapril, captopril and lisinopril with all interacting drugs were synthesized. Equimolar solutions of enalapril and interacting drugs were prepared in methanol. An equivolume solution of enalapril was mixed with each drug individually and the respective pH was adjusted either by 1-2 drops of ammonia or 0.1 N HCl. These mixtures were refluxed for three hours then filtered and left for crystallization at room temperature. Melting points and physical characteristics of these complexes were noted. Solubility of all these complexes was checked in different solvents: water, methanol, ethanol, chloroform and DMSO. A similar procedure was adopted for captopril and lisinoril.

2.3.1. Spectroscopic studies of complexes

2.3.1.1. Infrared studies

ACE inhibitors and their complexes were characterized by using a FT-IR spectrophotometer in the region 400-4000 cm^{-1}. The infrared spectra were recorded using a potassium bromide disc. ATR (attenuated total reflection) or smart performer accessory was used for the sample (minimum amount).

2.3.1.2. Proton NMR analysis

Proton ^1H NMR analysis was performed using a Bruker instrument in deuterated H_2O, chloroform and methanol using (TMS) tetramethyl silane as an IS (internal standard).

3. Results and discussion

3.1. Method development/validation by HPLC

Simple, cheap and very precise, HPLC was used for the determination of ACE inhibitors (captopril, enalapril and lisinopril) in the presence of different statins: ROS (rosuvastatin), ATR (atorvastatin) and SMV(simvastatin) in active ingredients as well as in formulations. It was developed according to guidelines ICH. All inhibitors with statins separated out in less than 10 mins without interference from any ingredients. The recovery of drugs was within the desired range (99-102%). These methods were validated according to ICH and the criteria for acceptance (accuracy/linearity/precision/specificity) and for system suitability were met. The methods can easily be used for quantitative analysis of ACE inhibitors and statins as single drugs or in formulations.

3.2. Interaction of ACE inhibitors with statins

Hyperlipidaemia and hypertension correlate with each other. They can effect coronary heart disease (CHD), because cardiovascular disease (CVD) is closely related to different factors,

http://dx.doi.org/10.5772/59491

such as hypertension (HT) or high cholesterol levels. Factors include family history, age, sex, and diabetes [60-66]. Co-administration of antihypertensive, lipid-lowering and antidiabetic drugs is used in the treatment [67-72]. The most commonly used combinations of diuretic (chlorthalidone, hydrochloroth-iazide, etc.) and an angiotensin II receptor antagonist to control hypertension, as well as with a statin (fluvastatin, simvastatin, etc.) to reduce the cholesterol [73]. Co-administration of an antihypertensive agent with statin is an effective therapeutic option for treatment of multiple cardiovascular risk factors, and especially for high blood pressure (BP) and LDL-C [74-78]. In addition, statins may improve the vasodilatation capacity of large arteries and may thus contribute to BP-lowering in patients treated with both an anti-hypertensive and a statin [79]. Hypercholesterolaemia is often accompanied by hypertension, an associated risk factor for coronary-artery disease (CAD) [80-82]. ACE inhibitors are effective for the management of hypertension, supraventricular arrhythmias and angina pectoris. Other antihypertensive drugs such as propranolol [83] and atenolol [84] also interact with HMG-CoA reductase inhibitor. In the light of the above results, ACE inhibitors may interact and effect a change in each other's availabilities. Methods were developed by HPLC for both ACE inhibitors and statins before starting interaction studies [85-88]. *In vitro"* interactions of ACE inhibitors with statins (atorvastatin, rosuvastatin, pravastatin and simvastatin) were studied in stimulated body environments utilizing the HPLC technique.

3.2.1. *Interaction of enalapril with statins using HPLC*

In vitro interactions of enalapril in the presence of statins drugs (rosuvastatin, atorvastatin and simvastatin) were observed in 1:1 ratio buffers of pH 4 and 7.4 at 37°C. Simultaneous determination of both interacting drugs was also developed, as described above. The results are summarized in Table 7 and Figures 1-3. There was no significant increase or decrease in the concentration of enalapril and interacting drugs at pH 4 and pH 7.4. When enalapril interacted with rosuvastatin, atorvastatin and simvastatin, concentration remained at nearly 99-103% at pH 4 and 99-107% at pH 7.4. Collectively, *in vitro* interaction of enalapril with rosuvastatin, atorvastatin and simvastatin using HPLC at pH 4 and pH 7.4 did not show any significant interactions.

Time	**% Availability at pH 4**						**% Availability at pH 7.4**					
min	**ENP**	**ROS**	**ENP**	**ATR**	**ENP**	**SIM**	**ENP**	**ROS**	**ENP**	**ATR**	**ENP**	**SIM**
0	100	100	98	98.3	99	99.8	100	99	99	99.99	99.02	99.97
30	100	100	99	99.3	100	101	99.78	99	98	100	99.9	99.9
60	99	100	104	98.3	99	101	98.99	95	98	102	99.99	100.3
90	100	101	100	99.4	100	102	102.6	106	106	101.8	100.3	100
120	100	100	104	99.4	101	102	99.79	106	104	101.9	101	101.3
150	100	100	101	99.4	100	103	98.93	106	105	102.6	101.3	102.1
180	100	100	99.7	102	101	102	102	106	107	106.5	102	103

Table 7. Percentage availability of enalapril and statins at pH 4 and 7.4 using HPLC

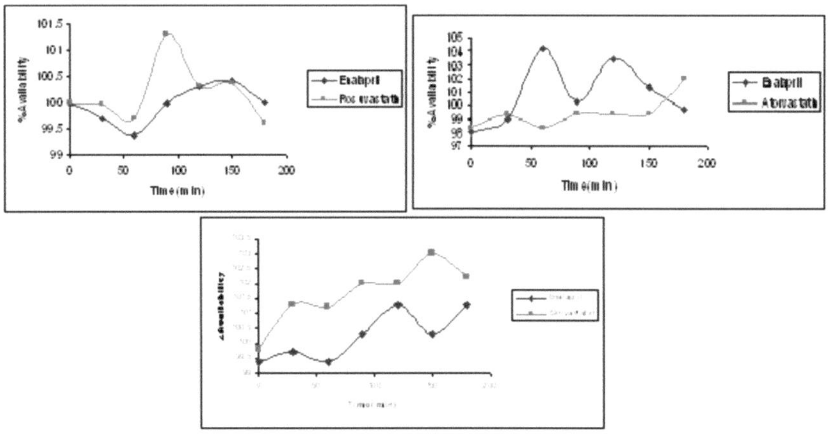

Figure 1. Percentage availability of enalapril and statins at pH 4

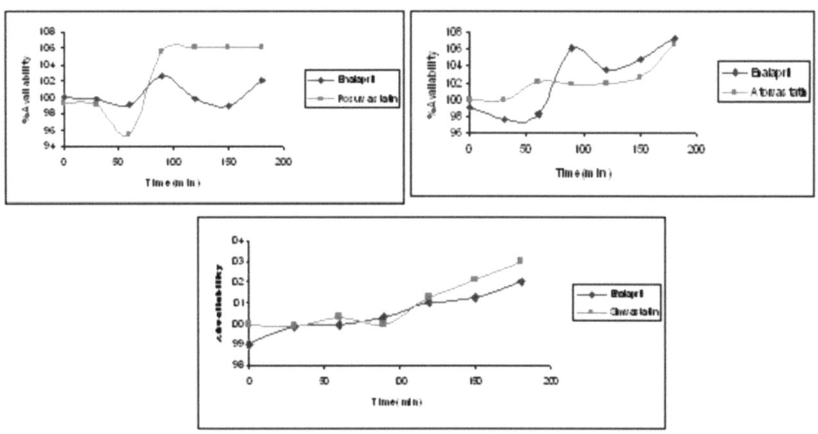

Figure 2. Percentage availability of enalapril and statins at pH 7.4

3.2.2. Interaction of captopril with statins using HPLC

In vitro interactions of captopril in the presence of statins drugs (rosuvastatin, atorvastatin and simvastatin) were observed in 1:1 ratio solutions at 37°C. Simultaneous determination of both interacting drugs was also developed, as described above. Interaction results (Table 8 and Figure 3) show that availability of all drugs was 100% at zero minutes; after that, availability of atorvastatin and simvastatin increased in ascending order, but the percentage availability of captopril decreased in the presence of atorvastatin and simvastatin and remained the same in the presence of rosuvastatin. The availability of atorvastatin and simvastatin was 173% and 115% after 180 min, respectively. Retardation effect was observed at availability of captopril of 97.8%, and 58.2% was available at the end of experiment. Rosuvastatin showed no effect on

http://dx.doi.org/10.5772/59491

captopril and availability of rosuvastatin and captopril at the end of experiment was 100% was 99.12%, respectively.

Time min	CAP	ROS	CAP	ATOR	CAP	SIM
0	100	100.4	100.3	100	100.7	100.3
30	100.2	100.4	100.3	101.5	100.36	100.23
60	100.3	100.3	101.3	100.3	62.1	105.3
90	100.2	99.98	100.2	102.2	67.3	108.2
120	99.9	99.69	100.2	160.8	59.3	110.3
150	100.3	99.87	98.9	162.1	59.3	113.6
180	100.2	99.12	97.8	173.1	58.2	115.6

Table 8. Percentage availability of captopril and statins using HPLC

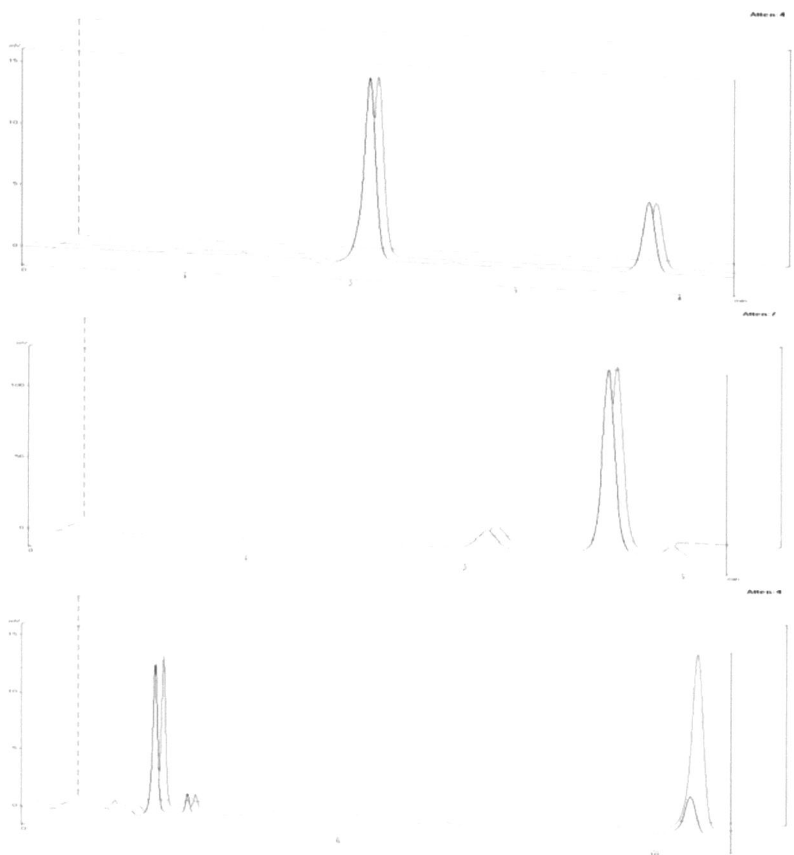

Figure 3. Chromatogram showing change in AUC of drugs. CAP+ATR, CAP+ROS and CAP+SIM (pink before and black after interaction).

3.2.3. Interaction of lisinopril with statins using HPLC

In vitro interactions of lisinopril in the presence of statin drugs (pravastatin, rosuvastatin and atorvastatin) were carried out in solution of 1:1 ratio at 37°C. Simultaneous determination of these interacting drugs was also developed as described above. Results of these interactions (Table 9 and Figure 4) show that when lisinopril interacted with pravastatin, rosuvastatin and atorvastatin its concentration remained in the range 100.3- 102%, 99.9-101.4% and 99.36-102% at 37°C. Pravastatin, rosuvastatin and atorvastatin amplified the availability of lisinopril, unaffected at 37 °C using HPLC. Availability of pravastatin and rosuvastatin after interaction almost stayed unchanged at 37 °C. Interactions of lisinopril in the presence of atorvastatin showed that availability of atorvastatin was enhanced, while that of lisinopril after interaction was unchanged. Collectively, *in vitro* interaction of lisinopril with rosuvastatin, atorvastatin and simvastatin using HPLC at 37 °C did not show any significant results.

Time min	LIS	PRA	LIS	ROS	LIS	ATOR
0	100.3	99.98	99.98	100.3	99.36	97.34
30	100.6	99.63	99.36	100.2	101.5	100.2
60	100.3	99.36	101	100.6	101.3	105.2
90	100.6	100.3	101	100.2	102.5	106.3
120	100.9	100.3	102.3	100.9	101.1	106.20
150	102.0	100.3	102.3	100.4	102.4	106.2
180	102.3	101.3	101.4	100.5	102.4	106.02

Table 9. Percentage availability of lisinopril and statins using HPLC

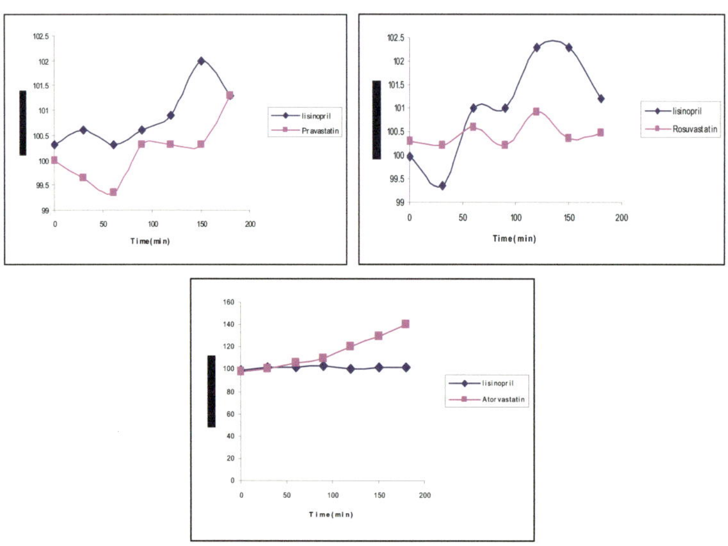

Figure 4. Percentage availability of lisinopril and statins

http://dx.doi.org/10.5772/59491

4. Conclusion

Interaction studies suggest that enalapril and lisinopril are not affected by statins but captopril changes the availability of drugs. *In vivo* studies are required to prove this relationship.

Author details

Safila Naveed*

Address all correspondence to: safila117@gmail.com

Faculty of pharmacy, Jinnah University for Women Karachi, Pakistan

References

[1] Bernstein KE, Martin BM, Edwards AS and Bernstein EA (1989) Mouse angiotensin-converting enzyme is a protein composed of two homologous domains, J. Biol. Chem., 264, 11945-11951.

[2] Soubrier F, Alhene-Gelas F, Hubert C, Allegrini J, John M, Tregear G and Corvol P (1988) Two putative active centres in human angiotensin I-converting enzyme revealed by molecular cloning, Proc. Natl. Acad. Sci., 85, 9386-9390.

[3] Ferreira SH (1965) A bradykinin-potentiating factor present in the venom of Bothrops jararaca, Brit. J. Pharmacol., 24, 163-169.

[4] Bakhle YS (1968) Conversion of angiotensin I to angiotensin II by cell free extracts of dog lung, Nature, 220, 919-21.

[5] Brunner HR, Laragh JH, Sealey JE, Gavras I and Vukovich RA (1974) An angiotensin converting enzyme inhibitor to identify and treat vasoconstrictor and volume factors in hypertensive patients, New Eng. J. Med., 291, 817-821.

[6] Hartsuck JA and Lipscomb WN (1971) *Carboxypeptidase A, In the Enzymes*, Vol 3, ed. P.D. Boyer., pp l-56, New York, Academic Press.

[7] Hofmann K and Bergmann M (1946) The specificity of carboxypeptidase, J. Biol. Chem., 134, 225-235.

[8] Quiocho F and Lipscomb WN (1971) Carboxypeptidase A, A protein and an enzyme, Adv. Protein. Chem., 25, l-78.

[9] Ferreira SH, Bartelt DC and Greene LJ (1970) Isolation of bradykinin potentiating peptides from Bothrops jararaca venom, Biochemistry, 9, 2583- 2593.

[10] Ondetti MA, Rubin B and Cushman DW (1977) Science, 196, 441-444.

[11] Maxwell RA and Eckhadt SB (1990) Captopril Drug Discovery, 19, 34.

[12] Cushman DW, Ondetti MA, Gordon EM, Natarajan S, Karanewsky DS, Krapcho J and Petrillo EW (1980) Rational Design and Biochemical utility of specific inhibitors, Journal of Cardiovascular Pharmacology: 7, S17-30.

[13] G a G(1996) *The Pharmacological Basis of Therapeutic*, 9th edition McGraw-Hill Press, New York p. 744.

[14] Fitz Gerald RJ, Murray BA and Walsh DJ (2004) Hypotensive peptides from milk proteins, J Nutr., 134, 980S-8S.

[15] Aloysius TN, Kelly C, Pierre R and Edward DS (2006) Synthesis and molecular modeling of a lisinopril-tryptophan analogue inhibitor of angiotensin I-converting enzyme. Bioorganic and Medicinal Chemistry Letters, 17(1), 4616-4619.

[16] Sweetman SC and M (2005) *The Complete Drug Reference,* Pharmaceutical Press, London & Chicago, 34th Ed., 900-901.

[17] Richard AH and Pamela CC (1977) *Illustrated Review Pharmacology*, Lippincott-Raven Publishers, Philadelphia, Revised ed., 151-162.

[18] Bertam GK (1998) *Basic and Clinical Pharmacology*, Appleton and Lange, Revised ed., 197-213 Stamford.

[19] Riley TN and De Ruiter J (1992) New drugs, U.S. Pharmacist., 17(3), 42-46.

[20] Riley TN and DeRuiter (1997) New Drugs, U.S. Pharmacist, 22(3)175-176.

[21] Leonetti G and Cuspidi C (1995) Choosing the right ACE inhibitor: A guide to selection, Drugs, 49, 516-535.

[22] Burris JF (1995) the expanding role of angiotensin-converting enzyme inhibitors in the management of hypertension, J. Clin. Pharmacol., 35, 337-342.

[23] The 1998 report of the Joint National Committee on the Detection, Evaluation and. Treatment of High Blood Pressure, Arch. Intern. Med., 1998; 148, 1023-1038.

[24] Borghi C and Ambrosioni E (1996) A risk-benefit arrestment of ACE inhibitor therapy post-myocardial infarction, Drug Safety, 14, 277-87.

[25] Murdoch DR and McMurray JJV (1998) ACE inhibitors in acute myocardial infarction, Hosp. Med., 59, 111-15.

[26] Deedwania PC (1990) Angiotensin converting enzyme inhibitors in congestive heart failure, Arch. Intern. Med., 150, 1798-1805.

[27] Jest P (1991) Angiotensin-converting enzyme inhibitors as a therapeutic potential in Bartter's syndrome, Eur. J. Clin. Pharmacol., 41, 303-5.

[28] 28 Okumura H, Nishimura E and Kariya S (2001) Angiotensin-converting enzyme (ACE), 121(3), 253-7.

[29] Anonymous (1994) Cough caused by ACE inhibitors, Drug Ther. Bull., 32(28)55-56.

[30] Ravid D (1994) ACE-inhibitors and cough: a prospective evaluation in hypertension and congestive heart failure, J. Clin. Pharmacol., 34, 1116-1120.

[31] Parish RC and Miller IJ (1992) Adverse effects of angiotensin-converting enzyme inhibitors: an update, Drug Safety, 7, 14-31.

[32] Cooper WO, Hernandez-Diaz S, Arbogast PG, Dudley JA, Dyer S and Gideon PS (2006) Major congenital malformations after first-trimester exposure to ACE inhibitors, N. 33 Engl. J. Med., 354(23), 2443-51.

[33] Molinaro G, Cugno M and Perez M (2002) Angiotensin-converting enzyme inhibitor-associated angioedema is characterized by a slower degradation of des-arginine(9)-bradykinin, J. Pharmacol. Exp. Ther., 303, 232-7.

[34] Verresen L (1990) Angiotensin-converting-enzyme inhibitors anaphylactoid reactions to high-flux membrane dialysis, Lan., 336, 1360-1362.

[35] Koopman PP, Van Megan T, Thien I and Gribrav FWJ (1989) The interaction between indomethacine and captopril or enalepril in normal volunteers, Journal of Internal Medicine, 226, 139-142.

[36] Bainbridge AD, MacFadyen RJ, Lees KR and Reid JL (1991) A study of the acute pharmacodynamic interaction of ramipril and felodipine in normotensive subjects, Br. J. Clin. Pharmacol., 31, 148-53.

[37] Casato M (1995) Granulocytopenia after combined therapy with interferone and angiotensin-converting enzyme inhibitors: evidence for a synergistic hematologic toxicity, Am. J. Med., 99, 386-91.

[38] Shionoiri H (1993) Pharmacokinetic drug interactions with ACE inhibitors, Clin. Pharmacokinet., 25(1), 20-58.

[39] Shionoiri H, Naruse M, Minamisawa K, Ueda S, Himeno H, Hiroto S, Takasaki I (1997) Fosinopril clinical pharmacokinetics and clinical potential, Clin. Pharmacokinet., 32(6), 460-80.

[40] D'Costa DF, Basu SK and Gunasekera NPR (1990) ACE inhibitors and Diuretics causing hypokalemia, B.J.C.P., 44, 26-7.

[41] Shionoiri H (1993) Pharmacokinetic drug interactions with ACE inhibitors, Clin. Pharmacokinet., 25(1), 20-58.

[42] 42 Mignat C and Unger T (1995) ACE-inhibitors: Drug interaction of clinical significance, Drug Safety, 12, 334-7.

[43] Good CB, McDermott L and McCloskey B (1995) Diet and serum potassium in patients on ACE inhibitors, JAMA, 274, 538.

[44] Baba T, Tomiyama T and Takebe K (1990) Enhancement by ACE inhibitors of first dose hypotension caused by an alpha1-blocker, N. Eng. J. Med., 322, 1237.

[45] Lee SC, Park SW and Kim DK (2001) Iron supplementation inhibits cough associated with ACE inhibitors, Hypertension, 38, 166-170.

[46] Campbell NR and Hasinoff BB (1991) Iron supplements, a common cause of drug interactions, Br. J. Clin. Pharmacol., 31, 251-255.

[47] Herings RMC (1995) Hypoglycemia associated with use of inhibitors angiogenesin converting enzyme, Lancet, 345, 1195-8.

[48] Morris AD (1997) ACE inhibitors' use is associated with hospitalization for severe hypoglycemia in patients with diabetes, Diabetes Care, 20, 1363-7.

[49] Gossmann J, Kachel HG, Schoeppe W and Scheuermann EH (1993) Anemia in renal transplant recipients caused by concomitant therapy with azathioprine angiotensin-converting enzyme inhibitors, Transplantation, 56, 585-9.

[50] Goldstein JL and Brown MS (1990) Regulation of the mevalonate pathway, Nature, 343, 425-430.

[51] Chester BG (2002) Polypharmacy in Elderly Patients with Diabetes, Diabetes Spectrum, 15, 240-248.

[52] Jones PH, Davidson MH, Stein EA, Bays HE, McKenney JM, Miller E, Cain VA and Blasetto JW (2003) Comparison of the efficacy and safety of rosuvastatin versus atorvastatin, simvastatin, and pravastatin across doses, Am. J. Cardiol., 92, 152-160.

[53] Caslake MJ, Stewart G, Day SP, Daly E, McTaggart F, Chapman MJ, Durrington P, Laggner P, Mackness M, Pears J and Packard CJ (2003) Phenotype-dependent and independent actions of rosuvastatin on atherogenic lipoprotein subfractions in hyperlipidaemia, Atherosclerosis,171, 245-253.

[54] 54 Engstrom G, Lind P, Hedblad B, Stavenow L, Janzon L and Lindgarde F (2002) Effects of cholesterol and inflammation-sensitive plasma proteins on incidence of myocardial infarction and stroke in men, Circulation, 105, 2632-2637.

[55] Dangas G, Smith DA, Unger AH, Shao JH, Meraj P, Fier C, Cohen AM, Fallon JT, Badimon JJ and Ambrose JA (2000) Pravastatin: an antithrombotic effect independent of the cholesterol lowering effect, Thromb Haemost., 83, 688-692.

[56] Honjo M, Tanihara H, Nishijima K, Kiryu J, Honda Y, Yue BY and Sawamura T (2002) Statin inhibits leukocyte-endothelial interaction and prevents neuronal death induced by ischemia-reperfusion injury in the rat retina, Arch. Ophthalmol., 120, 1707-1713.

[57] 67 Delanty N, Vaughan CJ and Sheehy N (2001) Statins and neuroprotection, Expert Opin. Investig. Drugs, 10, 1847-1853.

[58] Heart Protection Study Collaborative Group (2002) MRC/BHF Heart Protection Study of cholesterol lowering with simvastatin in 20,536 high-risk individuals: a randomised placebo-controlled trial, Lancet, 360, 7-22.

[59] Chong PH (2002) Lack of Therapeutic Interchangeability of HMG-CoA Reductase Inhibitors, Ann. Pharmacother., 36, 1907-1917.

[60] Poulter N (1999) Coronary heart disease is a multifactorial disease. Am. J. Hypertens., 12, 92S-95S.

[61] Lloyd-Jones DM, Evans JC and Larson MG (1999) Cross-classification of JNC VI blood pressure stages and risk groups in the Framingham Heart Study, Arch. Intern. Med., 159, 2206-2212.

[62] Wilson PW, Kannel WB, Silbershatz H and D'Agostino RB (1999) Clustering of metabolic factors and coronary heart disease, Arch. Intern. Med., 159, 1104-1109.

[63] Thomas F, Bean K and Guize L (2002) Combined effects of systolic blood pressure and serum cholesterol on cardiovascular mortality in young (<55 years) men and women, Eur. Heart J., 23, 528-535.

[64] Wood D, Durrington P and McInnes G (1998) Joint British recommendations on prevention of coronary heart disease in clinical practice, Heart, 80(Suppl. 2), S1-S29.

[65] Kannel WB (2000) Risk stratification in hypertension: New insights from the Framingham Study. Am. J. Hypertens., 13, 3S-10S.

[66] Grundy SM, Brewer HB, Cleeman JI, Smith SC and Lenfant C (2004) Definition of metabolic syndrome: Report of the National Heart, Lung, and Blood Institute/American Heart Association conference on scientific issues related to definition, Circulation, 109,433-438.

[67] Lars-Christian R, Elena B, Boguslaw O, Marianne W, Albert K and Philippe F (2008) Coadministration of Valsartan 160 and 320 mg and Simvastatin 20 and 40 mg in Patients with Hypertension and Hypercholesterolemia: A Multicenter, 12-Week, Double-Blind, Double-Dummy Parallel Group Study, Clinical Therapeutics, 30, 10.

[68] Cefalu WT (2008) Diabetic dyslipidemia and the metabolic syndrome, Diab. Metab. Synd. Clin. Res. Rev., 2, 208-222.

[69] Marcus AO (2000) Safety of drugs commonly used to treat hypertension, dyslipidemia, and type 2 diabetes (The Metabolic Syndrome): Part 1, Diabetes Technol. Ther., 2, 101-110.

[70] Grundy SM, Cleeman JI, Daniels SR, Donato KA, R Eckel H, Franklin BA, Gordon DJ, Krauss RM, Savage PJ, Smith SC, Spertus JA and Costa F (2005) Diagnosis and Management of the Metabolic Syndrome, Circulation, 112, 2735-2752.

[71] Plosker GL and Robinson DM (2008) Amlodipine/valsartan, fixed-dose combination in hypertension, Drugs, 68, 373.

[72] Jacobson TA (2004) Comparative pharmacokinetic interaction profiles of pravastatin, simvastatin, and atorvastatin when coadministered with cytochrome P450 inhibitors, Am. J. Cardiol., 94(9), 1140-6.

[73] Markham A and Goa KL (1997) Valsartan: A review of its pharmacology and therapeutic use in essential hypertension, Drugs, 54, 299-311.

[74] Pool JL, Glazer R, Chiang YT and Gatlin M (1999) Dose-response efficacy of valsartan, a new angiotensin II receptor blocker, J. Hum. Hypertens., 13, 275-281.

[75] Burnier M and Brunner HR (2000) Angiotensin II receptor antagonists, Lancet, 355, 637-645.

[76] Weir MR, Crikelair N and Levy D (2007) Evaluation of the dose response with valsartan and valsartan/hydrocholorothia- zide in patients with essential hypertension. J. Clin. Hypertens., 9, 103-112.

[77] Dorval JF, Anderson T and Buithieu J (2005) Reaching recommended lipid and blood pressure targets with amlodipine/atorvastatin combination in patients with coronary heart disease, Am. J. Cardiol., 95, S249-S253.

[78] Koh KK, Quon MJ and Han SH (2004) Additive beneficial effects of losartan combined with simvastatin in the treatment of hypercholesterol-emic, hypertensive patients, Circulation, 110, 3687-3692.

[79] Borghi C, Dormi A and Veronesi M (2002) Use of lipid-lowering drugs and blood pressure control in patients with arterial hypertension, J. Clin. Hypertens., 4, 277-285.

[80] Gotto Jr. AM (1998) Risk factor modification: rationale for management of dyslipidemia, American Journal of Medicine, 104, 6S-8S.

[81] Gould KL, Casscells SW, Buja LM and Goff DC (1995) Non-invasive management of coronary artery disease: Report of a meeting at the University of Texas Medical School at Houston, Lancet, 346, 750-753.

[82] Wood D (2001) Asymptomatic individuals' risk stratification in the prevention of coronary heart disease, British Medical Bulletin, 59, 3-16.

[83] Pan HY, Triscari J and DeVault AR (1991) Pharmacokinetic interaction between propranolol and HMG-CoA reductase inhibitor pravstatin and lovastatin, Br. J. Clin. Pharmacol., 31, 665-670.

[84] O'Riordan M (2005) ASCOT-LLA: Lower coronary event rates in patients treated with amlodipine and atorvastatin, Hypertension, Medscape, Medical News.

[85] Sultana N, Arayne MS and Safila Naveed (2010) Simultaneous Determination of Captopril and Statins in API, Pharmaceutical Formulations and in Human Serum by RP-

HPLC, J. Chin. Chem. Soc., 57, 378-383. [online] Available at: http://onlinelibrary.wiley.com/doi/10.1002/jccs.201000056/abstract

[86] Sultana N, Arayne MS and Safila N. (2011) Simultaneous Determination of Enalapril and Statins in Pharmaceutical Formulations by RP- HPLC, Chilean Chemical Society, 56(3), 734-737. [online] Available at:. http://www.scielo.cl/scielo.php?script=sci_arttext&pid=S0717-97072011000300003

[87] Sultana N, Arayne MS, Shah SN and Safila N. (2010) Simultaneous Determination of Prazosin, Atorvastatin, Rosuvastatin and Simvastatin in API, Dosage Formulations and Human Serum by RP-HPLC, Journal of the Chinese Chemical Society, 57(6), 1286-1292. [online] Available at: http://onlinelibrary.wiley.com/doi/10.1002/jccs.201000190/abstract

[88] Sultana N, Arayne MS and Safila N. (2011) Validated Method for the Simultaneous Determination of Lisinopril, Pravastatin, Atorvastatin and Rosuvastatin in API, Formulations and Human Serum by RP-HPLC, Chinese Journal of Chemistry, 29, 1216-1220. DOI: 10.1002/cjoc.201190226. [online] Available at: http://onlinelibrary.wiley.com/doi/10.1002/cjoc.201190226/abstract